ANNALS OF
THE NEW YORK ACADEMY
OF SCIENCES

Volume 919

EDITORIAL STAFF

Executive Editor
BARBARA M. GOLDMAN

Managing Editor
JUSTINE CULLINAN

Associate Editor
STEFAN MALMOLI

The New York Academy of Sciences
2 East 63rd Street
New York, New York 10021

THE NEW YORK ACADEMY OF SCIENCES
(Founded in 1817)

BOARD OF GOVERNORS, September 15, 1999 – September 15, 2000

BILL GREEN, *Chairman of the Board*
TORSTEN WIESEL, *Vice Chairman of the Board*
RODNEY W. NICHOLS, *President and CEO* [ex officio]

Honorary Life Governors
WILLIAM T. GOLDEN   JOSHUA LEDERBERG

JOHN T. MORGAN, *Treasurer*

Governors

D. ALLAN BROMLEY	LAWRENCE B. BUTTENWIESER	PRAVEEN CHAUDHARI
JOHN H. GIBBONS	RONALD L. GRAHAM	HENRY M. GREENBERG
ROBERT G. LAHITA	MARTIN L. LEIBOWITZ	JACQUELINE LEO
WILLIAM J. McDONOUGH	KATHLEEN P. MULLINIX	JOHN F. NIBLACK
SANDRA PANEM	RICHARD RAVITCH	RICHARD A. RIFKIND
	SARA LEE SCHUPF JAMES H. SIMONS	

ELEANOR BAUM, *Past Chairman of the Board*
HELENE L. KAPLAN, *Counsel* [ex officio]   PETER H. KOHN, *Secretary* [ex officio]

TOXICOLOGY FOR THE NEXT MILLENNIUM

ANNALS OF THE NEW YORK ACADEMY OF SCIENCES
Volume 919

TOXICOLOGY FOR THE NEXT MILLENNIUM

Edited by Robert J. Isfort and Joshua Lederberg

The New York Academy of Sciences
New York, New York
2000

Copyright © 2000 by the New York Academy of Sciences. All rights reserved. Under the provisions of the United States Copyright Act of 1976, individual readers of the Annals are permitted to make fair use of the material in them for teaching or research. Permission is granted to quote from the Annals provided that the customary acknowledgment is made of the source. Material in the Annals may be republished only by permission of the Academy. Address inquiries to the Permissions Department (editorial@nyas.org) at the New York Academy of Sciences.

Copying fees: For each copy of an article made beyond the free copying permitted under Section 107 or 108 of the 1976 Copyright Act, a fee should be paid through the Copyright Clearance Center, Inc., 222 Rosewood Drive, Danvers, MA 01923 (www.copyright.com).

⊖ The paper used in this publication meets the minimum requirements of the American National Standard for Information Sciences—Permanence of Paper for Printed Library Materials, ANSI Z39.48-1984.

Library of Congress Cataloging-in-Publication Data

Toxicology for the next millennium/ edited by Robert J. Isfort and Joshua Lederberg.
     p. cm. — (Annals of the New York Academy of Sciences, ISSN 0077-8923; v. 919)
"This volume is the result of a conference entitled Toxicology for the Next Millennium held by the New York Academy of Sciences on September 20–23, 1999, in Warrenton, Virginia"—Contents p.
    Includes bibliographical references and index.
    ISBN 1-57331-265-7 (cloth : alk. paper) — ISBN 1-57331-266-5 (pbk. : alk. paper)
     1. Toxicology—Congresses. 2. Toxicology—Technical innovations—Congresses. 3. Molecular toxicology—Congresses. I. Isfort, Robert J. II. Lederberg, Joshua. III. New York Academy of Sciences. IV. Series.

Q11.N5 vol. 919
[RA1191]
500 s—dc21
[615.9]   00-058423

GYAT / PCP
Printed in the United States of America
ISBN 1-57331-265-7 (cloth)
ISBN 1-57331-266-5 (paper)
ISSN 0077-8923

ANNALS OF THE NEW YORK ACADEMY OF SCIENCES

Volume 919
September 2000

TOXICOLOGY FOR THE NEXT MILLENNIUM

Editors and Conference Organizers
ROBERT J. ISFORT AND JOSHUA LEDERBERG

[This volume is the result of a conference entitled *Toxicology for the Next Millennium* held by the New York Academy of Sciences on September 20–23, 1999, in Warrenton, Virginia.]

CONTENTS

Introduction. *By* ROBERT J. ISFORT	ix
What's Important about Toxicology? *By* JOSHUA LEDERBERG	xi

Part I. Molecular Technologies

Use of Oligonucleotide Arrays to Analyze Drug Toxicity. *By* NAFTALI KAMINSKI, JOHN ALLARD, AND RENU A. HELLER	1
Analysis of Drug Pharmacology towards Predicting Drug Behavior by Expression Profiling Using High-Density Oligonucleotide Arrays. *By* JING-SHAN HU, MARK DURST, REINHOLD KERB, VIVI TRUONG, JING-TYAN MA, ELINA KHURGIN, DAVID BALABAN, THOMAS R. GINGERAS, AND BRIAN B. HOFFMAN	9

Part II. Cellular/Organismal Technologies

Development of Human Cell Lines from Multiple Organs. *By* JOHNG S. RHIM	16
Fluorometric High-Throughput Screening for Inhibitors of Cytochrome P450. *By* VAUGHN P. MILLER, DAVID M. STRESSER, ANDREW P. BLANCHARD, STEPHANIE TURNER, AND CHARLES L. CRESPI	26

Part III. Genomics/Proteomics

Quantitative Proteome Analysis: Methods and Applications. *By* RUEDI AEBERSOLD, BEATE RIST, AND STEVEN P. GYGI	33
Pharmaceutical Proteomics. *By* SANDRA STEINER AND N. LEIGH ANDERSON	48

Part IV. Computer Modeling/Bioinformatics

Gene Expression Microarray Data Analysis for Toxicology Profiling. *By* M. J. CUNNINGHAM, S. LIANG, S. FUHRMAN, J. J. SEILHAMER, AND R. SOMOGYI 52

In Silico Toxicology. *By* SAMUEL HOLTZMAN 68

Toxicity Testing: The FDA Perspective. *By* JANE E. HENNEY 75

Part V. Cancer

p53 Tumor Suppressor Gene: At the Crossroads of Molecular Carcinogenesis, Molecular Epidemiology, and Human Risk Assessment. *By* S. PERWEZ HUSSAIN, MONICA H. HOLLSTEIN, AND CURTIS C. HARRIS 79

Mechanisms of Cell Transformation in the Syrian Hamster Embryo (SHE) Cell Transformation System. *By* ROBERT J. ISFORT 86

Part VI. Neurotoxicology

Neurochemical Effects of Environmental Chemicals: *In Vitro* and *In Vivo* Correlations on Second Messenger Pathways. *By* PRASADA RAO S. KODAVANTI AND HUGH A. TILSON 97

Culture Models of Neurodegenerative Disease. *By* D. A. FIGLEWICZ, L. DONG, M. MLODZIENSKI, AND J. C. TURCOTTE 106

In Vitro Systems as Simulations of *In Vivo* Conditions: The Study of Cognition and Synaptic Plasticity in Neurotoxicology. *By* M. E. GILBERT 119

Part VII. Acute Toxicology

Transgenic Zebrafish as Sentinels for Aquatic Pollution. *By* MICHAEL J. CARVAN III, TIMOTHY P. DALTON, GARY W. STUART, AND DANIEL W. NEBERT 133

"Gene-Swap Knock-in" Cassette in Mice to Study Allelic Differences in Human Genes. *By* DANIEL W. NEBERT, TIMOTHY P. DALTON, GARY W. STUART, AND MICHAEL J. CARVAN III 148

The Use of Explant Lens Culture to Assess Cataractogenic Potential. *By* MICHAEL D. ALEO, MICHAEL J. AVERY, WILLIAM P. BEIERSCHMITT, CYNTHIA A. DRUPA, JAY H. FORTNER, ADAM H. KAPLAN, KIMBERLY A. NAVETTA, RICHARD M. SHEPARD, AND COLLEEN M. WALSH 171

In Vitro Percutaneous Absorption Models. *By* ROBERT L. BRONAUGH 188

In Vitro and Human Testing Strategies for Skin Irritation. *By* MICHAEL K. ROBINSON, ROSEMARIE OSBORNE, AND MARY A. PERKINS 192

Part VIII. Immunotoxicology

New Technologies to Prevent and Treat Contact Hypersensitivity Responses. *By* AKIRA TAKASHIMA, MARK MUMMERT, TOSHIYUKI KITAJIMA, AND HIROYUKI MATSUE 205

The Role of Tumor Necrosis Factor α in Chemical-Induced Hepatotoxicity. *By* MICHAEL I. LUSTER, PETIA P. SIMEONOVA, RANDLE M. GALLUCCI, ALEX BRUCCOLERI, MARK E. BLAZKA, BERRAN YUCESOY, AND JOANNA M. MATHESON 214

Aging and Resistance to *Trichinella spiralis* Infection following Xenobiotic Exposure. *By* ROBERT W. LUEBKE, CAREY B. COPELAND, AND DEBORA L. ANDREWS 221

Animal Models to Assess the Effects of Air Pollutants on Allergic Lung Disease. *By* MARYJANE K. SELGRADE, AMY L. LAMBERT, MARSHA D. W. WARD, AND M. IAN GILMOUR 230

Part IX. Developmental Toxicology

From Developmental Biology to Developmental Toxicology. *By* RUDI BALLING AND MARTIN HRABÉ DE ANGELIS 239

Molecular Genetic Control of Axis Patterning during Early Embryogenesis of Vertebrates. *By* GARY C. SCHOENWOLF 246

Genetic Basis of Susceptibility to Environmentally Induced Neural Tube Defects. *By* RICHARD H. FINNELL, JANEE GELINEAU–VAN WAES, GREGORY D. BENNETT, ROBERT C. BARBER, BOGDAN WLODARCZYK, GARY M. SHAW, EDWARD J. LAMMER, JORGE A. PIEDRAHITA, AND JAMES H. EBERWINE 261

Transient Modulation of Gene Expression in the Neurulation Staged Mouse Embryo. *By* E. SIDNEY HUNTER III AND PHILLIP HARTIG 278

Part X. Poster Papers

Queueing and Inventory Theory in Clinical Practice: Application to Clinical Toxicology. *By* C. P. ARUN 284

The "Rodent Carcinogen" Dilemma: Formidable Challenge for the Technologies of the New Millennium. *By* F. M. JOHNSON 288

Use of Bone Marrow Chimeras to Identify Cell Targets in the Immune System for the Actions of Chemicals. *By* THOMAS A. GASIEWICZ, T. SCOTT THURMOND, J. ERIN STAPLES, FRANCIS G. MURANTE, AND ALLEN E. SILVERSTONE 300

The Effects of Lead on PKC Isoforms. *By* ALDO A. COPPI, JACOB LESNIAK, DIANE ZIEBA, AND FRANCIS A. X. SCHANNE 304

Lead-Induced Activation of Protein Kinase C in Rat Brain Cortical Synaptosomes. *By* CHRISTOPHER D. TOSCANO AND FRANCIS A. X. SCHANNE .. 307

Reactivities of the Skin-Sensitization Test in Guinea Pig (GPMT) as a Function of Three Parameters: Induction Doses (MID), Challenge Doses (SCD), and Direct Exposures (DED). *By* SATOSHI KITAJIMA, JUNKO MOMMA, AND TOHRU INOUE 312

Toxicity of Ethylene Glycol Metabolites in Normal Human Kidney Cells. *By* K. E. MCMARTIN AND T. A. CENAC 315

Cadmium-Induced Bioaccumulation in the Selected Tissues of a Freshwater Teleost, *Oreochromis mossambicus (Tilapia)*. *By* A. USHA RANI 318

Concluding Remarks. *By* ROBERT J. ISFORT 321

Index of Contributors 323

Financial assistance was received from:

Major Funders
- THE PROCTER & GAMBLE COMPANY

Supporters
- COLGATE-PALMOLIVE COMPANY
- NATIONAL INSTITUTE OF ENVIRONMENTAL HEALTH SCIENCES, NIH
- PFIZER CENTRAL RESEARCH

Contributors
- CHEMICAL INDUSTRY INSTITUTE OF TOXICOLOGY
- ENTELOS, INCORPORATED
- EXELIXIS PHARMACEUTICALS, INCORPORATED
- SOCIETY OF TOXICOLOGY

The New York Academy of Sciences believes it has a responsibility to provide an open forum for discussion of scientific questions. The positions taken by the participants in the reported conferences are their own and not necessarily those of the Academy. The Academy has no intent to influence legislation by providing such forums.

Introduction

ROBERT J. ISFORT

Research Division, Procter & Gamble Pharmaceuticals, Cincinnati, Ohio, USA

Toxicology is the science of predicting and understanding adverse effects resulting from the exposure of organisms to chemical/physical/biological agents. As such, toxicologists must have a thorough understanding of both the toxic agent and the organism of interest in order to accurately predict and understand the results of exposure of the organism to the agent. Traditionally, the paradigm by which toxicologists work to acquire the necessary information needed to make such predictions has been through a case-study approach. This approach utilizes the analysis of the effects of exposure to single agents at the molecular, cellular, and organismal levels, thereby generating detailed understanding of the toxicity of individual agents. Analysis of an adequate number of agents allows a detailed history to be created, thus providing glimpses into common mechanisms of actions. This research paradigm is extremely effective in understanding agent-related effects that are important in developing a mechanism-based risk assessment. Unfortunately, this process does not readily lend itself to global predictions in a broad toxicological area, thereby leading to frustration during the development of molecular and cellular tools with widespread, agent-independent predicting capabilities.

Utilizing whole organisms, predicting the toxicity of agents has proceeded with relatively little change over the past century. The standard procedure involves dosing the animal to a maximum tolerated dose followed by observation of the organism for toxic effects. Several recent trends have converged that make the utilization of the traditional animal-based toxicological analysis difficult. First, economic factors including the large number and speed of development of novel chemicals have made large-scale animal studies impractical from both cost and timing standpoints. For example, analysis of carcinogenicity of a single chemical in a standard rodent bioassay takes approximately three years and costs over a million dollars. Second, societal pressures and ethical and regulatory restraints concerning the use of animals in toxicological evaluation have increased. Third, recognition that animal results, particularly at high dose levels, may not accurately predict human toxicity has led to uncertainty and an increase in the need for mechanistic-based analysis. These factors have increased the pressure to develop toxicological techniques that are fast, inexpensive, and mechanistically based, that minimize the use of animals, and that are more predictive than animals of the human response.

Recent developments in biological research have the potential to dramatically alter the way that toxicological evaluations are performed. First, the advent of molecular biology has allowed the researcher to understand the biological response to an agent at the molecular level, thus allowing alterations in specific molecular species to be measured with previously unknown precision. Also, by understanding the molecular mechanisms for specific types of toxicities, we can now begin to understand the underlying reasons of why toxicities occur with the potential to develop better tests to measure these toxicities. However, molecular understanding requires extensive research in order to better understand the system under study. Second, advances in our ability to culture specific cell types *in vitro*, including cells that remain metabolically active, have the potential to allow us to model whole organs in tissue culture systems. Third, the human genome analysis program, the genome analysis of a variety of additional organisms, and tissue-specific gene expression analysis will allow complete knowledge of all the genes that function in a particular tissue. This will allow identification of alterations in specific genes that occur during toxicological processes. Finally, computer modeling of complex biological systems has the potential to provide important insights into biological phenomena by allowing a single researcher to effectively review all the information known on any subject. In addition, computer modeling will allow investigators to predict processes by simulating, in virtual reality, the biological system being modeled, thereby allowing virtual perturbation of that system.

The convergence of all the above-discussed trends and technologies creates the potential for major advancements in toxicological research. More specifically, the application of modern technologies has the potential to provide more detailed and greater understanding of the convergent and underlying toxic effects of agents through the use of molecular, cellular, and computer technologies than the traditional, animal-based, case-history study approach to toxicology. However, application of these new technologies will have to be done using a paradigm that has proven successful in the past—namely, that of increased basic knowledge of the disease process followed by application of fundamental principles of the disease process to develop *in vitro* systems that measure markers of events that are central to the disease (global toxicological predictions). For example, the explosion in basic understanding of the neoplastic process, cellular biology, and genetics resulted in the discovery that cancer is a mutational disease of cells. This resulted in the design of tests that use, as their predictive indicators, markers that are central to the cancer development process. These markers are useful for determining the toxicity of a wide variety of agents, independent of the class or mechanism of toxicity of the agent. Applying a similar research scheme to the problems of neurotoxicity, acute toxicity, developmental toxicity, and immunotoxicity could greatly increase our ability to predict (using *in vitro* tools that measure alterations that are central to the disease process) the toxic potential of agents in these areas.

In conclusion, I hope everyone will view the technologies presented with an open mind and be ready and willing to ponder, discuss, and debate the impact that these technologies will have on the field of toxicology.

What's Important about Toxicology?

JOSHUA LEDERBERG
The Rockefeller University, New York, New York, USA

Often, the basic scientific issues involved in toxicology are obscured in previous debate. If we could use people like guinea pigs and freely test any number of individuals to see what the lethal dose of a substance is, we might not need scientific toxicology. This is neither desirable nor possible.

An alternative, animal testing, presents a number of problems. Above all, from a scientific perspective, the soundness of the extrapolation is very much in question, especially where results vary from one species to another. This suddenly puts us into some very hard and deep evolutionary and physiological territory. What rules govern expectations that what isn't toxic in an animal won't be toxic in a human? Keep in mind that we hardly ever use species that have a long life span. Why in the world should we think that a mouse getting along well after a year and a half should have any resemblance to a human outcome, especially when so many of the toxicities of concern are chronic over 20, 30, or even 40 years? Furthermore, there are variations in people.

How can we ensure that the enormous effort and expense that are put into the testing of products have any meaning whatsoever? As a discipline, toxicology has been burdened by all kinds of considerations. For many years, toxicologists were hired only by industrial groups and corporations to conduct LD50 tests, to verify to the world that the amount of a substance they were ramming down our throat, persuading us to buy, or polluting the environment with was well within the margins of safety when tested by the 50% lethal dose in various animal species. This is a grossly unsatisfactory situation from a technical, policy, or any other point of view.

At the same time, it presents exciting scientific challenges. As a geneticist, I stress the comparative aspects and try to understand why one species will differ from another. We should also reflect that the early development of biochemistry was very much bound up in how inhibitors worked. We had curare, used to make arrow dart poison, which is almost an invaluable agent in neurobiological studies. Much could be said for dozens of things that most people think of as toxicants, but that in the hands of biologists are very potent agents for dissecting chemical pathways, physiological actions, and so on. This continues to the present day, although since the 1940s we have had other modalities. Up to that time, almost the only method that we had of blocking metabolic pathways was inhibitors. Now, we have other options such as using genes to do the same thing.

Toxicology also played a very important role in understanding infectious disease. Many germs do their work through the secretion of toxins, which operate in a variety of ways that are described for other kinds of chemical substances. This has been a very interesting challenge in biology.

It is also important to bring new science into old regulations. This is something that I believe the FDA would be eager to do and they need scientific consensus to be able to do that; hence, a meeting of this kind is very helpful in that regard.

Subsequent areas of discussion include the following: the impact of advances in the field of toxicology for resolving debates about whether something is toxic and the degree of toxicity; the impact of metabolism on toxicity; advances in understanding the interaction of toxic substances; the policy dynamics of regulation; and the challenges to assessing risks of adverse drug reactions in new product development.

This particular conference was organized with a lot of assistance and advice from the Procter & Gamble Company. They have been beset by one other facet of the use of animals—namely, that a lot of people love animals and are distraught about how we might be torturing large numbers of animals for testing purposes. This meeting, in as good a way as I can think of, brought together a number of disciplines. These included genomics (a catchphrase for analytic work ultimately based on knowing what the sequence of information is in DNA and then how that is expressed), physiology, and neurobiology. Proteomics played a large role as well (the contrast between what we learn about the first-order measures of gene expression and RNAs and the further steps and discrimination about which proteins are actually going to be synthesized and will remain in the cell).

I also am impressed by how many times the New York Academy of Sciences has been the venue for conferences in this area. I attribute this to the Academy's historic role as a very good place for convergence of industrial and academic interests in a variety of areas, pharmaceuticals and pharmacology being among them. The Academy and its staff are to be highly commended, including Stefan Malmoli for his superb editorial skills.

Use of Oligonucleotide Arrays to Analyze Drug Toxicity

NAFTALI KAMINSKI,[a,b] JOHN ALLARD,[c] AND RENU A. HELLER[c]

[a]*Lung Biology Center and Cardiovascular Research Institute, University of California, San Francisco, California, USA*

[c]*Roche Bioscience, Palo Alto, California, USA*

ABSTRACT: The advent of oligonucleotide arrays allows the simultaneous analysis of the expression of thousands of genes. This powerful technology, highly dependent on advanced analysis tools, can transform the level of information currently available on the mechanisms underlying drug-related toxicity. It is now possible to analyze the global transcriptional response to a drug and determine the global pathways associated with the effects of this agent. This analysis can be performed on samples from patients that developed a toxic effect, on cells exposed to the toxic agent, and in animal models of toxicity. Especially useful is the comparison of transcriptional responses in animals susceptible to drug-induced disease with those of genetically modified animals that are resistant to this effect. This analytic strategy allows the delineation of specific mechanisms relevant and specific to drug-induced toxicity and thus might lead to novel therapeutic interventions in these toxic reactions.

INTRODUCTION

Oligonucleotide and cDNA arrays are novel and potent technologies. The use of array technology enables the global analysis of the expression of thousands of genes simultaneously.[1–3] Not only does this provide us with the global description of the transcriptional program underlying normal development and differentiation, but it can also potentially present us with a complete description of a disease state or of a toxic response.

So far, array technology has been successfully used in the analysis of the transcriptional responses in yeast and mammalian systems, describing and furnishing the responses to cell cycle progression,[4,5] serum and growth factors,[6] cytokines,[7] and caloric restriction.[8]

Drug toxic effects are often hard to comprehend: the inciting agent is frequently known; the result, the adverse effect, is known; however, the mechanisms determining this unwanted effect are at best partially defined, thus limiting the ability to prevent or treat toxicity. This is especially true for antineoplastic agents, where taking full advantage of their full therapeutic potential is limited by severe toxic side effects. In recent years, the abundance of sequence information derived from the var-

---

[b]Address for correspondence: Naftali Kaminski, Lung Biology Center, University of California, San Francisco, Box 0854, San Francisco, CA 94143. Voice: 415-206-5902; fax: 415-206-4123.

kamins@itsa.ucsf.edu

ious genome projects combined with the advances in array technology have made it possible to obtain detailed quantitative transcriptional analysis of these unwanted toxic effects. In the following pages, we will present several approaches to the use of array technology in toxicology and provide examples from our experiments in the mouse model of bleomycin-induced lung injury and fibrosis.

EXPERIMENTAL STRATEGIES

Genomic analysis of a known drug-related toxicity can be done at multiple levels (FIGURE 1). The most straightforward approach would be analyzing the transcriptional patterns in tissues and organs obtained from patients that developed the relevant toxic response. Although this approach can provide valuable data, it is clearly limited by several factors. The availability of human samples is limited; there are many organs, such as the brain, that are rarely, if at all, biopsied in live patients; and one has to depend upon the infrequent availability of postmortem samples. Even in organs that are more frequently sampled, such as the liver, kidney, or lung, the quantity of tissue obtained is not sufficient for analysis by the currently available methods. On top of that, the diversity of human samples complicates the analysis of experimental results. Patients come from different genetic backgrounds and present at different stages of the toxic process, thus making a comprehensive statement regarding the global transcriptional process very difficult. Often, investigators will claim that it is impossible to meet the statistical requirements for a minimal amount

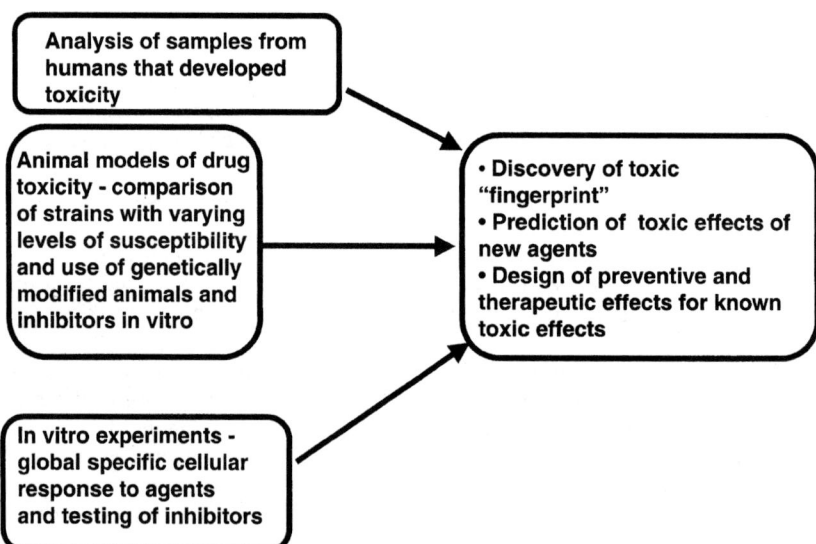

FIGURE 1. The various approaches to obtain a comprehensive transcriptional profile ideally involve not only one strategy, but the combined data obtained from large-scale gene expression analysis of human tissue, animal models of toxicity, and specific cell culture experiments.

of samples to detect a significant change. However, human samples will always have the central role of being the golden standard, that is, the real proof that a mechanism detected in another model is actually relevant.

A completely different approach is genomic analysis of the toxic effect of an agent *in vitro*. It is possible and very easy to expose biologically relevant cells in culture to the agents in question; one could, for example, expose keratinocytes to a cosmetic agent or hepatocytes to a known hepatotoxic agent and analyze the transcriptional response of these cells to various doses of the agent. This approach has several advantages. The experiments are usually simple and easy to analyze, and they are not confounded by cellular infiltration or multicellular interaction. It is relatively easy to standardize the experiments so that variability related to genetic backgrounds and different stages is minimized. Another advantage of this approach is discovery of the direct effects of an unmodified agent on cellular transcriptional response and the potential discovery of unknown mechanisms of action even in a well-characterized drug. This additional information may lead to better drug design and prevention of toxicity. Naturally, the limitations of *in vitro* experiments are clear; they represent a very isolated and artificial model for drug testing. Cells in culture behave phenotypically different than cells *in vivo*, the complex interactions present in a living organ are lacking, and the target cells *in vivo* might be completely different from those chosen for the experiments. However, this approach is valuable for specific questions emerging from *in vivo* studies and potentially in the future could prove as a useful tool for toxicity prediction by screening for a toxic expression "fingerprint" in response to a new compound.

A third possible approach is to utilize known animal models of drug toxicity. The advantages include all the advantages of using animal models of human disease and, in particular, the ability to study in a controlled environment and with minimal genetic variability the transcriptional programs in response to a drug in a single organ or in cell lines derived from the animal. Moreover, the effects of protective agents can be studied in detail at various stages of the toxic response, thus allowing for a full depiction of this response and its essential pathways. The disadvantages of this approach are relatively minor and involve the need to verify the findings in human tissues and the current limitation on the availability of arrays containing genomic data for animals other than mice and rats. Another advantage of using animals is the wide availability of strains with varying susceptibility to a toxic reaction, as well as genetically modified animals (transgenic animals) that may have altered responses to the drug in question. Comparison of the transcriptional response in multiple strains of mice with a differing reaction to a drug, or in mice susceptible to injury, with genetically identical mice in which a single molecule has been genetically modified to give an altered response to the same drug should provide valuable information regarding the toxic response.

None of these strategies is sufficient on its own. Ideally, one would have the advantage of using all three approaches and combining all the data in order to generate a comprehensive drug response transcriptional database. However, even the use of a single approach combined with information obtained by traditional methods might be extremely beneficial.

In the next chapter, we will present an example of our experiments in bleomycin-induced lung injury and fibrosis.

ANALYSIS OF BLEOMYCIN-INDUCED FIBROSIS

The use of bleomycin, an antineoplastic antibiotic commonly used in combination treatments of germ cell tumors, hematologic malignancies, and other malignant disorders, is limited by its pulmonary toxicity.[9] Risk factors for the development of bleomycin-induced lung toxicity include reduced kidney function, exposure to high oxygen concentration, and previous or concomitant thoracic radiotherapy.[9] Much of the information regarding the *in vivo* effects of bleomycin has been acquired using a well-characterized animal model in which lung injury and fibrosis are induced by a single intratracheal administration of the bleomycin.[10] In this model, bleomycin initially induces lung inflammation that is followed by progressive destruction of the normal lung architecture.[11] Studies of gene expression in this model have revealed activation of inflammatory pathways concomitant with upregulation of extracellular matrix proteins, downregulation of metalloproteases, and activation of tissue inhibitors of metalloproteases.[12–19] Some studies have suggested that the fibrotic effects of bleomycin are directly related to the initial inflammatory response.[11] All of these studies have analyzed one or a few genes at a time, thus providing little information about the coordinated patterns of gene expression involved in this toxic response. We have recently published a comprehensive profile of the pulmonary response to using Affymetrix oligonucleotide arrays (Genechip® Mu6500 set) containing probe sets for approximately 6000 murines.[20] Changes in gene expression were monitored after bleomycin treatment in wild-type 129 mice and in 129 mice homozygous for a null mutation of the integrin β6 subunit gene (β6$^{-/-}$)[20] (FIGURE 2). The phenotype of β6$^{-/-}$ mice is unique in that they develop inflammation, but not fibrosis, in response to bleomycin.[21] Of approximately 6000 genes analyzed, 1200–1600 genes were considered present in lung tissue by the Genechip® 3.1 criteria under each condition examined. There was statistically no significant difference between the number of genes considered present in any experimental condition. At baseline, the expression of 84 genes was substantially higher (>2-fold) in β6$^{-/-}$ mice than in β6$^{+/+}$ mice (17 by more than 4-fold), whereas expression of only 26 genes was substantially higher in β6$^{+/+}$ mice (3 by more than 4-fold). However, in response to bleomycin, more genes were induced in β6$^{+/+}$ mice than in β6$^{-/-}$ mice. When we analyzed the patterns of gene expression using hierarchical clustering,[22] we identified several very distinct clusters of genes.[20] The most interesting was a cluster that included genes encoding for proteins involved in extracellular matrix formation, cellular responses to matrix, and extracellular matrix degradation, as well as many TGFβ responsive genes. These genes were expressed at similar levels at baseline in wild-type and β6$^{-/-}$ mice; however, they were dramatically induced by bleomycin in wild-type mice, whereas being induced to a lesser degree in β6$^{-/-}$ mice.[20] These genes provided clues to critical steps in the development of fibrosis. Another cluster included genes that were expressed at higher levels at baseline in β6$^{-/-}$ mice and were also induced by bleomycin. After bleomycin, the absolute level of expression of most of the genes in this cluster was the same or higher in β6$^{-/-}$ mice as in wild-type mice. This cluster consisted mostly of genes known to encode for proteins involved in inflammatory responses. The distinction of two other clusters (namely, genes that were expressed at similar levels in wild-type and β6$^{-/-}$ mice at baseline and in response to bleomycin and genes that were preferentially induced by bleomycin in β6$^{-/-}$) demonstrated that the protection

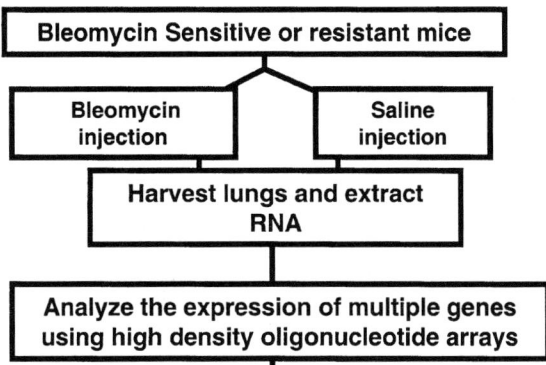

FIGURE 2. The various stages of the experimental design of the analysis of the lung transcriptional response to bleomycin are illustrated. Wild-type (sensitive) or genetically modified (sensitive) animals are subjected to bleomycin. Total RNA is extracted and used for preparation of biotin-labeled cRNA that is hybridized on the array. Patterns of gene expression are then analyzed and compared.

of $\beta 6^{-/-}$ mice from bleomycin-induced pulmonary fibrosis was not simply due to blunting of all cellular responses to the drug. An additional observation was the large number of genes whose expression was decreased after treatment with bleomycin. These genes have been previously largely ignored, although they could be as important in understanding pathogenesis as genes that are induced. The combined data obtained from these strains of mice enabled the depiction of distinct transcriptional modules for inflammation and fibrosis in bleomycin-induced lung injury. In addition, these experiments have provided an enormous amount of information regarding the specific induction of multiple genes, thus allowing the generation of new hypotheses related to bleomycin-induced injury.

DISCUSSION

In this paper, the possibilities embedded in the use of large-scale gene expression technologies in analysis of toxic responses are presented. Several experimental strategies, including global transcriptional analysis of human samples, *in vitro* studies, and comparison of multiple strains of mice with variable susceptibility to drug toxicity, are described.

The results of the analysis of the global transcriptional response to bleomycin that was provided as an example demonstrate the advantages of the latter approach. Several limitations need to be acknowledged and addressed. These methods only measure gene expression levels and they cannot directly identify proteins that participate in biologic responses solely or principally as a result of posttranslational modification. Nonetheless, the global changes in gene expression that are known to occur downstream of such modifications will probably be evident, thus allowing the design of a specific experiment to test this hypothesis. Another limitation is that global analysis of gene expression applied to complex multicellular organs or organisms provides a general expression pattern of the tissue, but is limited in distinguishing changes in transcriptional regulation from changes in cellular composition or from events in a particular cell type. In order to completely analyze and comprehend a toxic response, it is clear that one needs to combine all three experimental strategies previously mentioned, thus creating a complementary set of data that will allow the full understanding of a specific toxic response as well as overcoming the limitations mentioned. In the bleomycin example, we identified distinct groups of genes that are induced in association with the inflammatory and fibrotic responses to this drug and performed a detailed time course analysis. The complete description of the activities of hundreds of genes involved in the inflammatory response and tissue fibrosis induced by bleomycin defined a series of sequential genetic programs that could not have been determined with traditional methods of analysis on a select number of genes, thus proving the validity of this approach.[20] These findings provided a framework for designing interventions that could prevent the development or progression of lung injury fibrosis at various stages after bleomycin administration and may also be relevant to other fibrotic processes.

In conclusion, large-scale transcriptional analysis of tissue and cellular responses to a known toxic or potentially toxic agent using oligonucleotide or cDNA arrays is a valuable tool in toxicologic research. The combined use of multiple experimental approaches and multiple models of drug toxicity leads to a better understanding of the basic mechanisms of drug toxicity. The information and insight gained from the use of array technology in toxicology will lead to the advent of multiple efficient strategies to predict and prevent drug-related toxicity.

ACKNOWLEDGMENTS

The experiments described were done as a collaboration between Dean Sheppard's lab at the Lung Biology Center, University of California at San Francisco, and Renu Heller's lab at Roche Bioscience, Palo Alto, California. We wish to thank Dean Sheppard for his help and invaluable advice in developing the approaches mentioned in this paper.

REFERENCES

1. BROWN, P.O. & D. BOTSTEIN. 1999. Exploring the new world of the genome with DNA microarrays. Nat. Genet. **21:** 33–37.
2. DEBOUCK, C. & P.N. GOODFELLOW. 1999. DNA microarrays in drug discovery and development. Nat. Genet. **21:** 48–50.

3. LIPSHUTZ, R.J., S.P. FODOR, T.R. GINGERAS & D.J. LOCKHART. 1999. High density synthetic oligonucleotide arrays. Nat. Genet. **21:** 20–24.
4. CHU, S., J. DERISI, M. EISEN, J. MULHOLLAND, D. BOTSTEIN, P.O. BROWN & I. HERSKOWITZ. 1998. The transcriptional program of sporulation in budding yeast. Science **282:** 699–705.
5. SPELLMAN, P.T., G. SHERLOCK, M.Q. ZHANG, V.R. IYER, K. ANDERS, M.B. EISEN, P.O. BROWN, D. BOTSTEIN & B. FUTCHER. 1998. Comprehensive identification of cell cycle–regulated genes of the yeast *Saccharomyces cerevisiae* by microarray hybridization. Mol. Biol. Cell **9:** 3273–3297.
6. FAMBROUGH, D., K. MCCLURE, A. KAZLAUSKAS & E.S. LANDER. 1999. Diverse signaling pathways activated by growth factor receptors induce broadly overlapping, rather than independent, sets of genes [see comments]. Cell **97:** 727–741.
7. DER, S.D., A. ZHOU, B.R.G. WILLIAMS & R.H. SILVERMAN. 1998. Identification of genes differentially regulated by interferons α, β, or γ using oligonucleotide arrays. Proc. Natl. Acad. Sci. U.S.A. **95:** 15623–15628.
8. LEE, C.K., R.G. KLOPP, R. WEINDRUCH & T.A. PROLLA. 1999. Gene expression profile of aging and its retardation by caloric restriction. Science **285:** 1390–1393.
9. FRASER, R.S.P., P.J.A. FRASER & R.G. PARE. 1994. Pulmonary disease caused by drugs, poisons, and inhaled toxic gases and aerosols. *In* Synopsis of Diseases of the Chest, p. 754. Saunders. Philadelphia.
10. SNIDER, G.L., J.A. HAYES & A.L. KORTHY. 1978. Chronic interstitial pulmonary fibrosis produced in hamsters by endotracheal bleomycin: pathology and stereology. Am. Rev. Respir. Dis. **117:** 1099–1108.
11. SHEN, A.S., C. HASLETT, D.C. FELDSIEN, P.M. HENSON & R.M. CHERNIACK. 1988. The intensity of chronic lung inflammation and fibrosis after bleomycin is directly related to the severity of acute injury. Am. Rev. Respir. Dis. **137:** 564–571.
12. ZHAO, Y., S.L. YOUNG & J.C. MCINTOSH. 1998. Induction of tenascin in rat lungs undergoing bleomycin-induced pulmonary fibrosis. Am. J. Physiol. **274:** L1049–L1057.
13. SWIDERSKI, R.E., J.E. DENCOFF, C.S. FLOERCHINGER, S.D. SHAPIRO & G.W. HUNNINGHAKE. 1998. Differential expression of extracellular matrix remodeling genes in a murine model of bleomycin-induced pulmonary fibrosis. Am. J. Pathol. **152:** 821–828.
14. SHAHZEIDI, S., B. MULIER, B. DE CROMBRUGGHE, P.K. JEFFERY, R.J. MCANULTY & G.J. LAURENT. 1993. Enhanced type III collagen gene expression during bleomycin induced lung fibrosis. Thorax **48:** 622–628.
15. SHAHZEIDI, S., P.K. JEFFERY, G.J. LAURENT & R.J. MCANULTY. 1994. Increased type I procollagen mRNA transcripts in the lungs of mice during the development of bleomycin-induced fibrosis. Eur. Respir. J. **7:** 1938–1943.
16. SANTANA, A., B. SAXENA, N.A. NOBLE, L.I. GOLD & B.C. MARSHALL. 1995. Increased expression of transforming growth factor beta isoforms (beta 1, beta 2, beta 3) in bleomycin-induced pulmonary fibrosis. Am. J. Respir. Cell Mol. Biol. **13:** 34–44.
17. LUCEY, E.C., H.Q. NGO, A. AGARWAL, B.D. SMITH, G.L. SNIDER & R.H. GOLDSTEIN. 1996. Differential expression of elastin and alpha 1 (I) collagen mRNA in mice with bleomycin-induced pulmonary fibrosis. Lab. Invest. **74:** 12–20.
18. LASKY, J.A., L.A. ORTIZ, B. TONTHAT, G.W. HOYLE, M. CORTI, G. ATHAS, G. LUNGARELLA, A. BRODY & M. FRIEDMAN. 1998. Connective tissue growth factor mRNA expression is upregulated in bleomycin-induced lung fibrosis. Am. J. Physiol. **275:** L365–L371.
19. HOYT, D.G. & J.S. LAZO. 1988. Alterations in pulmonary mRNA encoding procollagens, fibronectin, and transforming growth factor–beta precede bleomycin-induced pulmonary fibrosis in mice. J. Pharmacol. Exp. Ther. **246:** 765–771.
20. KAMINSKI, N., J. ALLARD, J.F. PITTET, F. ZOU, M.J.D. GRIFFITHS, D. MORRIS, X. HUANG, D. SHEPPARD & R.A. HELLER. 2000. Global analysis of gene expression in pulmonary fibrosis reveals distinct programs regulating lung inflammation and fibrosis. Proc. Natl. Acad. Sci. U.S.A. **97:** 1778–1783.
21. MUNGER, J.S., X. HUANG, H. KAWAKATSU, M.J. GRIFFITHS, S.L. DALTON, J. WU, J.F. PITTET, N. KAMINSKI, C. GARAT, M.A. MATTHAY, D.B. RIFKIN & D. SHEPPARD. 1999.

The integrin alpha v beta 6 binds and activates latent TGF beta 1: a mechanism for regulating pulmonary inflammation and fibrosis. Cell **96:** 319–328.
22. EISEN, M.B., P.T. SPELLMAN, P.O. BROWN & D. BOTSTEIN. 1998. Cluster analysis and display of genome-wide expression patterns. Proc. Natl. Acad. Sci. U.S.A. **95:** 14863–14868.

Analysis of Drug Pharmacology towards Predicting Drug Behavior by Expression Profiling Using High-Density Oligonucleotide Arrays

JING-SHAN HU,[a,b] MARK DURST,[a] REINHOLD KERB,[c] VIVI TRUONG,[a]
JING-TYAN MA,[a] ELINA KHURGIN,[a] DAVID BALABAN,[a]
THOMAS R. GINGERAS,[a] AND BRIAN B. HOFFMAN[c]

[a]*Affymetrix, Incorporated, 3380 Central Expressway,
Santa Clara, California 95051, USA*

[c]*Department of Medicine, Stanford University and VA Medical Center,
Palo Alto, California 94304, USA*

> ABSTRACT: An important aspect of the drug development process is prediction of efficacious and toxic side effects. Profiling of mRNA expression is a powerful approach to analyze the molecular phenotype of cells under various conditions, for example, in response to stimulation by compounds. We attempt to explore the approach of using expression profiling to identify patterns or fingerprints that are correlated with specific drug properties or behaviors. Identification of such expression patterns may also lead to revelation of the potential action mechanism of drugs and fingerprints indicative of certain drug efficacy or side effects. We describe here a strategy that was used to identify a set of genes whose differential expression pattern correlates with activation mode and target specificity of a specific group of drug compounds.

INTRODUCTION

The process of drug discovery and development is lengthy and costly. It typically involves the stages of target identification, target validation, lead discovery, lead optimization, preclinical studies, and subsequent clinical trials, including phase I study to evaluate drug safety and toxicity, small-scale phase II, and large-scale phase III studies to evaluate drug efficacy. Many lead compounds fail due to unexpected toxicity or lack of efficacy in late stages of the drug development process. This is often due to incomplete knowledge and understanding about the drug properties, including all their molecular targets and action mechanisms, some of which may be the basis of unpredicted adverse effects or insufficient efficacy. The traditional standard methods to evaluate drug efficacy and toxicity *in vitro* and in animal models are limited to a number of known assays, which sometimes are not sufficient to reveal every aspect of the drug properties. A more thorough approach to survey and reveal the molecular consequences of the drug compounds in the target cells will help a

[b]jing-shan_hu@affymetrix.com

great deal in understanding better the potential side effects and efficacy *in vitro* during early stages of the process of drug discovery and development.

Over the past few years, tremendous advance has been made in deciphering the sequence information of a large portion of human genes. Accompanying this is the development of powerful and versatile microarray technologies to simultaneously monitor mRNA expression levels of these genes using high-density arrays of oligonucleotide or complementary DNAs. These advances provide a particularly efficient way of understanding the molecular phenotype of cells at a genome-wide scale in terms of the activity of the genes and their mRNA expression levels. We hypothesize that pharmaceutical compounds targeted to cells will induce characteristic changes in mRNA expression patterns as a result of affecting specific pathways downstream of the molecular targets of the compounds. Thus, the mode of action and efficacious or toxic side effects of the compounds may be reflected in these characteristic changes in mRNA expression. Profiling of the mRNA expression using microarray technology allows us to determine at genome-wide scale the molecular response of the cells to drug compounds—therefore, to survey more thoroughly the properties and effects of novel compounds on target cells. To explore the approach of using expression profiling to identify patterns or fingerprints that can help predict specific drug effects or behaviors, we aimed to correlate known drug properties with expression patterns that are likely to be the signature for a specific drug property.

DRUG TREATMENT AND EXPRESSION PROFILING

In order to correlate certain drug properties with expression patterns, it is necessary to have enough compounds that can be grouped into different property categories. The more compounds sharing the same property, the more accurately this property can be correlated to the same expression patterns induced by these compounds. There are a large number of agonist and antagonist drugs that are targeted to adrenergic receptors. The pharmacological and biochemical properties of these compounds are well understood and can serve as a good model system for this purpose. As shown in FIGURE 1, their target specificity can be basically classified into three major receptor categories, $\alpha 1$, $\alpha 2$, and β receptors, mediated through three distinct biochemical pathways. Since vascular smooth muscle cells express all three receptors and are a major target cell type of these adrenergic compounds, we used human primary aortic smooth muscle cells as the target cells to investigate changes in mRNA expression patterns induced by these compounds. Human primary cells may serve as a better *in vitro* system to mimic the human *in vivo* cellular response than other human cell lines or nonhuman systems.

To determine the optimal time point for drug treatment, we initially treated human aortic smooth muscle cells at 1, 4, 8, and 24 h time intervals with 10 µM norepinephrine, a full agonist activating $\alpha 1$, $\alpha 2$, and β receptors. By comparing the number of genes differentially expressed after the stimulation, we decided to use the 8 h time interval for the treatment with all the other drugs since gene expression changes induced at this time were relatively more significant than at the 4 h and 24 h time points. The number of genes changed in expression at the 1 h time point was comparable with that at 8 h. However, we were concerned that some of the genes changed at this time point may be too transient to be easily reproducible and some may not

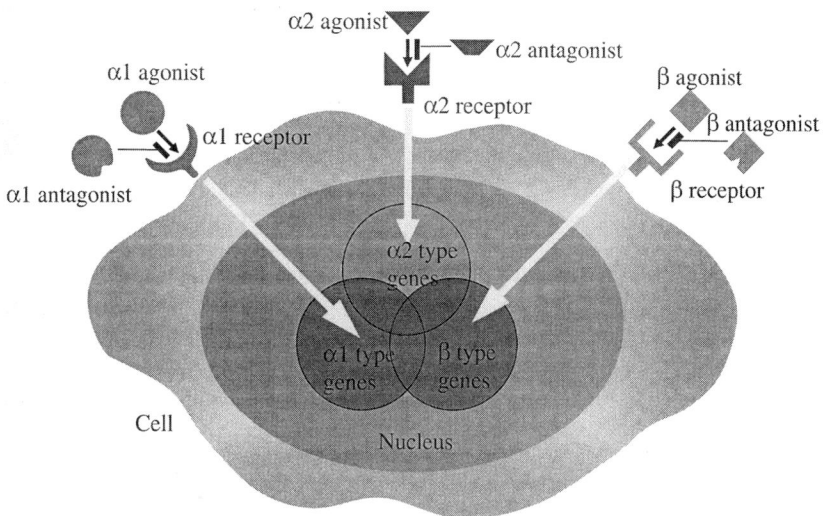

FIGURE 1. Schematic diagram of the activation mode, target specificity, and signaling pathways of compounds targeted to adrenergic receptors.

TABLE 1. List of compounds used to treat cells and their properties

Treatment compounds	Target specificity	Activation mode
Control at 0 h		(0)
Control at 8 h		(0)
Chlorethyclonidine	$\alpha 1$	(−)
Phentolamine	$\alpha 1, 2$	(−)
Norepinephrine	$\alpha 1, 2, \beta$	(−)
SKF39315-C	$\alpha 1, 2$	(+)
SKF1015237-C	$\alpha 2$	(+)
Yohimbine	$\alpha 2$	(−)
Angiotensin II	AT	(?)
Atenolol	$\beta 1$	(−)
Metropolol	$\beta 1$	(−)
Ritodrine	$\beta 2$	(+)
SKF60210-C	$\beta 2$	(+)
Terbutaline	$\beta 2$	(+)
Dopamine	dopamine, α, β	(?)
SKF85174	dopamine	(+)
Epinephrine + Timolol	$\beta 1, 2, \alpha 1, 2$	(+/−)
Norepinephrine + Timolol	$\alpha 1, 2, \beta 1$	(+/−)

NOTE: The sign (0) in activation mode stands for no expected effect, (+) for agonist effect, (−) for antagonist effect, (?) for nonadrenergic receptor involved effect, and (+/−) for combinatory effect of agonist plus antagonist.

necessarily be directly relevant to specific drug action, such as c-fos. Therefore, we treated cells for 8 h with other compounds as listed in TABLE 1 at the concentration of 10 µM. These compounds include agonists and antagonists targeted for α1, α2, and β adrenergic receptors, as well as angiotensin II targeted to angiotensin II receptors. Total RNAs were isolated from cells before the treatment and from cells treated with these compounds and vehicle as a control using an RNeasy kit supplied by QIAGEN. Using the GeneChip® high-density oligonucleotide array of Affymetrix as described previously,[1,2] we monitored the mRNA expression of approximately 6000 human full-length genes from UniGene, GeneBank, and TIGR databases with total RNAs. Duplicate profiles were obtained by hybridizing samples labeled at different times using the same total RNA to different lots of GeneChip® arrays.

EXPRESSION PROFILE ANALYSIS

A gene expression profile contains the hybridization results analyzed by the GeneChip® expression Analysis Suite Version 3.0, including the intensity of the mRNA expression and the fold change of expression levels. The analysis also applies a decision matrix based on the hybridization behavior of all 20 pairs of oligonucleotide probes for each gene. These matrices are used to determine if the gene is expressed above a threshold level (called Present by Absolute Call decision matrix) and changed/differentially expressed above a threshold level (called Increase or Decrease by Difference Call decision matrix). Based on this analysis algorithm and decision matrix, we observed on average that only about 30 genes (0.5%) were called changed by 2-fold or more (increase or decrease) between control and drug-treated samples (TABLE 2). This is the same as the difference between control duplicates presumably caused by the background noise, indicating that the drug treatment induced a very small number of genes to have significant expression changes, indistinguishable from noise based on a single experiment. When using duplicate experiments to analyze the change, however, the average number of genes changed reproducibly in agonist treatments was around 10, or five times as many as in control duplicates (TABLE 2). Therefore, duplicating the experiment can allow the specific changes to stand out from the background differences that usually are caused by random noise and are less likely to be reproducible.

Since the change in gene expression stimulated by drug treatment is very subtle, it would be very difficult to identify common gene expression changes shared by compounds with similar properties from such a small number of genes *significantly* changed. Therefore, expression changes that were less significant need to be included in data analysis using a statistical approach to explore patterns correlated with a drug property.

TABLE 2. Number of genes with significant expression changes of 2-fold or greater as detected by the Difference Call decision matrix as increase or decrease

	Average change/single exp.	Average reproducible change
Agonist vs. control	~30 genes (~0.5%)	~10 genes
Control 2 vs. control 1 (noise level)	~30 genes (~0.5%)	~2 genes

IDENTIFYING GENE SETS BY STATISTICAL APPROACH FOR CLUSTERING

Genes that cannot be detected to be expressed at significant levels or cannot be stimulated to change significantly in response to drug treatment are not relevant in identifying expression change patterns. Thus, we filtered out genes that were never called "increased or decreased" or "present" in any of the drug treatments, according to the expression analysis decision matrices. After these two filtering processes, 1434 genes were kept. To discover gene expression patterns, we attempted to identify gene sets that can be used to cluster drug compounds into different groups based on two properties—their activation mode (agonists versus antagonists) and their target specificity ($\alpha 1$, $\alpha 2$ or β receptors).

It was found that standard clustering software[3] (such as found in the statistical package S-Plus from Mathsoft [www.mathsoft.com] used for most of the analysis in this example) was still swamped by noise in the large number of genes. Further reduction in the number of genes was required. A variety of techniques were tried to isolate a smaller number of genes that might show differences in behavior between the agonist and antagonist treatments. For instance, genes for which the fold change variable had the highest variance across the different treatments were selected for cluster analysis. With the top-ranked 75 most variable genes, the compound can be clustered into separate subgroups correlated with their activation mode and, to a cer-

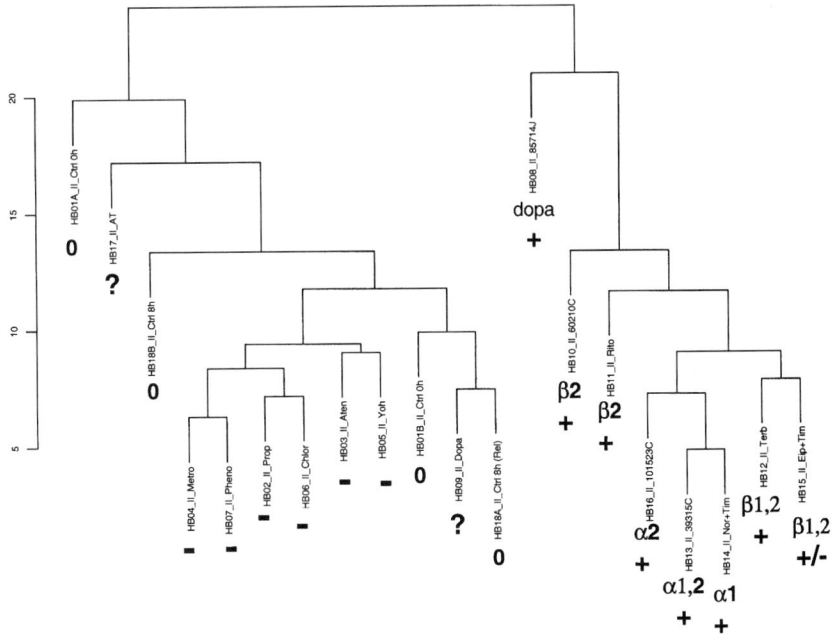

FIGURE 2. Hierarchical clustering of compounds based on the expression fold changes of the 75 most variable genes in response to the compound treatments. The sign (0) stands for no expected effect, (+) for agonist effect, (–) for antagonist effect, (?) for nonadrenergic receptor involved effect, and (+/–) for combinatory effect of agonist plus antagonist.

tain extent, target specificity as well (FIG. 2). The clustering with 75 genes was significantly better than with much smaller (25, 50) or larger (100, 200, 250) numbers of top-ranked gene sets. These 75 genes may be an expression fingerprint that can potentially be used to classify the activation mode and possibly target specificity of other compounds targeted to adrenergic receptors.

In the second statistical approach, 35 genes whose fold change variable behaved most differently between the agonist and antagonist treatments were examined. The distance used was the Kolmogorov-Smirnov (K-S) distance[4] between two empirical distributions, which works as follows. At any threshold value for fold change, it could be determined what fraction of the fold change values were below it and above it for either the agonist or antagonist populations. The K-S distance is the largest difference (across all possible thresholds) between the fractions for the agonists and antagonists. This measure provided slightly more consistent differentiation among the populations. For data visualization, we used the standard technique of principal components.[5] In this technique, an ordered set of orthogonal variables is constructed to explain the most variation in the data with the fewest number of variables. The single linear combination of the variables (the 35 genes with highest K-S distance) that has the highest variance is the first principal component. The highest-variance linear combination orthogonal to the first principal component is the second principal component, and so forth. We computed and graphed the first two principal components on a plot. We were able to see patterns in the data (FIG. 3), including the separation that permitted clustering for most of the agonists (squares) versus antagonists (circles), except for two drugs. It is likely that some of the 35 genes used in principal component analysis are not relevant to the agonist versus antagonist behavior, causing the aforementioned two drugs to fall into a cluster different from most

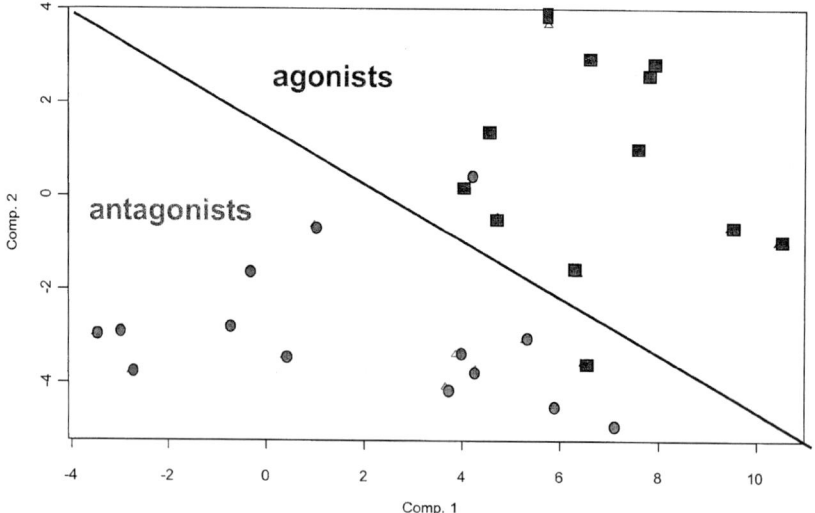

FIGURE 3. Plot of the agonists and antagonists based on the first two principal components derived from the expression fold changes of the 35 selected genes in response to the compound treatment.

of the drugs with the same activation mode. Since agonists and antagonists can be clustered primarily into two groups based on the expression behavior of these 35 genes in response to agonists versus antagonists, these 35 genes can be potentially used as another candidate fingerprint gene set to predict the activation mode of new compounds in the same category.

CONCLUSIONS

The hierarchical clustering analysis based on the behavior of the most variable genes showed that these compounds can be classified into separate groups correlated with their activation mode and, to a certain extent, the target specificity as well. By the Kolmogorov-Smirnov (K-S) distance and principal component analysis, a set of genes have been identified whose expression changes correlated with the activation properties of the compounds targeted at adrenergic receptors. Agonists and antagonists can be classified primarily into two different groups based on the behavior of this set of genes. These two groups of genes can be potentially used as fingerprints for predicting the activation mode or target specificity properties of the compounds. This approach may be extended to identifying expression patterns correlated with specific toxic properties of compounds, which may be used as fingerprints for prediction of drug toxicity. This study suggests that specific gene expression patterns correlated with certain drug effects and behavior can be identified through expression profiling using appropriate statistical analysis approaches.

REFERENCES

1. WODICKA, L. et al. 1997. Genome-wide expression monitoring in *Saccharomyces cerevisiae*. Nat. Biotechnol. **15:** 1359–1367.
2. LOCKHART, D.J. et al. 1996. Expression monitoring by hybridization to high density oligonucleotide arrays. Nat. Biotechnol. **14:** 1675–1680.
3. JOHNSON, R.A. & D.W. WICHERN. 1988. Applied Multivariate Statistical Analysis. Second edition. Prentice–Hall. Englewood Cliffs, New Jersey.
4. WILCOX, R. 1998. Kolmogorov-Smirnov test. *In* Encyclopedia of Biostatistics. Volume 3, pp. 2174–2176. Wiley. New York.
5. GABRIEL, K.R. 1971. The biplot graphical display of matrices with applications to principal component analysis. Biometrika **58:** 453–467.

Development of Human Cell Lines from Multiple Organs

JOHNG S. RHIM

Center for Prostate Disease Research, Uniformed Services University of the Health Sciences, Bethesda, Maryland 20814, USA

ABSTRACT: While the majority of carcinogenesis studies have relied on the use of rodent cells in culture, experimental models to define the role of carcinogenic agents in the development of cancers must be established by using a variety of human cells. Unlike rodent cells, normal human cells in culture rarely undergo spontaneous transformation and have generally proven to be resistant to neoplastic transformation by carcinogens. Remarkable progress has been made during the past decade in human cell transformation systems. Malignant transformation of human cells in culture has been achieved by a stepwise process: immortalization and conversion of the immortalized cells to tumorigenic cells. One of the critical initial events in the progression of normal human cells to tumor cells is the escape from cellular senescence, with few exceptions; normal human cells require immortalization to provide a practical system for carcinogenesis studies. Different cell types require different conditions and transforming agents to achieve a useful cell line. The current state of the art in immortalization of human cells will be presented.

Knowledge of the mechanisms of carcinogenesis in human cells will have obvious implications on strategies for cancer therapy and cancer prevention. Since the development of cancer is a multistage process that generally takes several years, opportunities exist to stabilize, reverse, and inhibit the preneoplastic stages. While the majority of carcinogenesis studies have relied on the use of rodent cells in culture, experimental models to define the role of carcinogenic agents in the development of cancer must be established by using a variety of human cells.

Unlike rodent cells, normal human cells in culture do not or rarely undergo spontaneous transformation and have generally proven to be resistant to neoplastic transformation by carcinogens.[1] For initial studies, a flat, nontumorigenic clonal line (TE85 clone F-5) originally derived from human osteosarcoma cells was used. This cell system was found to be very useful for viral and chemical carcinogenesis since nonproducer Kirsten murine sarcoma virus (Ki-MSV) transformed human cells[2] and chemically transformed human cells[3] have been derived using this cell system. Since most human cancers are of epithelial origin, it is important to obtain a better understanding of this cell type. We used primary human foreskin epidermal keratinocytes to ascertain whether prototype RNA (Ki-MSV) or DNA (Ad12-SV40 hybrid virus) tumor viruses could confer the malignant phenotype to normal primary human epithelial cells. In doing so, we were able to develop for the first time an *in vitro* multistep model suitable for the study of human epithelial cell carcinogenesis.[4] Remarkable progress has been made during the past decade in human cell transformation systems. Malignant transformation of human cells in culture has been achieved by a stepwise process: immortalization and conversion of the immortalized cells to tumorigenic cells. One of the critical initial events in the progression of normal human cells to tumor cells is the escape from cellular senescence, with few exceptions; normal human cells require immortalization to provide a practical system for carcinogenesis studies. Different cell types require different conditions and transforming agents to achieve a useful cell line. The current state of the art in immortalization of human cells will be presented.

IMMORTALIZED HUMAN OSTEOSARCOMA CELLS FOR CARCINOGENESIS STUDY

In the 1970s, there were no human cell lines available to study human cell carcinogenesis. Many attempts were made to transform normal human cells to the neoplastic state without success. Initial successful transformation was achieved in human tumor cells. The nontumorigenic established human osteosarcoma (HOS) clonal (TE85 clone F-5) line was used. This cell system was found to be very useful for chemical and viral carcinogenesis in as much as the first chemically transformed neoplastic human cells and the only nonproducer human transformed cells were derived using this cell system. The HOS cell line, derived originally from aneuploid human osteosarcoma, exhibits a flat morphology, grows densely, forms small colonies in agar, and is nontumorigenic in nude mice. When treated with N-methyl-N'-nitro-N-nitrosoguanidine (MNNG), a potent carcinogen, the cells acquire an altered phenotype, grow as aggregates, form large colonies in agar, and are tumorigenic in nude mice. In addition to MNNG, cell lines derived by treatment with 7,12-dimethylbenzo(α) anthracene (DMBA) and 3-methylcholanthrene (3-MC), as well as by infection with Ki-MSV, have similar properties. The conversion of the nontumorigenic parent HOS line to differing degrees of tumorigenicity following treatment with carcinogenic agents thus provides an *in vitro* model for studying additional genetic alteration involved in tumor progression. These chemically treat-

TABLE 1. Human osteosarcoma clonal (HOS) cells and their transformants

Cell designation	Cell description	Remarks
HOS (TE85 Cl F-5)	Human osteogenic sarcoma clonal cells	p53 (low)
KHOS/NP	Nonproducer cells from Ki-MSV transformed HOS cells	Rescuable sarcoma genome (+)
MNNG/HOS	MNNG transformed HOS cells	*met* (+), p53 (high)
DMBA/HOS	DMBA transformed HOS cells	
Revertant 240S	Revertant from KHOS cells	
S$^+$ L$^-$ HOS	Sarcoma-positive, leukemia-negative HOS cells induced by Mo-MSV	
RSV/HOS	RSV-SR transformed HOS cells	
Revertant 312H	Revertant from KHOS cells	
3-MC/312H	3-MC transformed 312H cells	Activated H-*ras*, p53 (high)
DMBA/312H	DMBA transformed 312H cells	p53 (high)
DU/HOS	Depleted uranium (DU) transformed cells	

ed malignantly transformed HOS cell lines were later found to be useful for studying activated oncogenes and tumor suppressor genes. In fact, MNNG/HOS cells contain activated *met* oncogenes, and 3-MC-HOS contains activated H-*ras* oncogenes. These two oncogenes are thus far the only reported activated oncogenes from chemically transformed human cells. Recently, the transforming potential of depleted uranium, a dense heavy metal used primarily in military applications, has been shown in this HOS cell line[5] (TABLE 1).

IMMORTALITY

Normal human cells in culture have a limited life span, beyond which the cells cease to proliferate, enlarge in size, and undergo a process termed cellular senescence, which results in cell death. Immortalization of human cells by physical and chemical carcinogens has rarely been achieved, and then often with nonreproducible success. Immortalization also can be achieved in cells infected or transfected with certain viral genes; however, this occurred infrequently and only after continuous cell passing (TABLE 2). While immortality is not sufficient for neoplastic transformation, most immortalized cells have an increased sensitivity for spontaneous, carcinogen-induced, or oncogene-induced neoplastic progression. Therefore, escape from senescence can be a preneoplastic change that predisposes a cell to neoplastic conversion. Although immortalization of human cells is an initial key step in neoplastic progression, the mechanisms underlying this event are poorly understood—for example, cellular senescence by which a powerful tumor suppression occurs.[6] Immortalization possibly results from recessive gene mutations and clonal selection associated with carcinogen treatment or prolonged culturing. Besides chemicals, physical agents, and viral genes as immortalizing agents, the importance of negative regulators of cell growth (tumor suppressor genes, Rb, and p53), their inactivation, their genomic instability, and recently the reactivation of a telomerase have been considered in the molecular mechanisms of human cell immortalization.[7,8]

In contrast to rodent cells, the establishment of immortal cell lines that arose spontaneously from normal human cell cultures, without carcinogen treatment, has been rarely reported (TABLE 2). However, spontaneously immortalized human cell lines may be expected to increase in the future, as has been seen in the rapidly increasing number of carcinoma cell lines established by improved cell culture methodology. For example, cells from human mammary carcinoma had been among the most difficult human tumor-derived cells to grow in culture and, therefore, very few primary mammary tumor cell lines were available for study. Development of improved medium now permits us to grow normal and tumor mammary epithelial cells. Although a recent report showed that epithelial cells from patients with Li-Fraumeni syndrome are relatively easy to immortalize,[9] there have been only a few reports on the immortalizing of human cells, spontaneously or by chemical or physical agents (TABLE 2). Once the cells are immortalized using DNA virus such as SV40, adenovirus, papilloma viruses, and recently human telomerase catalytic component (hTERT),[10] they are relatively easy to transform into neoplastic cells, most by *ras* oncogenes, but also by using chemicals or physical agents. These results indicate that the immortalization process is a critical initial and rate-limiting step for transformation of human cells *in vitro*, and immortalized and nontumorigenic human

TABLE 2. Immortalized human cells

Cells	Immortalizing agents	Cells	Immortalizing agents
Fibroblast	SV40, SV40T, SV40 ori, SV40tsA	Kidney	Ad5 DNA
	X ray		Nickel
	v-myc		v-src
	Spontaneous		
	hTERT (telomerase)	Thyroid	SV40, tsSV40, SV40 ori
Epithelia			Ad12S & 135 EIA
Foreskin	SV40, SV40 DNA	Colon	SV40
	Ad12-SV40	Liver	SV40
	Ad12S-EIA DNA	Tracheal gland	Ad12-SV40
	HPV-16, 18, 31, 33 DNA	Oral cavity	SV40
	Spontaneous (HaCat)		HPV-18 DNA
Bronchus	v-H-*ras*	Lentinal gland	SV40
	Ad12-SV40		Ad12-SV40
Breast	Spontaneous (MCF-10, Li-FS)	Cornea	Ad12-SV40
	Mutated p53 (273his)	Ocular ciliary	SV40
	BP (benzopyrene)	Prostate	SV40
	HPV-16 DNA		HPV-18
Ureter	SV40	Melanocyte	SV40
Cervix	HPV-16 & 18 DNA	Endometrial stroma	tsSV40

cells may be useful for detecting and characterizing cellular genes that can contribute to the malignant transformation of human cells.

IMMORTALIZATION OF HUMAN CELLS BY INFECTION WITH AD12-SV40 VIRUS

Because the majority of human tumors are of epithelial origin, it is important to study the epithelial cell system. Human epidermal keratinocytes appear to constitute choice target cells for investigation of *in vitro* transformation of human epithelial cells because of the existence of defined culture conditions allowing their propagation or differentiation. Indeed, the human epidermal keratinocyte system has been one of the most important *in vitro* epithelial cell systems for the study of cellular transformation. When we began our studies, there had been a few reports describing altered growth and differentiation of human keratinocytes following SV40 infection and SV40 DNA transection, but the tumorigenicity of the altered cells was not demonstrated. We used primary human foreskin epidermal keratinocytes to ascertain if prototypic RNA (Ki-MSV) or DNA (Ad12-SV40 hybrid virus) tumor viruses could induce the malignant phenotype. In doing so, we were able to develop for the first time an *in vitro* multistep model suitable for the study of human epithelial cell carcinogenesis.[4] Neither control nor Ki-MSV-infected human epithelial cultures could be propagated serially beyond two or three subcultures. In contrast, infection of primary cultures of human epidermal cells with Ad12-SV40 virus led to the appearance

TABLE 3. Characteristics of human epidermal keratinocytes (HEK) transformed by virus, oncogene, chemicals, and X ray

	Stage of carcinogenesis				
Cells	Primary	Immortalization agent	Transformation agent	Growth in soft agar	Tumorigenicity in nude mice
Primary HEK	+			−	−
K-HEK	Ki-MSV			−	−
RHEK-1	−	Ad12-SV40		−	−
K-RHEK-1	−	Ad12-SV40	Ki-MSV	+	+
pSV$_2$ ras RHEK-1	−	Ad12-SV40	v-H-ras	+	+
M-RHEK-1	−	Ad12-SV40	MNNG	+	+
N-RHEK-1	−	Ad12-SV40	4NQO	+	+
X-RHEK-1	−	Ad12-SV40	X ray (2X)	+	+

NOTE: Nude mice were inoculated with 10^7 cells.

of actively growing colonies by weeks 3 to 4. By week 6, SV40 tumor (T) antigen was detected in the infected cultures by indirect immunofluorescence staining. A number of cell lines were obtained by limiting dilution from colonies that proliferated. All lines, but one, released Ad12-SV40 virus, as indicated by the induction of a cytopathic effect in Vero cells. A nonproducer line, designated RHEK-1, was characterized. The RHEK-1 line had a flat epithelial morphology, showed a number of epithelial cell markers, and was not tumorigenic in nude mice (TABLE 2), although in some cases regressing small cystic nodules containing epidermoid cells appeared at the site of inoculation. Analysis by immunoprecipitation and sodium dodecyl sulfate–polyacrylamide gel electrophoresis (SDS-PAGE) revealed that both large T and small t antigens of SV40 were expressed in this human epithelial cell line. Thus, the SV40 T/t antigens could be responsible for inducing and maintaining the growth properties of the RHEK-1 cell line. This "flat" nonproducer cell line has proven useful for studying multistage carcinogenesis.

This line was sensitive to Ki-MSV infection, chemical carcinogens,[11] X ray,[12] and a variety of retroviruses[13] and by transfection with an activated human *ras* oncogene (TABLE 2). Besides the human epidermal cell described, we were able to successfully establish lines from primary culture by Ad12-SV40 virus infection of human bronchial epithelial cells,[14] human salivary gland,[15] nasal polyp epithelial cells from cystic fibrosis (CF) patients,[16] normal and CF bronchial epithelial cells,[17] human lens cells,[18] and human prostate epithelial cells[19] (TABLE 3).

EFFICIENT IMMORTALIZATION OF HUMAN CELLS BY HUMAN PAPILLOMAVIRUS 16 E6-E7 RETROVIRUSES

The establishment of immortalized human cell lines has proven to be more difficult than the establishment of rodent cell lines. The reason is not fully understood; likely factors include growth requirements for human cells, more difficulty in induc-

TABLE 4. Human cell types immortalized by HPV-16 E6-E7

Epithelia	Smooth muscle
Foreskin	Artery
Cervix	Uterus
Breast	Umbilical cord
Kidney	
Ovary	Hepatocytes
Bronchus	
Ureter	Melanocyte
Oral cavity	
Middle ear	Endothelia
Prostate	Umbilical cord
	Artery
Fibroblast	
Skin	

ing DNA into human cells, and greater genetic stability of human cells. DNA tumor viruses such as SV40 and adenovirus have efficiently transformed rodent cells. However, their utility in human cells is limited by the fact that viral infection results in a productive infection; thus, human cells transformed by DNA tumor viruses continue to release virus as described. To overcome these problems, many investigations have introduced the DNA viral oncogenes into cells. However, this is not an easy task to achieve since different cell types required different conditions and transforming agents to achieve a useful cell line. For example, strontium phosphate transfection has been successfully used to immortalize human neonatal prostatic epithelial cells using plasmid containing the SV40 early region genes,[20] but has failed when used on adult cells.[21] We have succeeded in immortalizing adult human prostate epithelial cells by polybrene-induced DNA transfection of plasmid containing an origin-defective SV40 genome together with a plasmid carrying the neomycin resistance gene.[22] Polybrene, in conjunction with dimethyl sulfoxide (DMSO) shock, has been shown to increase the frequency of DNA transfection of mammalian cells, including human epidermal keratinocytes, as compared with the frequency obtained with calcium phosphate–mediated transfection.[23]

To circumvent problems of inefficient delivery of genes into the cells and to avoid the use of differentiation-promoting agents, such as the effect of calcium on epithelial cells, Galloway et al.[24] constructed a series of recombinant amphotropic retroviruses by using the LXSN vector and the PA 317 packaging cell line.[25] Recent data have shown that use of the amphotropic retroviruses[24] to transduce HPV-16 E6-E7 into human cells has permitted the establishment of a wide variety of established human cell lines from many types of epithelia, as well as from other cells[24] (TABLE 4). Although the HPV-16 E6 or E7 alone was known to be sufficient to immortalize certain human cells,[26–30] only E6-E7 efficiently immortalized most cells. Human keratinocytes were immortalized by HPV-16 E7, but attempts to immortalize with E6 were not successful.[27,28] HPV-16 E6 alone was sufficient to immortalize breast epithelium.[29] A notable exception was bladder epithelium, which was reported to be immortalized efficiently by either E6 or E7.[26]

Cell lines immortalized by HPV-16 genes were nontumorigenic in nude mice and retained most of the phenotypes of primary cells. In a very few cell lines, prolonged passage of the cells in culture led to the generation of tumorigenic lines.[31] Analysis of these cell lines showed no alterations in HPV gene expression, but additional karyotypic changes were noted.[32] One interesting change was the loss of DCC expression in tumorigenic clones.[33] Importantly, ecotropic expression of DCC in the tumorigenic clones suppressed their tumorigenicity.[34] These observations are consistent with the long latency seen to be associated with the development of cervical cancer *in vivo*, and they suggest that the role of HPV is to allow the continued proliferation of cells and that additional non-HPV events are required for the development of malignancy.

As described, integration of DNA encoding the HPV-18 E6-E7 into the genome of cultured primary human cells of different origin leads to a high efficiency of immortalization.[24,35–40] The mechanism underlying this process is not fully understood, although it appears to involve an interaction between the E6-E7, the cellular tumor suppressor protein p53, and the retinoblastoma (Rb) gene product. These interactions are expected to result in disturbance of the normal cell cycle control, leading to the immortalization.[41] A key factor other than p53, Rb, and cellular oncogenes in the establishment of immortalized cells may be the reactivation of a telomerase.[7,8] An important factor in the genetic instability associated with immortalization of cells may be the stability of telomere sequences as recently reported.[42]

CONCLUSIONS

In vitro human cell models are critical for defining the mechanisms of carcinogenesis and for testing preventive and therapeutic regimens. Ideal human cell models should retain the phenotypes of primary cells. It has been known that human cells in culture rarely undergo spontaneous transformation and are remarkably resistant to experimentally induced tumorigenicity. However, as shown here, primary human cells now can be efficiently immortalized and can be transformed into tumorigenic cells. The immortalization and transformation of cultured human cells has far reaching implications for both cell and cancer biology. Human cell transformation studies will increase our understanding of the mechanisms underlying carcinogenesis and differentiation. The neoplastic process can now be studied in a model human cell culture system. The accompanying biochemical and genetic changes, once identified, will help define the relationship between malignancy and differentiation. Thus, the role of carcinogenic agents in human carcinogenesis is presently being defined using a variety of human cells as experimental model systems.

ACKNOWLEDGMENTS

I would like to acknowledge my main collaborators involved in the different phases of this work: R. Huebner, P. Arnstein, E. Weisburger, W. Nelson-Rees, G. Jay,

K. Sanford, S. A. Aaronson, C. Harris, M. Durst, W. Peterson, A. Dritschillo, B. Hukku, M. Webber, and D. Peehl.

REFERENCES

1. RHIM, J.S. 1993. Neoplastic transformation of human cells *in vitro*. Crit. Rev. Oncog. **4**: 313–335.
2. RHIM, J.S., H.Y. CHO & R.J. HUEBNER. 1975. Nonproducer cells of murine sarcoma virus transformed human cells. Int. J. Cancer **15**: 23–29.
3. RHIM, J.S., D.P. PARK, P. ARNSTEIN, R.J. HUEBNER, E.K. WEISBURGER & W.A. NELSON-REES. 1975. Transformation of human cells in culture by N-methyl-N'-nitro-N-nitrosoguanidine. Nature **256**: 751–753.
4. RHIM, J.S., G. JAY, P. ARNSTEIN, F.M. PRICE, K.K. SANFORD & S.A. AARONSON. 1985. Neoplastic transformation of human epidermal keratinocytes by AD12-SV40 and Kirsten sarcoma viruses. Science **227**: 1250–1252.
5. MILLER, A.C., W.F. BLAKELY, D. LIVENGOOD, T. WHITAKER, J. XU, J.W. EJNIK, M.F. HAMILTON, E. PARKETTE, T.S. JOHN, H.M. GERSTENBERG & H. HSU. 1998. Transformation of human osteoblast cells to the tumorigenic phenotype by depleted uranium uranyl chloride. Environ. Health Perspect. **106**: 465–471.
6. O'BRIEN, W., G. STENMANU & R. SAGER. 1986. Suppression of tumor growth by senescence in virally transformed human fibroblasts. Proc. Natl. Acad. Sci. U.S.A. **83**: 8659–8663.
7. SHAY, J.W., W.E. WRIGHT & H. WERBINI. 1991. Defining the molecular mechanisms of human cell immortalization. Biochim. Biophys. Acta **1072**: 1–7.
8. ALLSOPP, R.C., E. CHANG, M. KASHEFI-AAZAM, E.I. ROAGAEV, M.A. PIATYSZEK, J.W. SHAY & C.B. HARLEY. 1995. Telomere shortening is associated with cell division *in vitro* and *in vivo*. Exp. Cell Res. **220**: 194–200.
9. SHAY, J.W., G. TOMLINSON, M.A. PIATYSZEK & L.S. GOLLAHON. 1995. Spontaneous *in vitro* immortalization of breast epithelial cells from a patient with Li-Fraumeni syndrome. Mol. Cell. Biol. **15**: 425–432.
10. MORALES, C.P., S.E. HOLT, M. QUELLETTE, K.J. KAUR, Y. YAN, K.S. WILSON, M.A. WHITE, W.E. WRIGHT & J.W. SHAY. 1999. Absence of cancer-associated changes in human fibroblasts immortalized with telomerase. Nat. Genet. **21**: 115–118.
11. RHIM, J.S., J. FUJITA, P. ARNSTEIN & S.A. AARONSON. 1986. Neoplastic conversion of human epidermal keratinocytes by adenovirus 12–SV40 virus and chemical carcinogens. Science **232**: 385–388.
12. THRAVES, P., Z. SALEHI, A. DRITSCHILLO & J.S. RHIM. 1990. Neoplastic transformation of immortalized human epidermal keratinocytes by ionizing radiation. Proc. Natl. Acad. Sci. U.S.A. **87**: 1174–1177.
13. RHIM, J.S., T. KAWAKAMI, J. PIERCE, K. SANFORD & P. ARNSTEIN. 1988. Cooperation of v-oncogenes in human epithelial cell transformation. Leukemia **2**(151S): 1598.
14. REDDEL, R., Y. KE, B.I. GERWIN, M. MCMENAMIN, J.F. LECHNER, R.T. SU, D.E. BRASH, J.B. PARK, J.S. RHIM & C.C. HARRIS. 1988. Transformation of human bronchial epithelial cells by infection with SV40 or adenovirus 12–SV40 hybrid virus, or transfection via strontium phosphate coprecipitation with a plasmid containing SV40 early region genes. Cancer Res. **48**: 1904–1909.
15. SCHOLTE, B.J., J. BIJMAN, A.T. HOOGEVEEN, R. WILLENSE, J.S. RHIM & W.M. VAN DER KAMP. 1989. Immortalization of nasal polyp epithelial cells from cystic fibrosis patients. Exp. Cell Res. **182**: 559–571.
16. ZEITLIN, P.L., L. LU, J.S. RHIM, G. CUTTING, G. STETTEN, K.A. KIEFFER, R. CRAIG & W.B. GUZZINO. 1991. A cystic fibrosis bronchial epithelial cell line: immortalization by Ad12-SV40 infection. Am. J. Respir. Cell Mol. Biol. **4**: 313–319.
17. CHOPRA, D.P., G.W. TAYLOR, P. MATHIEU, B. HUKKU & J.S. RHIM. 1991. Immortalization of human tracheal gland epithelial cells by adenovirus 12–SV40 virus. In Vitro Cell. Dev. Biol. **27A**: 763–765.

18. ANDLEY, U.P., J.S. RHIM, L.T. CHYLACK & T.P. FLEMING. 1994. Propagation and immortalization of human lens epithelial cells in culture. J. Invest. Ophthalmol. Vis. Sci. **35:** 3094–3102.
19. WEBBER, M.M., D. BELLO, H.K. KLEINMAN, D.D. WANTINGER, D.E. WILLIAMS & J.S. RHIM. 1996. Prostate specific antigen and androgen receptor induction and characterization of an immortalized adult human prostate epithelial cell line. Carcinogenesis **17:** 1751–1755.
20. KAIGHN, M.E., R.R. REDDEL, J.F. LECHNER, D.M. PEEHL, R.F. CAMALIER, D.E. BRASH, U. SAFFIOTTI & C.C. HARRIS. 1989. Transformation of human neonatal prostate epithelial cells by strontium phosphate transfection with a plasmid containing SV40 early region genes. Cancer Res. **49:** 3050–3056.
21. CUSSENOT, O., P. BERTHON, R. BERGER, I. MOWSZOWICZ, A. FAILE, F. HOJMAN, P. TEILLAC, A. LE DUC & F. CALVO. 1991. Immortalization of human adult normal prostatic epithelial cells by liposomes containing large T-SV40 gene. J. Urol. **146:** 881–886.
22. LEE, M.S., E. GARKOVENKO, J.S. YUN, P.C. WEIJERMAN, D.M. PEEHL, L.S. CHEN & J.S. RHIM. 1994. Characterization of adult human prostatic epithelial cells immortalized by polybrene-induced DNA transfection with a plasmid containing an origin-defective SV40 genome. Int. J. Oncol. **4:** 821–830.
23. RHIM, J.S., J.B. PARK & G. JAY. 1989. Neoplastic transformation of human keratinocytes by polybrene-induced DNA-mediated transfer of an activated oncogene. Oncogene **4:** 1403–1409.
24. GALLOWAY, D.A., C.L. HALBERT, G.W. DEMERS, S.A. FOSTER, R.A. BHANTON, D. MEDRICK, A. KLINGELHUTZ & J.K. MCDOUGALL. 1996. Use of amphotropic retroviruses expressing human papillomavirus 16 E6 and E7 to determine the consequences of acute expression of the viral oncogenes and to establish immortalized human cell lines. Radiat. Oncol. Invest. **3:** 315–319.
25. MILLER, A.D. 1992. Retroviral vectors. Curr. Top. Microbiol. Immunol. **158:** 1–24.
26. REZNIKOFF, C.A., C.D. BELAIR, E. SAVELIEVA, Y. ZHAI, K. PFEIFER, T. YEAGER, K.J. THOMPSON, S. DEVERIES, C. BINDLEY, M.A. NEWTON, G. SCKHON & F. WALDMAN. 1994. Long-term genome stability and minimal genotypic and phenotypic alterations in HPV-16 E7, but not E6 immortalized human uroepithelial cells. Genes Dev. **8:** 2227–2240.
27. HALBERT, C.L., G.W. BEMERS & D.A. GALLOWAY. 1991. The E7 gene of human papillomavirus type 16 is sufficient for immortalization of human epithelial cells. J. Virol. **65:** 473–478.
28. HASHIDA, T. & S. YASUMOTO. 1991. Induction of chromosome abnormalities in mouse and human epidermal keratinocytes by the human papillomavirus type 16 E7 oncogene. J. Gen. Virol. **72:** 1569–1577.
29. WAZER, D.E., X.L. LIU, Q. CHU, Q. GAO & V. BAND. 1995. Immortalization of distinct human mammary epithelial cell types by human papillomavirus 16 E6 or E7. Proc. Natl. Acad. Sci. U.S.A. **92:** 3687–3681.
30. SHAY, J.W., W.E. WRIGHT, D. BRASISKYTE & B.A. VAN DER HAEGE. 1993. E6 of human papillomavirus type 16 can overcome the M1 stage of immortalization in human mammary epithelial cells, but not in human fibroblasts. Oncogene **8:** 1407–1413.
31. HURLIN, P.J., P. KAUR, P.P. SMITH, N. PEREZ-REYES, R.A. BLANTON & J.K. MCDOUGALL. 1991. Progression of human papillomavirus type 18–immortalized human keratinocytes to a malignant phenotype. Proc. Natl. Acad. Sci. U.S.A. **88:** 570–574.
32. SMITH, P.P., C.L. FRIEDMAN, E.M. BRYANT & J.K. MCDOUGALL. 1992. Viral integration and fragile sites in human papillomavirus-immortalized human keratinocyte cell lines. Genes Chromosomes Cancer **5:** 150–157.
33. KLINGELHUTZ, A.J., P.P. SMITH, L.R. GARRETT & J.K. MCDOUGALL. 1993. Alteration of the DCC tumor-suppressor gene is transformed by nitrosomethylurea. Oncogene **8:** 95–99.
34. KLINGELHUTZ, A.J., L. HEDRICK, K.R. CHO & J.K. MCDOUGALL. 1995. The DCC gene suppresses the malignant phenotype of transformed human epithelial cells. Oncogene **10:** 1581–1586.
35. WILLEY, J.C., A. BROUSSAND, A. SLEEMI, W. BENNETT, P. CERUTI & C.C. HARRIS. 1991. Immortalization of normal human bronchial epithelial cells by human papillomavirus 16 or 18. Cancer Res. **51:** 5370–5377.

36. PECOKARO, G., D. MORGAN & W. DEFENDI. 1989. Differential effects of human papillomavirus type 6, 16, and 18 DNAs on immortalization and transformation of human cervical epithelial cells. Proc. Natl. Acad. Sci. U.S.A. **86:** 563–567.
37. DURST, M., R.T. DZARLIEVA-PETRUSEUSKA, P. BOUKAMP, N.E. FUSNIG & L. GISSMANN. 1986. Molecular and cytogenetic analysis with human papillomavirus type 16 DNA. Oncogene **1:** 251–256.
38. TSAO, S.W., S.C. MOK, E.G. FEY, J.A. FLETCHER, T.S.K. WAN, E.C. CHEW, M.G. MUTO, R.E. KNAPP & R.B. BERKOWITZ. 1995. Characterization of human ovarian surface epithelial cells immortalized by human papillomaviral oncogenes (HPV-E6E7 ORF's). Exp. Cell Res. **218:** 499–507.
39. PEREZ-REYES, N., C.L. HALBERT, P.P. SMITH, E.P. BENDITT & J.K. MCDOUGALL. 1992. Immortalization of primary human smooth muscle cells. Proc. Natl. Acad. Sci. U.S.A. **89:** 1224–1228.
40. LAZARO, C.A., C. YU, N. FANSTO & J.A. RHIM. 1999. Efficient establishment of human hepatocyte cell lines from multiple individuals: significance for studying the biotransformation of chemical carcinogens. Presented at the *In Vitro* Transformation Meeting of the International Congress of Radiation Research, Cork, Ireland, July 24, 1999.
41. VOUSDEN, K. 1993. Interactions of human papillomavirus transforming proteins with products of tumor suppressor genes. FASEB J. **7:** 872–879.
42. KLINGELHUTZ, A.J., S.A. BARBER, P.P. SMITH, K. DYER & J.K. MCDOUGALL. 1994. Restoration to telomeres in human papillomavirus-immortalized human anogenital epithelial cells. Mol. Cell. Biol. **14:** 961–969.

Fluorometric High-Throughput Screening for Inhibitors of Cytochrome P450

VAUGHN P. MILLER,[a] DAVID M. STRESSER, ANDREW P. BLANCHARD, STEPHANIE TURNER, AND CHARLES L. CRESPI

GENTEST Corporation, Woburn, Massachusetts 01801, USA

ABSTRACT: Rapid screening for cytochrome P450 inhibitors is part of the current paradigm for avoiding development of drugs likely to give clinical pharmacokinetic drug-drug interactions and associated toxicities. We have developed microtiter plate–based, direct, fluorometric assays for the activities of the principal human drug-metabolizing enzymes, CYP1A2, CYP2C8, CYP2C9, CYP2C19, CYP2D6, and CYP3A4, as well as for CYP2A6, which is an important enzyme in environmental toxicology. These assays are rapid and compatible with existing high-throughput assay instrumentation. For CYP1A2, CYP2C8, CYP2C9, CYP2C19, and CYP2D6, the potency of enzyme inhibition (IC_{50}) is consistent regardless of the probe substrate or assay method employed. In contrast, CYP3A4 inhibition for an individual inhibitor shows significant differences in potency (>300-fold) depending on the probe substrate being used. We have investigated these differences through the use of several structurally distinct fluorescent substrates for CYP3A4 and several classical substrate probes (e.g., testosterone, nifedipine, and midazolam), with a panel of known, clinically significant, CYP3A4 inhibitors. The use of multiple probe substrates appears to be needed to characterize the inhibition potential of xenobiotics for CYP3A4.

INTRODUCTION

Adverse reactions due to drug-drug interactions have become a serious concern for pharmaceutical companies, doctors, and the public as patients. In such an interaction, the new drug entity (NDE) inhibits the metabolism of a comedication. As a result, the circulating concentrations of the comedication are increased and, if the comedication has a narrow therapeutic index, an adverse toxic reaction can occur. An NDE that causes drug-drug interactions can be more time-consuming and costly to develop, can suffer decreased market acceptance, and in some cases can lead to product withdrawal. For example, shortly after approval, Posicor[1] (mibefradil) was withdrawn from the marketplace due to drug-drug interactions at the level of cytochrome P450 metabolism. Testing for drug-drug interactions has been the subject of a recent FDA guidance document.[2] These commercial and regulatory pressures have created a need to move this testing into the lead optimization phase of drug development.

The majority of drug-drug interactions are metabolism-based, that is, two or more drugs competing for metabolism by the same enzyme, and the majority of these

---

[a]Address for correspondence: GENTEST Corporation, 6 Henshaw Street, Woburn, MA 01801. Voice: 781-935-5115 ×2208; fax: 781-938-8644.
vpmiller@gentest.com

interactions involve cytochrome P450.[3,4] The cytochrome P450 system is a superfamily of membrane-bound, heme-containing, mixed-function oxygenases that are a principal enzyme system for the metabolism of drugs. Cytochromes P450 principally function to introduce oxygen into a molecule to increase the hydrophilicity of the product and hence the ease with which the product can be eliminated from the body. These enzymes are expressed in many tissues, but in mammals are found at the highest levels in liver. Liver and many other tissues contain several different cytochrome P450 forms with different substrate specificities.

There are 11 xenobiotic-metabolizing cytochromes P450 that are expressed in a typical human liver (CYP1A2, CYP2A6, CYP2B6, CYP2C8/9/18/19, CYP2D6, CYP2E1, and CYP3A4/5). Comprehensive reviews of each of the cytochrome P450 subfamilies have been recently published.[5] A subset of these enzymes, CYP1A2, CYP2C8, CYP2C9, CYP2C19, CYP2D6, and CYP3A4, appear to be responsible for the metabolism of most drugs.[6,7] The importance of these enzymes in drug metabolism is due to their mass abundance (e.g., CYP3A4 is the most abundant P450 in human liver) and their preference for chemical structures commonly found in drugs (e.g., CYP2D6 preferentially binds and metabolizes drugs with basic amine functionalities). In addition, several of these enzymes (e.g., CYP2C9, CYP2C19, and CYP2D6) are polymorphic in humans, with a significant percentage of the population either lacking the enzyme or carrying a variant form.[8–10]

The rationale for *in vitro* screens is the single enzyme paradigm for drug-drug interactions. In this paradigm, if an NDE inhibits the metabolism of one probe substrate for an enzyme, then it is assumed that it inhibits all substrates of that enzyme. Therefore, potential drug-drug interactions can be tested on an enzyme-by-enzyme basis with a limited number of probe substrates. The classical approach for *in vitro* cytochrome P450 inhibition analysis is to use a drug as a probe substrate and measure inhibition over a range of substrate and inhibitor concentrations. Quantitative measures of inhibition potential, apparent K_i or IC_{50} at a given substrate concentration, are calculated. In lead optimization, a higher throughput mode of operation, it is not always necessary to determine an apparent K_i or IC_{50}. For example, as an initial screen, a single inhibitor concentration can be tested as a means to identify potent (<1 µM) and/or weak inhibitors (>50 µM). More detailed analyses would be performed in follow-up testing.

Traditionally, analysis of the metabolism of a drug probe substrate usually involves HPLC separations that are, by definition, not high throughput. A number of improvements and refinements to the assay methodology have been reported. For example, Rodrigues *et al.*[11–13] have used a radiolabeled drug molecule and measured the formation of the radiolabeled metabolites, either formaldehyde or acetaldehyde. The simple sample workup (e.g., charcoal extraction) facilitates parallel processing in a multiwell plate. Similarly, Wynalda and coworkers[14] have reported the use of radiolabeled substrates with a rapid HPLC analysis.

Much higher data acquisition rates (true high throughput) can be achieved by using direct, fluorometric cytochrome P450 substrates in a multiwell plate format. Recently, we have developed microtiter plate–based, fluorometric assays for the activities of the principal drug-metabolizing P450 enzymes.[15] These assays are based on cytochrome P450–catalyzed *O*-dealkylation reactions that generate an easily detectable fluorescent product. The cytochrome P450 enzymes can be introduced into the assay as single, cDNA-expressed enzymes or as enzyme mixtures (i.e., tissue fractions such as human liver microsomes). If tissue fractions are to be used, the probe substrate must be selectively metabolized by the enzyme of interest and not by other enzymes.

NEW ASSAY METHODS

Since our initial reports, a number of new substrates and refinements in the assay methodology have been achieved. The purpose of these refinements was to increase the signal-to-noise ratio in the assay, which allowed a reduction in the amount of enzyme necessary to obtain a robust signal. A summary of the current fluorometric assay conditions and kinetics is shown in TABLE 1. These conditions are based on a reaction volume of 200 µL per microtiter plate well. (Note: The most recent information regarding this assay can be found at the following internet web site: www.gentest.com.)

All relevant enzyme preparations now contain the cytochrome P450 redox partner, cytochrome b_5. Cytochrome b_5 stimulates the rates of metabolite formation for some cytochromes P450. For example, incorporation of cytochrome b_5 into the CYP2C9 and CYP2C19 microsome preparations increased the rates of 7-ethoxy-3-cyanocoumarin (CEC) metabolism by 4- to 6-fold. This allows a reduction in the amount of enzyme needed in the assay. The presence or absence of cytochrome b_5 does not affect the observed IC_{50} values.

We have optimized the buffer concentration for each enzyme assay. The optimal concentrations are listed in TABLE 1. Optimization of the buffer concentrations has increased metabolite formation by 20–50% for CYP2C9, CYP2C19, and CYP3A4.

New, novel substrates have been developed. These include (1) 3-[2-(N,N-Diethyl-N-methylammonium)ethyl]-7-methoxy-4-methylcoumarin (AMMC) as a substrate for CYP2D6. Relative to the original substrate, CEC, AMMC has a 3-fold better signal-to-noise ratio per unit enzyme. AMMC O-demethylation is CYP2D6-selective in human liver microsomes (CEC is not enzyme selective). Therefore, this substrate can be used with either cDNA-expressed CYP2D6 or human liver microsomes (HLM). However, the low CYP2D6 content in HLM requires the use of high protein concentrations. (2) 7-Benzyloxyquinoline (BQ) and 7-benzyloxy-4-trifluoromethyl-coumarin (BFC) as substrates for CYP3A4. Relative to the original substrate, 7-benzyloxyresorufin (BzRes), both BQ and BFC have higher aqueous solubility and BFC has a 15-fold better signal-to-noise ratio per unit enzyme. Both BQ and BFC are highly selective for CYP3A in HLM. These substrates can be readily used with either cDNA-expressed CYP3A4 or HLM as an enzyme source. (3) O-Benzyl-fluorescein benzyl ester (dibenzylfluorescein or DBF) as a substrate for several enzymes. The benzyl ether of DBF is removed through cytochrome P450 catalysis. Following ester hydrolysis by sodium hydroxide, the fluorescent product, fluorescein, is easily detected and quantitated. DBF is the first fluorescent substrate reported for CYP2C8. DBF is a structurally diverse fluorescent substrate for CYP3A4 that complements other substrates in assessing the inhibition potential of this enzyme's complicated kinetics (see discussion below). DBF is also a useful substrate for CYP2C9 and CYP2C19, providing greater sensitivity than the previously reported coumarin derivatives.

TABLE 1. Summary of assay conditions and kinetics

	Cytochrome P450 enzyme				
	CYP1A2	CYP2A6	CYP2C8	CYP2C9	
Substrate	CEC 5 μM	Coumarin 3 μM	DBF 1 μM	MFC 75 μM	DBF
Enzyme quantity	0.5 pmol	1.0 pmol	4.0 pmol	1.0 pmol	2 pmol
Buffer	100 mM KPO$_4$ pH 7.4	100 mM Tris pH 7.5	50 mM KPO$_4$ pH 7.4	25 mM KPO$_4$ pH 7.4	25 mM KPO$_4$ pH 7.4
Apparent K_m	3.5 μM	1.2 μM	1.0 μM	78 μM	0.8 μM
Apparent V_{max}	3.4 min^{-1}	33 min^{-1}	0.4 min^{-1}	2.1 min^{-1}	0.1 min^{-1}
Incubation time	15 min	15 min	30 min	45 min	30 min

	Cytochrome P450 enzyme			
	CYP2C19	CYP2D6	CYP3A4		
Substrate	CEC 25 μM	DBF	AMMC 1.5 μM	BzRes 50 μM	7-BQ 40 μM	BFC 50 μM	DBF 1 μM
Enzyme quantity	0.5 pmol	1 pmol	1.5 pmol	3.0 pmol	3.0 pmol	1.0 pmol	0.5 pmol
Buffer	50 mM KPO$_4$ pH 7.4	50 mM KPO$_4$ pH 7.4	100 mM KPO$_4$ pH 7.4	200 mM KPO$_4$ pH 7.4			
Apparent K_m	29 μM	1.6 μM	1 μM	38 μM	38 μM	>200 μM	1.0 μM
Apparent V_{max}	0.016 min^{-1}	1.0 min^{-1}	1 min^{-1}	0.3 min^{-1}	44 min^{-1}	1.5 min^{-1} @ 40 μM	22 min^{-1}
Incubation time	30 min	30 min	30 min	30 min	30 min	30 min	10 min

Finally, the standard CYP2A6 coumarin hydroxylase assay[16] has been modified into a microtiter plate–based format.

CORRELATION OF IC_{50} VALUES

For CYP1A2, CYP2C9, CYP2C19, and CYP2D6 enzymes, we have observed a good correlation between IC_{50} values obtained with traditional methods and with the fluorometric substrates.[17] This has been observed both retrospectively with a panel of 20 established inhibitors and in follow-up traditional testing of potential NDEs that showed high potency in the fluorometric assays. Similarly, Palamanda *et al.*[18] have found that, for 62 compounds, IC_{50} values determined with cDNA-expressed CYP2D6 and the original fluorescent substrate for CYP2D6 (CEC) were in good agreement with IC_{50} values determined with dextromethorphan and HLM. However, for 9 of the 62 compounds, the difference between the two systems was more than 5-fold and the authors recommend follow-up testing using traditional methodology in HLM.

INTERPRETATION OF DATA WITH CYP3A4

The good correlation in IC_{50} values among fluorometric substrates and traditional substrates for CYP1 and CYP2 enzymes does not extend to CYP3A4. We have investigated these differences through the use of several structurally distinct fluorescent substrates for CYP3A4 and several classical substrate probes (e.g., testosterone, nifedipine, and midazolam), with a panel of known, clinically significant, CYP3A4 inhibitors (TABLE 2). This enzyme demonstrates marked substrate specificity in IC_{50} values among different probe substrates (both traditional substrates and fluorometric substrates). The average sensitivity of the fluorescent probe substrates to inhibition is BFC > BzRes and DBF > BQ. The poor correlation between substrates cannot be easily attributed to differences in experimental conditions. For example, all substrates were used at a concentration around the apparent K_m, and the enzyme was often present at identical concentrations. When BQ and BFC were used to determine IC_{50} values with HLM and cDNA-expressed CYP3A4, the IC_{50} values obtained with cDNA-expressed CYP3A4 and HLM were in good agreement. Therefore, these differences in IC_{50} values appear not to be related to the source of enzyme.

Human CYP3A4 has been demonstrated to simultaneously bind and metabolize multiple compounds in its active site.[19] Cooperativity, activation, and complex inhibition kinetics[20,21] are much more common with CYP3A4 than with enzymes of the CYP1 and CYP2 families. For example, a common probe substrate for CYP3A4, testosterone, does not inhibit, but activates or stimulates BzRes and BQ dealkylation. At this time, the full extent of the substrate dependence in CYP3A4 inhibition is unknown and additional research is needed. Given the variability seen with CYP3A4 and different substrate/inhibitor pairs, there will always be a significant level of uncertainty in interpreting the results of screening for CYP3A4 inhibition. A prudent approach would be to use multiple CYP3A4 probe substrates in a screening mode and follow-up studies with likely comedications. If a single substrate must be used, BFC appears to be the most conservative choice.

TABLE 2. CYP3A4 IC$_{50}$ correlations (r^2)

	Testosterone	BQ	BFC	DBF	Midazolam	Nifedipine
BzRes	0.42	0.71	0.63	0.77	0.18	0.73
Testosterone		0.85	0.93	0.85	0.66	0.85
BQ			0.90	0.94	0.43	0.92
BFC				0.94	0.59	0.96
DBF					0.45	0.98
Midazolam						0.73

NOTE: All values are log-transformed.

CONCLUSIONS

Novel experimental designs like the development of sensitive fluorometric assays for cytochromes P450 have increased the throughput to assess the potential for xenobiotics to inhibit these enzymes—a mechanism for clinical drug-drug interactions and associated toxicities. Inhibition results (IC$_{50}$ values) with these fluorometric methods are in general agreement with results obtained with traditional methods. This methodology is simple and compatible with existing high-throughput screening instrumentation, providing a rapid means to assess the potential for drug candidates to inhibit cytochromes P450.

The complexity of CYP3A4 inhibition analysis indicates that the use of a single substrate is inappropriate. Therefore, it is desirable to identify additional fluorometric CYP3A4 substrates and an appropriate approach for decision making based on the results of experiments with multiple substrates.

REFERENCES

1. MULLINS, M.E., B.Z. HOROWITZ, D.H.J. LINDEN, G.W. SMITH, R.L. NORTON & J. STUMP. 1998. Life-threatening interactions of mibefradil and beta-blockers with dihydropyridine calcium channel blockers. J. Am. Med. Assoc. **280**: 157.
2. FDA. 1997. Drug metabolism/drug interaction studies in the drug development process: studies *in vitro*. *In* Guidance for Industry. United States FDA.
3. MURRAY, M. 1992. P450 enzymes: inhibition mechanism, genetic regulation, and effects of liver disease. Clin. Pharmacokinet. **23**: 132.
4. GUENGERICH, F.P. 1997. Role of cytochrome P450 enzymes in drug-drug interactions. *In* Drug-Drug Interactions: Scientific and Regulatory Perspectives, p. 7. Academic Press. San Diego.
5. IOANNIDES, C. 1996. Part II. Cytochrome P450 families/subfamilies. *In* Cytochromes P450: Metabolic and Toxicological Aspects, p. 77. CRC Press. New York.
6. SPATZENEGGER, M. & W. JAEGER. 1995. Clinical importance of hepatic cytochrome P450 in drug metabolism. Drug Metab. Rev. **27**: 397.
7. RENDIC, S. & F.J. DI CARLO. 1997. Human cytochrome P450 enzymes: a status report summarizing their reactions, substrates, inducers, and inhibitors. Drug Metab. Rev. **29**: 413.
8. GONZALEZ, F.J., R.C. SKODA, S. KIMURA, M. UMENO, U.M. ZANGER, D.W. NEBERT, H.V. GELBOIN, J.P. HARDWICK & U.A. MEYER. 1988. Characterization of the common genetic defect in humans deficient for debrisoquine metabolism. Nature (Lond.) **331**: 442.

9. WRIGHTON, S.A., J.C. STEVENS, G.W. BECKER & M. VANDENBRANDEN. 1993. Isolation and characterization of human liver cytochrome P450 2C19: correlation between 2C19 and S-mephenytoin 4'-hydroxylase. Arch. Biochem. Biophys. **306:** 240.
10. FURUYA, H., P. FERNANDEZ-SALGUERO, W. GREGORY, H. TABER, A. STEWARD, F.J. GONZALEZ & J.R. IDLE. 1995. Genetic polymorphism of CYP2C9 and its effect on warfarin maintenance dose requirement in patients undergoing anticoagulation therapy. Pharmacogenetics **5:** 389.
11. RODRIGUES, A.D., M.J. KUKULKA, B.W. SURBER, S.B. THOMAS, J.Y. UCHIC, G.A. ROTERT, G. MICHAEL, B. THOME-KROMER & J.M. MACHINIST. 1994. Measurement of liver microsomal cytochrome P450 (CYP2D6) using [O-methyl-^{14}C]-dextromethorphan. Anal. Biochem. **219:** 309.
12. RODRIGUES, A.D., M.J. KUKULKA, E.M. ROBERTS, D. OUELLET & T.R. RODGERS. 1996. (O-Methyl C-14) naproxen O-demethylase activity in human liver microsomes—evidence for the involvement of cytochrome P4501A2 and P4502C9/10. Drug Metab. Dispos. **24:** 126.
13. RODRIGUES, A.D., B.W. SURBER, Y. YAO, S.L. WONG & E.M. ROBERTS. 1997. [O-Ethyl-^{14}C]-phenacetin O-deethylase activity in human liver microsomes. Drug Metab. Dispos. **25:** 1097.
14. WYNALDA, M.A. & L.C. WIENKERS. 1997. Assessment of potential interactions between dopamine receptor agonists and various human cytochrome P450 enzymes using a simple *in vitro* inhibition screen. Drug Metab. Dispos. **25:** 1211.
15. CRESPI, C.L., V.P. MILLER & B.W. PENMAN. 1997. Microtiter plate assays for inhibition of human, drug-metabolizing cytochromes P450. Anal. Biochem. **248:** 188.
16. YAMANO, S., J. TATSUNO & F.J. GONZALEZ. 1990. The CYP2A3 gene product catalyzes coumarin 7-hydroxylation in human liver microsomes. Biochemistry **29:** 1322–1329.
17. CRESPI, C.L., V.P. MILLER & B.W. PENMAN. 1998. High throughput screening for inhibition of cytochrome P450 metabolism. Med. Chem. Res. **8:** 457.
18. PALAMANDA, J.R., L. FAVREAU, C-C. LIN & A.A. NOMEIR. 1998. Validation of a rapid microtiter plate assay to conduct cytochrome P450 2D6 enzyme inhibition studies. Drug Discovery Today **3:** 466.
19. KORZEKWA, K.R., N. KRISHNAMACHURY, M. SHOU, A. OGAI, R.A. PARISE, A.E. RETTIE, F.J. GONZALEZ & T.S. TRACY. 1998. Evaluation of atypical cytochrome P450 kinetics with two-substrate models: evidence that multiple substrates can simultaneously bind to the cytochrome P450 active sites. Biochemistry **37:** 4137.
20. WANG, R.W., D.J. NEWTON, T.D. SCHERI & A.Y.H. LU. 1997. Human cytochrome P4503A4-catalyzed testosterone 6(beta)-hydroxylation and erythromycin N-demethylation: competition during catalysis. Drug Metab. Dispos. **25:** 502.
21. UENG, Y-F., T. KUWABARA, Y.J. CHUN & F.P. GUENGERICH. 1997. Cooperativity in oxidation catalyzed by cytochrome P450 3A4. Biochemistry **36:** 370.

Quantitative Proteome Analysis
Methods and Applications

RUEDI AEBERSOLD, BEATE RIST, AND STEVEN P. GYGI

Department of Molecular Biotechnology, University of Washington, Seattle, Washington 98195, USA

ABSTRACT: With the completion of a rapidly increasing number of complete genomic sequences, much attention is currently focused on how the information contained in sequence databases might be interpreted in terms of the structure, function, and control of biological systems. Quantitative proteome analysis, the global analysis of protein expression, has been proposed as a method to study steady-state gene expression and perturbation-induced changes. Here, we discuss the rationale for quantitative proteome analysis, highlight the limitations in the current standard technology, and introduce a new experimental approach to quantitative proteome analysis.

INTRODUCTION

The investigation of the structure, function, and control of biological processes and systems defines a significant part of biological and medical research. Traditionally, such investigations have been essentially reductionist in nature. A process, biochemically, pharmacologically, or genetically dissected, was reconstructed from the knowledge gained from the detailed analysis of the individual components.

The genomics revolution has changed the paradigm for the comprehensive analysis of biological processes and systems. It is a hypothesis of genomic analysis that biological processes and systems can be identified if global, quantitative gene expression patterns from cells or tissues representing different states are compared. To test this hypothesis, it is essential that methods for the global, quantitative measurement of gene expression are being developed and applied.

Several methods, including serial analysis of gene expression (SAGE),[1] oligonucleotide and cDNA arrays,[2,3] and large-scale sequencing of expressed sequence tags (ESTs), have been developed to globally measure gene expression at the mRNA level. The discovery of posttranscriptional mechanisms that control the rate of synthesis and half-life of proteins suggests that the mRNA level for a particular gene might not accurately reflect the amount of the respective protein expressed and that therefore the direct measurement of protein expression is also essential for the genome-wide analysis of biological processes and systems.

The global analysis of gene expression at the protein level is now also termed proteomics. The standard method for quantitative proteome analysis combines protein separation by high-resolution two-dimensional (IEF/SDS-PAGE) gel electrophoresis (2DE) with mass spectrometric (MS) or tandem mass spectrometric (MS/MS) identification of selected protein spots detected in the 2D gel by specific protein staining. Important technical advances in 2D gel electrophoresis and protein mass spectrometry have made this approach to proteome analysis more sensitive, reproducible, and of higher throughput.[4] Specific advances include the introduction of immobilized pH gradient (IPG), isoelectric focusing (IEF), extended gradient IPG-IEF (zoom gels), computerized imaging, spot detection/isolation, and protein digestion systems,[5] and the development of automated, mass spectrometry–based protein analytical systems.[6,7] Collectively, these developments have created an integrated technology in which several thousand protein species can be separated and detected in a single operation and hundreds of the detected proteins can be identified in a highly automated fashion.

Evaluating the level of expression of the proteins from the yeast *S. cerevisiae* that have been identified to date in large-scale protein analysis studies,[8–10] we made the surprising observation that the population of identified proteins is extremely biased for high expression.[8] This is in spite of the fact that the number of observed features in a 2D gel of a total yeast cellular lysate can approach the number of yeast proteins that are expected to migrate within the useful separation range of the gels. This indicates that the 2DE/MS approach to proteome analysis is fundamentally limited in its ability to detect and analyze low abundance proteins and that the number of protein spots detected is a poor indicator for the number of genes expressed in the cell from which the sample originated. Because of these limitations, the current standard approach to proteome analysis (2DE/MS/MS) is predominantly being used for the detection of marker proteins, the expression of which correlates with a specific physiological or pathologic state of a cell or tissue.[11,12] The mechanistic or functional analysis of biological systems using the proteome approach has been much more limited, mainly because only a subset of the expressed proteins is generally detected. To extend the use of the proteomics approach towards the comprehensive analysis of biological systems and pathways, general or selective protein enrichment procedures or alternative approaches to quantitative proteome analysis are required. In the following, we discuss the rationale for quantitative proteome analysis, highlight the limitations of the current standard technology, and introduce a new experimental approach to quantitative proteome analysis. Since essentially all the methods for proteome analysis are based on mass spectrometric identification of proteins, we first briefly summarize the current relevant techniques.

RESULTS AND DISCUSSION

Protein Identification by Mass Spectrometry and Tandem Mass Spectrometry

Mass spectrometry provides the means to unambiguously identify proteins. The commonly used different methods have been described in detail elsewhere[4] and are therefore only briefly summarized here. In one technique called mass mapping or peptide mass fingerprinting, a pure protein is reduced to specific peptide fragments by digestion with a protease such as trypsin. The masses of the resulting peptides are measured in a mass spectrometer. The resulting list of masses can be compared to a theoretical list of masses from a protein database. High mass accuracy along with matching multiple peptide fragment masses derived from the same protein result in protein identification.

A second technique can identify proteins by collecting amino acid sequence information and then correlating this information with protein sequence databases. A second stage of mass spectrometry is required and thus the technique is called tandem mass spectrometry (MS/MS). Similar to mass mapping, the pure protein is reduced to smaller peptide fragments by proteolysis, and peptide masses are determined in the first stage of mass analysis in a mass spectrometer. In addition, the tandem mass spectrometer selects (either automatically or controlled by the operator) the mass of a specific peptide ion for a second stage of mass spectrometry. The peptide is selectively energized and collided with an inert gas [collision-induced dissociation (CID)] with the goal of inducing on average only a single peptide bond breakage per molecule. The resulting masses from fragmenting the peptide contain the amino acid sequence information for the peptide. Such data can become quite complicated because at least two ion series representing sequencing inward from both the N and C termini are present in the spectrum. For this reason, sophisticated computer algorithms have been developed to aid in sequence identification based on CID spectra.[13,14] This technique results in sequence information being generated for many peptides from a protein and, thus, the redundant and unambiguous identification of the protein from the database. In addition, this technique can readily identify the precise amino acid location of a myriad of posttranslational modifications, the best known being phosphorylation.[15]

When used with a matrix-assisted laser desorption time-of-flight mass spectrometer, peptide mass mapping has the advantage of being extremely fast, simple, and sensitive. The technique, however, is not well suited for the analysis of protein mixtures and generally only works in cases in which the complete protein sequence is known. In addition, the identification is frequently inconclusive because not all measured masses can be assigned to the sequence of the known protein.

The major disadvantages to protein identification by tandem mass spectrometry are that it is experimentally more complex and slower and has a lower throughput. However, the technique has the tremendous advantage that it can readily be applied to the analysis of protein mixtures.[16,17] Furthermore, the technique works with partial databases such as ESTs. Finally, the technique is more conclusive because of the redundancy of sequence information collected from multiple peptides derived from the same protein.

Rationale for Quantitative Proteome Analysis

With recent technical advances including the development of differential display PCR,[18] cDNA microarray and DNA chip technology,[2,19] and SAGE,[1,2,19,20] it is now feasible to establish global and quantitative mRNA expression maps of cells and tissues of species for which the sequence of all the genes or the complete genome is known. The presence of posttranscriptional mechanisms controlling the amount of protein expressed, including those that control the translation rate[21] and protein and mRNA half-lives,[22] led us to predict that quantitative mRNA transcript measurements are generally insufficient for predicting the quantity of the expressed, corresponding proteins. To test this hypothesis, we determined the correlation between the mRNA and protein levels for a group of genes expressed in exponentially growing cells of the yeast *Saccharomyces cerevisiae*.[8] Protein expression levels were quantified by metabolic labeling of the yeast proteins to a steady state, followed by

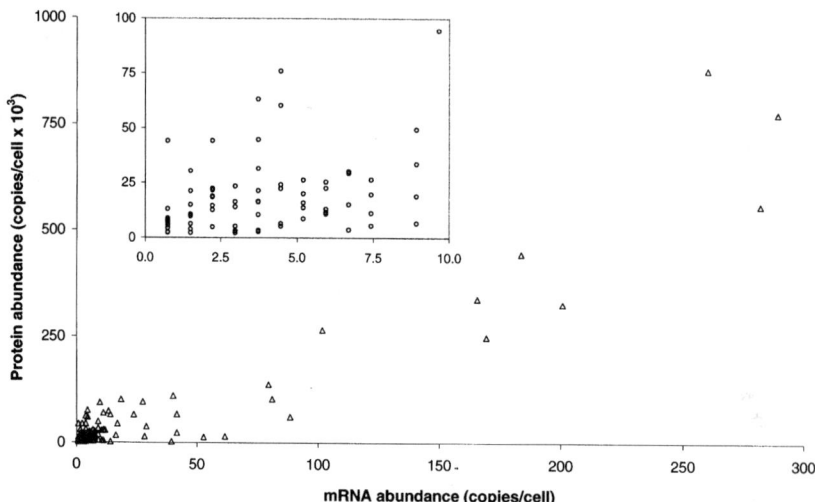

FIGURE 1. Correlation between protein and mRNA levels for 106 genes in yeast growing at log phase with glucose as a carbon source. mRNA and protein levels were calculated as described in the text. The data represent a population of genes with protein expression levels visible by silver staining on a 2D gel chosen to include the entire range of molecular weights, isoelectric focusing points, and staining intensities. The inset shows the low-end portion of the main figure. It contains 69% of the original data set. The Pearson product moment correlation for the entire data set was 0.935. The correlation for the inset containing 73 proteins (69%) was 0.356.

2D gel electrophoresis and liquid scintillation counting of selected, separated protein species. Specific proteins were identified by in-gel tryptic digestion of spots with subsequent analysis by microcapillary high-performance liquid chromatography–tandem mass spectrometry (μLC-MS/MS) and sequence database searching.[8,15,23,24] The corresponding mRNA transcript levels were calculated from SAGE frequency tables obtained from the same yeast strain grown under the same conditions that were employed for the protein quantitation experiment.[20]

The correlation between mRNA and protein levels for the more than 100 species selected in this study is shown in FIGURE 1. For the entire set of genes, there was a general trend of increased mRNA levels resulting in increased protein levels. The Pearson product moment correlation coefficient for the whole data set was 0.935. This number is highly biased by a relatively small number of genes with very large protein and message levels. A more representative subset of the data is shown in the inset of FIGURE 1. It shows message levels below 10 copies/cell and includes 70% of the data set used in the study. The Pearson product moment correlation coefficient for this data set was 0.356. This weak correlation is further evident by the observation that levels of protein expression coded for by mRNA with comparable abundance varied by as much as 30-fold and that the mRNA levels coding for protein with comparable expression levels varied by as much as 20-fold. This study,[8] for the first time, correlated the mRNA transcript and protein expression levels of a relatively large number of genes expressed in cells representing the same state. Similar conclusions were reached in another study that was performed under less controlled experimental conditions.[25] It is apparent that the observed correlation is not sufficiently high to allow for protein levels to be predicted by mRNA levels. We therefore conclude that quantitative proteome analysis is an essential component of any comprehensive analysis of biological systems.

The 2DE/MS/MS Technology Is Transparent to Proteins of Low Abundance

The current standard approach to quantitative proteome analysis is based on the separation of proteins by 2DE and the subsequent identification of specific separated and detected protein spots by MS or MS/MS, followed by sequence database searching.[8,26] The method is sequential, labor-intensive, and difficult to automate. It can, however, provide precise quantitation[27] at the level of the 2D gel and is well suited

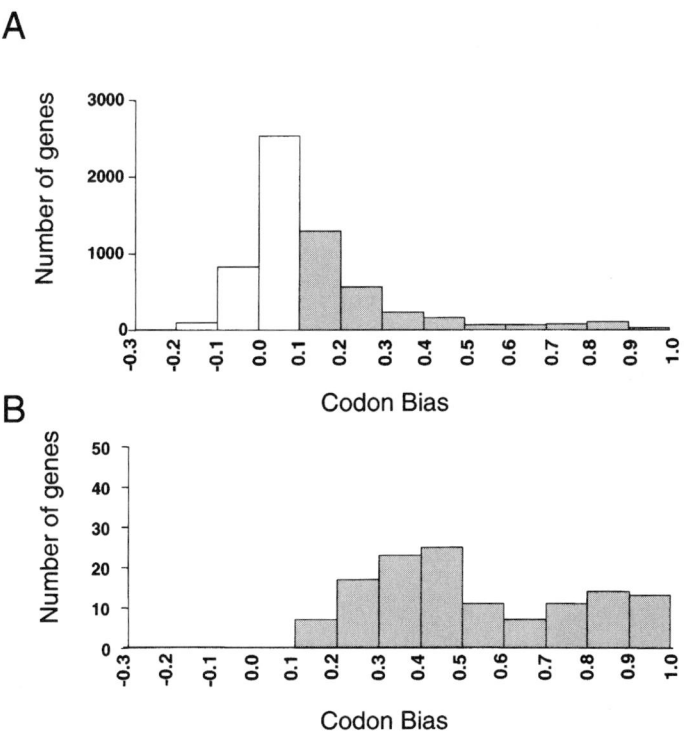

FIGURE 2. Current proteome analysis technology utilizing 2D gel electrophoresis without preenrichment samples mainly highly expressed proteins. Genes encoding highly expressed proteins generally have large codon bias values. (**A**) Distribution of the yeast genome (more than 6000 genes) based on codon bias. The interval with the largest frequency of genes is 0.0 to 0.1 with more than 2500 genes. (**B**) Distribution of the genes identified from proteins in this study based on codon bias. No genes were detected in this study with codon bias values less than 0.1.

to reveal subtle, relative changes in protein expression, clusters of concurrently regulated proteins, and additional features that affect the electrophoretic mobility of proteins, including posttranslational protein processing and modifications. The number of features observed if total yeast lysates are separated by high-resolution 2DE can approach the number of genes identified in the yeast genome (>2000 protein spots/gel and 4000–5000 expressed genes). However, a comparison of the proteins identified in three relatively large published protein identification studies[8–10] indicates a significant overlap in the list of proteins identified in each study. The proteins in each one of the studies were independently and presumably randomly sampled among the detected spots. The observed large overlap suggests that the number of samples (expressed genes detected by 2DE) is much smaller than the approximately 6000 genes present in the yeast genome. To assess to what extent the 2DE protein pattern obtained from a total yeast lysate represents the proteome of this microorganism, we related protein expression levels from proteins detected by silver staining to the predicted expression levels of all the open reading frames (ORFs) in the yeast genome (FIG. 2).

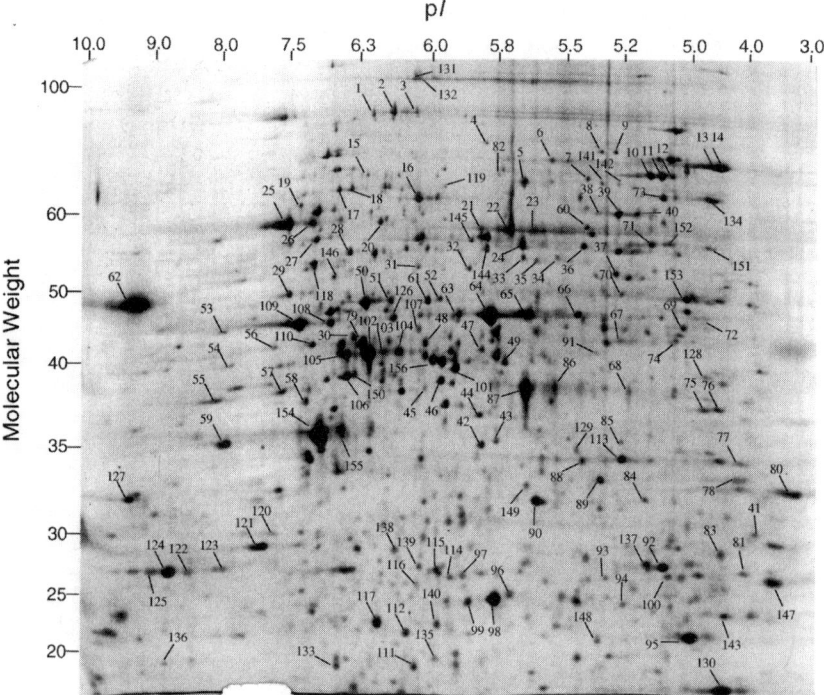

FIGURE 3. Two-dimensional silver-stained gel of yeast proteins. Proteins from 50 µg of total yeast lysate were separated in the first dimension (horizontal) by isoelectric focusing and then in the second dimension (vertical) by molecular weight sieving. Protein spots (156) were chosen to include the entire range of molecular weights, isoelectric focusing points, and staining intensities. Spots were excised, and the corresponding protein(s) identified by mass spectrometry and database searching.

Prediction of the level of protein expression was based on the codon bias of the respective genes. The codon bias indicates the propensity for a gene to utilize the same codon to encode an amino acid, even though other codons would insert the identical amino acid into the growing polypeptide chain.[28,29] Its value varies between −0.3 and 1.0, and it has further been found empirically that highly expressed proteins have large codon bias values (>0.2) and proteins expressed at low levels have low codon bias values (<0.1).[30] The codon bias distribution for all the yeast ORFs is indicated in FIGURE 2A and the codon bias distribution of the proteins analyzed by 2DE, silver staining, and MS/MS is indicated in FIGURE 2B. Comparison of the distributions in panels A and B indicates that the population of proteins analyzed by the standard 2DE/MS/MS proteome analysis technique is highly biased towards the most highly expressed proteins. This was in spite of the fact that the staining intensities of the proteins included in the study spanned the entire range of detected intensities (FIG. 3).

In an attempt to increase the detectability of low abundance proteins in total cell lysates separated by 2DE, we expanded the separation range of the gels in the IEF dimension and applied significantly higher amounts (10-fold) of total protein to each gel. The proteins detected by silver staining in the arbitrarily selected rectangular area (FIG. 4) were identified as described above and the codon bias values were cal-

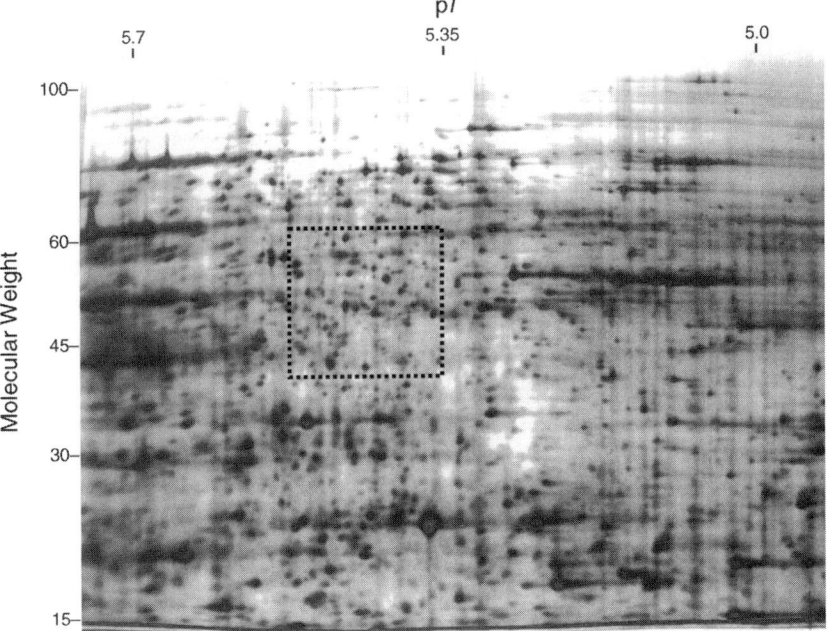

FIGURE 4. Narrow-range 2D gel (IEF pH range: 4.5–5.5) of total yeast lysate. Proteins were separated as in FIGURE 3, except that 500 μg of total yeast lysate was applied to the first dimension strip. The resulting gel has more than 2000 visible spots within a narrow 0.7 pH unit first dimension. Fifty protein spots within the area designated by the square were excised, and the corresponding protein(s) identified by mass spectrometry and database searching.

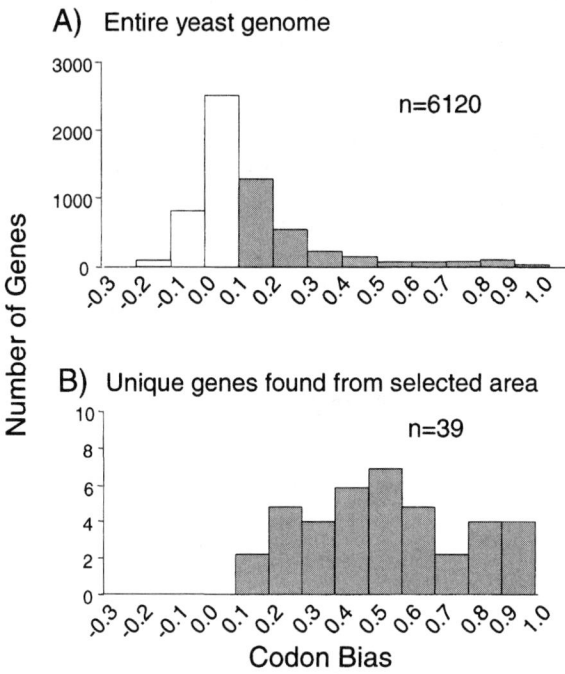

FIGURE 5. Comparison of codon bias values from the entire genome with those found in the selected area from FIGURE 4. Genes encoding highly expressed proteins generally have large codon bias values. **(A)** Distribution of the yeast genome based on codon bias. The interval with the largest frequency of genes is 0.0 to 0.1 with more than 2500 genes. **(B)** Distribution of the genes identified from protein spots in the selected area. No genes were detected in this study with codon bias values less than 0.1.

culated for each of the identified proteins. The distribution of codon bias values is displayed and compared to predicted codon bias distribution for all yeast genes in FIGURE 5. The data indicate that the use of 2D gels with extended separation range and increased sample load improved the detection of proteins of somewhat moderate abundance, but that the low abundance proteins characterized by codon bias values < 0.1 (more than one-half of the genes in the yeast genome) were still generally undetectable. We therefore conclude that the current proteome technology, used without sample preenrichment, is not suitable for the global detection of proteins expressed by cells and that the construction of complete, quantitative proteome maps based on the 2DE/MS/MS approach will be very challenging, even for relatively simple, unicellular organisms.

A Novel Method for Quantitative Proteome Analysis

To address the limitations inherent in the 2DE/MS/MS method to proteome analysis, we have developed a new experimental strategy. It is designed to provide rela-

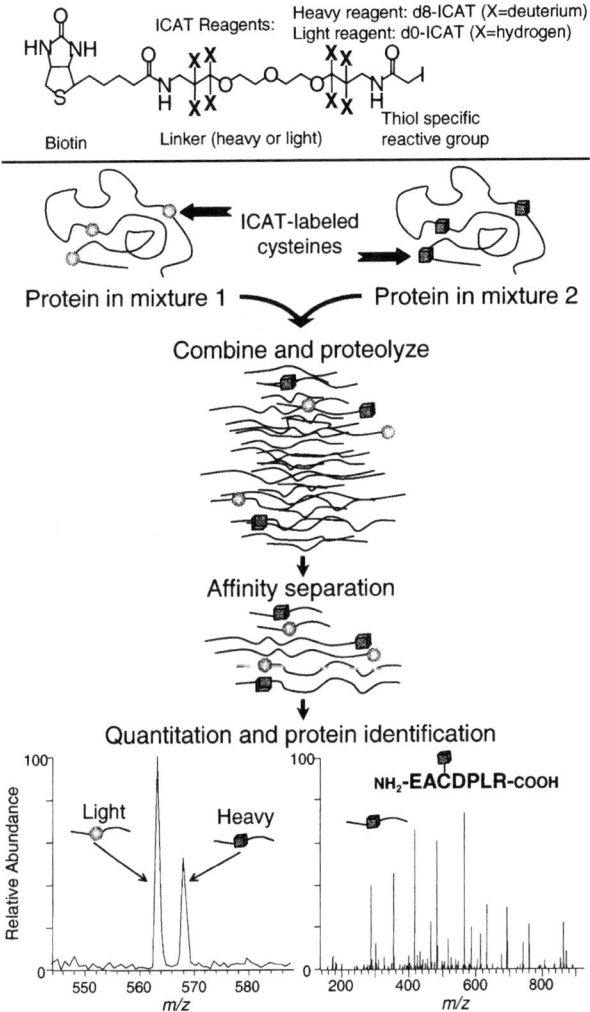

FIGURE 6. Schematic representation of the ICAT strategy for measuring quantitative gene expression at the protein level. See text for details.

tive quantitative information of the same protein in different samples and to rapidly and conclusively identify the components of a mixture, even if they are of low abundance. This method is based on a class of new chemical reagents termed isotope coded affinity tags (ICAT) and MS/MS.[16]

The ICAT strategy is schematically illustrated in FIGURE 6 and data obtained from the quantitative analysis of a protein mixture containing six proteins at known, different ratios is shown in TABLE 1. Protein mixtures 1 and 2 are treated after reduction with the sulfhydryl-specific ICAT reagent (FIG. 6, top). The reagents exist in two

TABLE 1. Sequence identification and quantitation of the components of a protein mixture in a single analysis

Gene name[a]	Peptide sequence identified	Observed ratio (d0/d8)[b]	Mean ± SD	Expected ratio (d0/d8)[c]	% error
LCA_BOVIN	ALC#SEK	0.94	0.96 ± 0.06	1.00	4.2
	C#EVFR	1.03			
	FLDDLTDDIMC#VK	0.92			
OVAL_CHICK	ADHPFLFC#IK	1.88	1.92 ± 0.06	2.00	4.0
	YPILPEYLQC#VK	1.96			
BGAL_ECOLI	LTAAC#FDR	1.00	0.98 ± 0.07	1.00	2.0
	IGLNC#QLAQVAER	0.91			
	IIFDGVNSAFHLWC#NGR	1.04			
LACB_BOVIN	WENGEC#AQK	3.64	3.55 ± 0.13	4.00	11.3
	LSFNPTQLEEQC#HI	3.45			
G3P_RABIT	VPTPNVSVVDLTC#R	0.54	0.56 ± 0.02	0.50	12.0
	IVSNASC#TTNC#LAPLAK	0.57			
PHS2_RABIT	IC#GGWQMEEADDWLR	0.32	0.32 ± 0.03	0.33	3.1
	TC#AYTNHTVLPEALER	0.35			
	WLVLC#NPGLAEIIAER	0.30			

NOTE: # = ICAT-labeled cysteinyl residue.
[a]Gene names are according to Swiss Prot nomenclature (www.expasy.ch).
[b]Ratios were calculated for each peptide as shown in FIGURE 7.
[c]Expected ratios were calculated from the known amounts of proteins present in each mixture.

forms: isotopically light (d0) and isotopically heavy (d8). The heavy and light forms are used to derivatize the proteins in samples 1 and 2, respectively. The cysteinyl residues derivatized with the heavy and light ICAT reagents are represented in the two mixtures by spheres and squares, respectively. After treatment with the ICAT reagents, the samples are mixed. At this point, any optional fractionation technique can be performed to enrich for low abundance proteins or to reduce the complexity of the mixture, while the relative quantities are maintained. The combined protein sample is then proteolyzed and the ICAT-tagged peptides are selectively enriched by avidin-biotin affinity chromatography. These peptides are separated and analyzed by microcapillary HPLC-ESI-MS/MS. The relative ion intensities of the two differentially isotopically tagged forms of a specific peptide indicate their relative abundance. Such pairs of tagged peptides are easily detected because they essentially coelute from the column and because of the eight mass units difference encoded in the ICAT tag that is detected in the mass spectrometer. Every other scan is devoted to fragmenting and then recording sequence information about an eluting peptide (MS/MS spectrum). The protein from which this peptide originated is then identified by searching a sequence database with the recorded MS/MS spectrum. The procedure thus provides the relative quantitation and identification of the components of protein mixtures in a single analysis. For illustration purposes in FIGURE 6, only a single protein is shown in each mixture. However, the method is identically applicable for identifying proteins from a complex mixture.

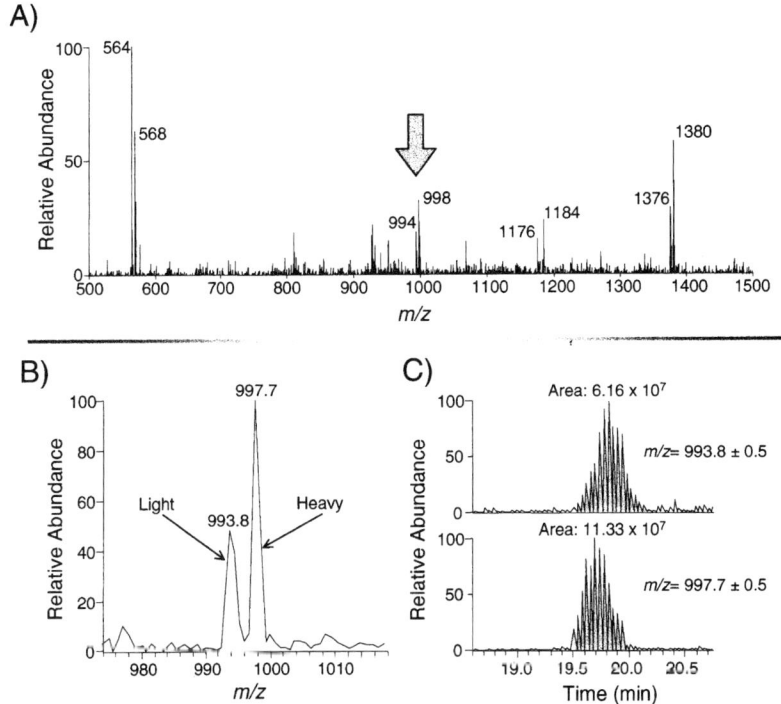

FIGURE 7. ICAT quantitative analysis of a protein from the mixture in TABLE 1. **(A)** Full-scan (500–1500 *m/z*) mass spectrum at time 19.76 min of the microcapillary μLC-MS and μLC-MS/MS mixture analysis. Shown are at least 4 different peptide doublets eluting from the column. Each doublet corresponded to ICAT-labeled peptides of identical sequence. The mass spectrometer operated in a dual mode, switching back and forth on alternating scans between measuring the ion intensities of all the eluting peptide peaks (MS mode) and recording the sequence information (MS/MS or tandem MS mode) generated by selectively fragmenting a peptide ion from the previous scan. The mass-to-charge (*m/z*) ratio difference between peptides is dependent on the charge state (number of hydrogen ions) and is typically either 4.0 or 8.0 (mass difference of 8 daltons and a charge state of 1 or 2, respectively). **(B)** Expanded view of the full-scan mass spectrum showing the ion abundances for each species of an ICAT-labeled peptide eluting from the column at 19.76 min. **(C)** Reconstructed ion chromatograms for the peptide ions measured in panel B. The ratio of the calculated areas (0.54) was used to determine the relative peptide concentrations in the two mixtures. Peaks appear serrated because every other scan was devoted to an MS/MS spectrum as shown in FIGURE 8A.

To illustrate the new method, two mixtures consisting of the same six proteins at known, but different, concentrations were prepared and analyzed. The protein mixtures were labeled, combined, and treated as schematically illustrated in FIGURE 6. The isolated, tagged peptides were quantified and sequenced in a single combined μLC-MS and μLC-MS/MS experiment on an electrospray ionization ion trap mass spectrometer. All six proteins were unambiguously identified and accurately quantified (TABLE 1). Multiple tagged peptides were encountered for each protein. The mean differences between the observed and expected quantities for the six proteins ranged between 2% and 12%.

The entire process is further illustrated for a single peptide pair in FIGURE 7. A single scan of the mass spectrometer operated in MS mode is shown in FIGURE 7A. Four pairs of peptide ions characterized by the ICAT-encoded mass differential are detected in this scan and indicated with their respective mass-to-charge (m/z) values. Pairs of ICAT-labeled peptides can differ in measured m/z values depending on the nominal peptide charge (i.e., the number of hydrogen ions acquired during the electrospray ionization process), but will be typically either eight for singly charged ions or four for doubly charged ions. The scan shown was acquired in 1.3 s. Over the

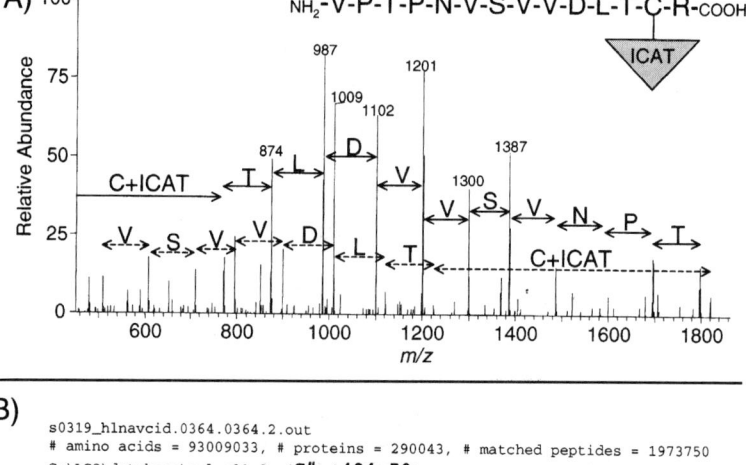

FIGURE 8. ICAT sequence identification of the peptide quantitated in FIGURE 7, derived from glyceraldehyde-3-phosphate dehydrogenase. Shown is the identification of the amino acid sequence from the peptide for which the abundance was measured in FIGURE 7C. (**A**) Tandem mass spectrum derived by collision-induced dissociation of the $[M+2H]^{2+}$ precursor, m/z 998. Fragment ions in the spectrum represent mainly single-event preferential cleavage of peptide bonds, resulting in sequence information recorded from both the N and C termini of the peptide simultaneously. The one-letter code for encountered amino acids is shown. The ICAT modification remained fairly stable and attached to the cysteinyl residue. (**B**) Database search output file for the above spectrum. The recorded sequence information was computer-searched with the Sequest program[13] against the OWL nonredundant database containing 290,043 protein entries[31] with cysteinyl residues modified by the mass of either the light or heavy ICAT reagent. The best-matching peptide was from glyceraldehyde-3-phosphate dehydrogenase and was a tryptic peptide with a modified cysteinyl residue.

course of the 1-h chromatographic elution gradient, more than 1200 such scans were automatically recorded. FIGURE 7B shows an expanded view of the mass spectrum around the ion pair with m/z ratios of 993.8 and 977.7, respectively. Coelution and a detected mass differential of four units potentially identifies the ions as a pair of doubly charged ICAT-labeled peptides of identical sequence (mass difference of eight and a charge state of two). FIGURE 7C shows the reconstructed ion chromatograms for these two species. The relative quantities were determined by integrating the contour of the respective peaks. The ratio (light/heavy) was determined as 0.54 (TABLE 1). The peaks in the reconstructed ion chromatograms appear serrated because in every second scan the mass spectrometer switched between the MS and the MS/MS modes to collect sequence information (CID mass spectrum) of a selected peptide ion. These CID spectra were used to identify the protein from which the tagged peptides originated. FIGURE 8A shows the CID spectrum recorded from the peptide ion with $m/z = 998$ (marked with an arrow in FIG. 7A). Database searching with this CID spectrum identified the protein as glyceraldehyde-3-phosphate dehydrogenase (FIG. 8B), which was a component of the protein mixture.

Several features of the ICAT strategy are immediately apparent. First, at least two peptides were detected from each protein in the mixture. Therefore, both quantitation and protein identification can be redundant. Second, the identified peptides all contained at least one tagged cysteinyl residue. The presence of the relatively rare cysteinyl residue in a peptide adds an additional powerful constraint for database searching. Third, tagging and selective enrichment of cysteine-containing peptides significantly reduced the complexity of the peptide mixture generated by the concurrent digestion of six proteins. For this protein mixture, the complexity was reduced from 293 potential tryptic peptides to 44 tryptic peptides containing at least one cysteinyl residue. Fourth, the peptide samples eluted from the avidin affinity column are directly compatible with analysis by µLC-MS/MS.

CONCLUSIONS

In this manuscript, we have argued that, in the emerging postgenomic era, technologies that can quantitatively, globally, and automatically measure gene expression at the protein level are essential for the comprehensive analysis of biological processes and systems. We have documented the limitations of the current standard method, 2DE/MS/MS, for large-scale protein analysis with respect to the analysis of low abundance proteins. While this approach has been successfully used to detect and characterize marker proteins that are idiotypic for a specific physiologic or pathologic state of a cell or tissue, it appears that the 2DE/MS/MS approach is unsuitable to detect, identify, and quantify every protein in a sample, a task that seems necessary for the comprehensive analysis and eventual mathematical description of biological processes and systems. We therefore have proposed a new method based on the ICAT reagents. This method promises to detect, quantify, and identify all proteins in a sample, irrespective of their levels of expression. We anticipate that the new ICAT strategy will provide broadly applicable means for the quantitative cataloging and comparison of expressed proteins in a variety of normal, developmental, and disease states.

ACKNOWLEDGMENTS

This work was supported in part by the NSF Science and Technology Center for Molecular Biotechnology, NIH Grant Nos. T32HG00035 and RR11823, a grant from the Merck Genome Research Institute, and a fellowship to B. Rist from the Swiss National Science Foundation.

REFERENCES

1. VELCULESCU, V.E., L. ZHANG, B. VOGELSTEIN & K.W. KINZLER. 1995. Serial analysis of gene expression. Science **270:** 484–487.
2. SHALON, D., S.J. SMITH & P.O. BROWN. 1996. A DNA microarray system for analyzing complex DNA samples using two-color fluorescent probe hybridization. Genome Res. **6:** 639–645.
3. CHEE, M., R. YANG, E. HUBBELL, A. BERNO, X.C. HUANG, D. STERN, J. WINKLER, D.J. LOCKHART, M.S. MORRIS & S.P. FODOR. 1996. Accessing genetic information with high-density DNA arrays. Science **274:** 610–614.
4. PATTERSON, S.D. & R. AEBERSOLD. 1995. Mass spectrometric approaches for the identification of gel-separated proteins. Electrophoresis **16:** 1791–1814.
5. HOUTHAEVE, T., H. GAUSEPOHL, K. ASHMAN, T. NILLSON & M. MANN. 1997. Automated protein preparation techniques using a digest robot. J. Protein Chem. **16:** 343–348.
6. WALSH, B.J., M.P. MOLLOY & K.L. WILLIAMS. 1998. The Australian Proteome Analysis Facility (APAF): assembling large scale proteomics through integration and automation. Electrophoresis **19:** 1883–1890.
7. FIGEYS, D., S.P. GYGI, G. MCKINNON & R. AEBERSOLD. 1998. An integrated microfluidics tandem mass spectrometry system for automated protein analysis. Anal. Chem. **70:** 3728–3734.
8. GYGI, S.P., Y. ROCHON, B.R. FRANZA & R. AEBERSOLD. 1999. Correlation between protein and mRNA abundance in yeast. Mol. Cell. Biol. **19:** 1720–1730.
9. SHEVCHENKO, A., O.N. JENSEN, A.V. PODTELEJNIKOV, F. SAGLIOCCO, M. WILM, O. VORM, P. MORTENSEN, A. SHEVCHENKO, H. BOUCHERIE & M. MANN. 1996. Linking genome and proteome by mass spectrometry: large-scale identification of yeast proteins from two-dimensional gels. Proc. Natl. Acad. Sci. U.S.A. **93:** 14440–14445.
10. BOUCHERIE, H., F. SAGLIOCCO, R. JOUBERT, I. MAILLET, J. LABARRE & M. PERROT. 1996. Two-dimensional gel protein database of *Saccharomyces cerevisiae*. Electrophoresis **17:** 1683–1699.
11. ANDERSON, N.L. & N.G. ANDERSON. 1998. Proteome and proteomics: new technologies, new concepts, and new words. Electrophoresis **19:** 1853–1861.
12. HAYNES, P.A., S.P. GYGI, D. FIGEYS & R. AEBERSOLD. 1998. Proteome analysis: biological assay or data archive? Electrophoresis **19:** 1862–1871.
13. ENG, J., A.L. MCCORMACK & J.R. YATES. 1994. An approach to correlate tandem mass spectral data of peptides with amino acid sequences in a protein database. J. Am. Soc. Mass Spectrom. **5:** 976–989.
14. MANN, M. & M. WILM. 1994. Error-tolerant identification of peptides in sequence databases by peptide sequence tags. Anal. Chem. **66:** 4390–4399.
15. GYGI, S.P., D.K.M. HAN, A.C. GINGRAS, N. SONENBER & R. AEBERSOLD. 1999. Protein analysis by mass spectrometry and sequence database searching: tools for cancer research in the post-genomic era. Electrophoresis **20:** 310–319.
16. GYGI, S.P., B. RIST, S.A. GERBER, F. TURECEK, M.H. GELB & R. AEBERSOLD. 1999. Quantitative analysis of protein mixtures using isotope coded affinity tags. Nat. Biotechnol. In press.
17. LINK, J., J. ENG, D.M. SCHIELTZ, E. CARMACK, G.J. MIZE, D.R. MORRIS, B.M. GARVIK & J.R. YATES. 1999. Direct analysis of large protein complexes using mass spectrometry. Nat. Biotechnol. **17:** 676–682.

18. LIANG, P. & A.B. PARDEE. 1992. Differential display of eukaryotic messenger RNA by means of the polymerase chain reaction. Science **257**: 967–971.
19. LASHKARI, D.A., J.L. DERISI, J.H. MCCUSKER, A.F. NAMATH, C. GENTILE, S.Y. HWANG, P.O. BROWN & R.W. DAVIS. 1997. Yeast microarrays for genome-wide parallel genetic and gene expression analysis. Proc. Natl. Acad. Sci. U.S.A. **94**: 13057–13062.
20. VELCULESCU, V.E., L. ZHANG, W. ZHOU, B. VOGELSTEIN, M.A. BASRAI, D.E. BASSETT & K.W. KINZLER. 1997. Characterization of the yeast transcriptome. Cell **88**: 243–251.
21. HARFORD, J.B. & D.R. MORRIS. 1997. Post-transcriptional Gene Regulation. Wiley–Liss. New York.
22. VARSHAVSKY, A. 1996. The N-end rule: functions, mysteries, uses. Proc. Natl. Acad. Sci. U.S.A. **93**: 12142–12149.
23. SHEVCHENKO, A., M. WILM, O. VORM & M. MANN. 1996. Mass spectrometric sequencing of proteins from silver-stained polyacrylamide gels. Anal. Chem. **68**: 850–858.
24. LINK, A.J., L.G. HAYS, E.B. CARMACK & J.R. YATES III. 1997. Identifying the major proteome components of *Haemophilus influenzae* type–strain NCTC 8143. Electrophoresis **18**: 1314–1334.
25. ANDERSON, L. & J. SEILHAMER. 1997. A comparison of selected mRNA and protein abundances in human liver. Electrophoresis **18**: 533–537.
26. DUCRET, A., I. VANOOSTVEEN, J.K. ENG, J.R. YATES & R. AEBERSOLD. 1998. High throughput protein characterization by automated reverse-phase chromatography/electrospray tandem mass spectrometry. Prot. Sci. **7**: 706–719.
27. GYGI, S.P. & R. AEBERSOLD. 1998. *In* 2-D Protocols for Proteome Analysis. Humana Press. Totowa, New Jersey.
28. URLINGER, S., K. KUCHLER, T.H. MEYER, S. UEBEL & R. TAMP'E. 1997. Intracellular location, complex formation, and function of the transporter associated with antigen processing in yeast. Eur. J. Biochem. **245**: 266–272.
29. KURLAND, C.G. 1991. Codon bias and gene expression. FEBS Lett. **285**: 165–169.
30. GARRELS, J.I., C.S. MCLAUGHLIN, J.R. WARNER, B. FUTCHER, G.I. LATTER, R. KOBAYASHI, B. SCHWENDER, T. VOLPE, D.S. ANDERSON, F.R. MESQUITA & W.E. PAYNE. 1997. Proteome studies of *Saccharomyces cerevisiae*: identification and characterization of abundant proteins. Electrophoresis **18**: 1347–1360.
31. BLEASBY, A.J., D. AKRIGG & T.K. ATTWOOD. 1994. OWL—a non-redundant composite protein sequence database. Nucleic Acids Res. **22**: 3574–3577.

Pharmaceutical Proteomics

SANDRA STEINER[a] AND N. LEIGH ANDERSON

Large Scale Proteomics Corporation, Rockville, Maryland, USA

ABSTRACT: Genomics and proteomics are today well established in drug discovery and, in combination with combinatorial chemistry and high-throughput screening, are helping to bring forward an unprecedented number of potential lead compounds. To avoid the generation of bottlenecks downstream in drug development, increasing pressure is arising to integrate these technologies into the development environment. Proteomics has demonstrated proof-of-concept in toxicology as shown by a number of successful applications in mechanistic toxicology and lead selection. The "technology wave" is now starting to impact the clinical phase of drug development. Expected benefits are optimized clinical trials based on the availability of biologically relevant markers of drug efficacy and safety.

INTRODUCTION

In recent years, a number of technology developments have had a profound impact on the drug discovery process. The exponential growth in genomics and proteomics capabilities and the subsequent generation of large amounts of novel information have facilitated an unprecedented number of potential new drug targets. Advances in combinatorial chemistry resulting in a nearly unlimited availability of compound libraries, in combination with constant improvements in high-throughput screening (HTS) technologies, have resulted in unprecedented numbers of potential lead compounds. A consequence of this technology-driven acceleration of drug discovery is the creation of bottlenecks downstream in drug development. Thus, increasing pressure is currently arising to integrate genomics and proteomics approaches in the development environment to introduce a similar boost to drug development. The implementation of proteomics in safety assessment has actually advanced beyond the proof-of-concept stage as demonstrated by a significant number of studies performed by our laboratory and by other investigators.

PROTEOME PROFILING TO OBTAIN INSIGHTS INTO MECHANISMS AND PATHWAYS OF TOXICITY

Insights into molecular mechanisms and knowledge of biological pathways involved in toxic responses are an asset for the interpretation of adverse drug effects and contribute to an accurate risk assessment for humans. There is abundant evidence that links can be established between the up- or downregulation of specific

---

[a]Address for correspondence: S. Steiner, Large Scale Biology Corporation, 9620 Medical Center Drive, Rockville, MD 20850-3338. Voice: 301-424-5989; fax: 301-762-4892.
sandra.steiner@lsbc.com

pathways and the morphological manifestation of toxic endpoints, as shown for example with the chemically diverse group of peroxisome proliferating compounds.[1,2] We have studied the liver effects of a set of strong peroxisome proliferators (PP; agonists of the nuclear receptor PPARα) and a nonproliferator (an analogue of one of the PPs tested having similar pharmacological potency) in mice and demonstrated three distinct proteome signature patterns.[3] The patterns that could be distinguished corresponded to (i) PPARα agonist activity, (ii) animal age (30 days difference in age at sacrifice between 5- and 35-day treatment groups), and (iii) action of the non-PP compound by a different mechanism. These results provided support for a unified receptor-based mechanism controlling the main PP response, but demonstrate that individual responsive genes can show quite different dose-response curves. More than 100 proteins showed significant changes following PP treatment, and multiple sensitive markers were identified in this project. Based on the assumption that impairments of biological pathways (as visualized in proteome signature patterns) precede potential morphological manifestations, proteins showing coherent changes following treatment with PPs are likely to be early markers for stimuli that eventually result in proliferation of peroxisomes.

Proteomics was the key to new insights into the molecular mechanisms involved in cyclosporine A (CsA) nephrotoxicity.[4,5] The use of CsA, a potent immunosuppressant, is limited by its kidney toxicity. In kidney proteome patterns from CsA-treated rats, we showed a profound downregulation of the calcium binding protein, calbindin D28, an intracellular calcium buffer and transport protein. Its near absence in the kidneys of CsA-treated animals provides an explanation for the accumulation of calcium in the tubules and consequent tubular toxicity. A subsequent SAR study showed that the downregulation of calbindin was closely associated with immunosuppressant activity[6] and that its downregulation also occurred in humans showing CsA-related nephrotoxicity. Prior to the proteome study, the link in relationship between CsA kidney toxicity and calbindin D28 downregulation was not known.

PROTEOME PROFILING AND LEAD SELECTION

The selection of lead compounds is a critical step in the drug development process with profound downstream consequences. The selection pressure favors compounds with a wide therapeutic window, as defined by high pharmacological potency in combination with low toxicity. Estimation of therapeutic windows in light of the limited data sets typically available for compounds at the late discovery/early development phase is often similar to guesswork. Thus, information residing in proteome profiles produced from lead candidates can be essential to support compound prioritization decisions.

We used proteome profiling as a basis to select protein markers linked to compound efficacy or toxicity and demonstrated the possibility of using these markers for lead prioritization.[7] A compound studied in this context was SDZ PGU 693, a hypoglycemic agent found to induce hepatocellular hypertrophy in the rat. Liver proteome profiling of treated rats showed the induction of several microsomal proteins, including NADPH cytochrome P-450 reductase and cytochrome b5, indicative of microsomal proliferation and induction of the P-450 enzyme system causing hepatocellular hypertrophy. Decreases were evident in a series of mitochondrial proteins such as F_1ATPase-alpha subunit and cytosolic liver fatty acid binding protein suggesting a downregulation of the mitochondrial liver fatty acid metabolism, likely reflecting the pharmacological action of the compound. These data demonstrate that the liver proteome of treated rats revealed protein markers indicative for both SDZ PGU efficacy and toxicity. Markers for both endpoints were selected from these profiles and high-throughput protein assays set up to screen follow-up compounds to assess an estimate of their therapeutic window.

Similarly, efficacy and toxicity markers for "statin"-class cholesterol-lowering compounds were selected using proteome analysis. We found that agents acting to alter blood cholesterol (e.g., the statin HMG-CoA reductase inhibitors, cholestyramine, and high-cholesterol diets) change the abundances of several proteins in rat liver.[8] Most strongly affected is a protein identified as HMG-CoA synthase, a critical enzyme of the cholesterol synthesis pathway. Based on these data, HMG-CoA synthase can be used as an intracellular reporter of the pathway's performance. The statins, but not cholestyramine, also induce a peroxisomal enoyl hydratase-like protein, which was identified as a sensitive marker for peroxisome proliferation (representing in this case an undesirable side effect). The ratio between these efficacy and toxicity markers is different for different members of the marketed statin drugs, indicating their likely pharmacological inequivalence.

A study that we performed with etomoxir resulted in the observation that drug-induced liver steatosis is linked to the expression of a protein considered to be adipocyte-specific.[9] The liver toxicity of etomoxir, an inhibitor of carnitine palmitoyl transferase developed as a potential antidiabetic, was found to involve induction of the "adipocyte differentiation–related protein" (ADRP). This protein appears to be associated with lipid droplets that accumulate in the hepatocytes following treatment with etomoxir and demonstrates that at least one gene product previously considered specific to the adipocyte is induced in hepatocytes by the drug. ADRP may serve as an early toxicity marker for impaired lipid metabolism and lipid accumulation in liver.

CONCLUSIONS AND PERSPECTIVES

The basic methodology of safety evaluation has changed little during the past decades. Toxicity in laboratory animals has been evaluated primarily by using hematological, clinical chemistry, and histological parameters as indicators of organ damage. There is an emerging number of studies proving the unique value of global approaches such as proteome analysis to obtain crucial insights into mechanisms of toxicity and to pave the way towards predictive toxicology. All these data justify the expectation that the integration of proteomics and genomics into state-of-the-art toxicology will significantly advance the safety assessment of new drugs.

It becomes obvious that the impact of these new technologies will continue downstream into the development process and will extend from the preclinical to the clinic phase. As a consequence, former bottlenecks may disappear and new ones may appear and will need to be addressed. One of these is apparent today and arises from the necessity to obtain proof-of-concept of new drug candidates in humans as early as possible. Phase II and III clinical trials are the most expensive studies in the drug development process and failures at this stage may be fatal (both to the drug and, unfortunately, occasionally to patients). The possibility to perform early proof-of-concept trials is greatly dependent on the availability of appropriate markers for drug efficacy and safety. Markers of this kind need to be easily accessible in biological fluids such as serum or urine to guarantee the possibility for frequent monitoring (which makes them likely to be proteins or peptides). The detection and validation of such markers are far from trivial tasks, and technologies such as proteomics, allowing one to mine serum, urine, and other biological fluids for relevant markers, are expected to be key players in this effort. Pressure is also growing to improve the selection of patient populations for clinical trials. Genomics and proteomics are expected to occupy central roles in the efforts to stratify patient populations. Finally, a vast amount of biologically highly relevant data will cycle back from the development to the discovery end, generating a continuous impulse that will stimulate the drug pipeline.

REFERENCES

1. REDDY, J.K. & D.L. AZARNOFF. 1980. Hypolipidemic hepatic peroxisome proliferators form a novel class of chemical carcinogens. Nature **283**: 397–398.
2. DREYER, C., G. KREY, H. KELLER, F. GIVEL, G. HELFTENBEIN & W. WAHLI. 1992. Control of the peroxisomal β-oxidation pathway by a novel family of nuclear hormone receptors. Cell **68**: 879–887.
3. ANDERSON, N.L., R. ESQUER-BLASCO, F. RICHARDSON, P. FOXWORTHY & P. EACHO. 1996. The effects of peroxisome proliferators on protein abundances in mouse liver. Toxicol. Appl. Pharmacol. **137**: 75–89.
4. AICHER, L., D. WAHL, A. ARCE, O. GRENET & S. STEINER. 1998. New insights into cyclosporine A nephrotoxicity by proteome analysis. Electrophoresis **19**: 1998–2003.
5. STEINER, S., L. AICHER, J. RAYMACKERS, L. MEHEUS, R. ESQUER-BLASCO, N.L. ANDERSON & A. CORDIER. 1996. Cyclosporine A mediated decrease in the rat renal calcium binding protein calbindin-D 28kDa. Biochem. Pharmacol. **51**: 253–258.
6. AICHER, L., G. MEIER, A. NORCROSS, J. JAKUBOWSKI, M.C. VARELA, A. CORDIER & S. STEINER. 1997. Decrease in kidney calbindin-D as a possible mechanism mediating CsA and FK-506-induced calciuria and tubular mineralization. Biochem. Pharmacol. **53**: 723–731.
7. ARCE, A., L. AICHER, D. WAHL, R. ESQUER-BLASCO, N.L. ANDERSON, A. CORDIER & S. STEINER. 1998. Changes in the liver proteome of female Wistar rats treated with the hypoglycemic agent SDZ PGU 693. Life Sci. **63**: 2243–2250.
8. ANDERSON, N.L., R. ESQUER-BLASCO, J-P. HOFMANN & N.G. ANDERSON. 1991. A two-dimensional gel database of rat liver proteins useful in gene regulation and drug effects studies. Electrophoresis **12**: 907–930.
9. STEINER, S., D. WAHL, B.L.K. MANGOLD, R. ROBISON, J. RAYMACKERS, L. MEHEUS, N.L. ANDERSON & A. CORDIER. 1996. Induction of the adipose differentiation–related protein in liver of etomoxir treated rats. BBRC **218**: 777–782.

Gene Expression Microarray Data Analysis for Toxicology Profiling

M. J. CUNNINGHAM,[a] S. LIANG, S. FUHRMAN, J. J. SEILHAMER, AND R. SOMOGYI

Incyte Pharmaceuticals, Incorporated, Palo Alto, California 94304, USA

> ABSTRACT: When dealing with thousands of genes, all potentially interesting, it is desirable to rank the genes according to their degree of participation in a physiological process. Therefore, genes with the highest Shannon entropy and ERL can be selected as the best toxicity target candidates, permitting preclinical scientists to focus their research and resources on those genes.

INTRODUCTION

The preclinical phase of pharmaceutical drug development comprises efficacy testing and safety assessment of the new chemical entities (NCEs) prior to regulatory submission. Most NCEs fail in this phase. Previously, the bottleneck for drug discovery and development occurred in the drug discovery phase with limited numbers of drug targets available. With the advent of genomic technologies and advanced combinatorial chemistry, large numbers of compounds and drug targets are now available, moving the bottleneck to the discovery and preclinical border (lead compound selection and optimization). To help alleviate this backup, new alternative technologies, such as gene expression microarrays, have become available. Microarrays can often determine the expression of up to 10,000 genes and are currently being used on an investigational basis to help prioritize lead compounds by screening for efficacy and safety. Since experiments from the arrays can result in 10^6 data points or more, the challenge is how to handle the vast amount of data and how best to visualize the observed trends.

The following study was designed to obtain gene expression values from rats treated with different toxic agents and to compare different data analysis methods so as to address this challenge. Three known unrelated rat hepatotoxins were chosen: benzo(a)pyrene (BP), acetaminophen (APAP), and clofibrate (CLO). BP is a known rodent and probable human carcinogen.[1] It is metabolized by several forms of cytochrome P450 (1A1, 1A2, 2B1, 2C9, 3A4) and associated enzymes to both activated and detoxified metabolites.[2–5] In most tissues, the ultimate metabolite is the bay-region diol epoxide, benzo(a)pyrene-7,8-diol-9,10-epoxide (BPDE). BPDE-DNA adducts have been shown to persist in rat liver for up to 56 days post-dose with the treatment regimen of 10 mg/kg body weight (bw) given 3 times per week for 2 weeks.[6] It has recently been shown that the BPDE-DNA adducts preferentially

---

[a]Address for correspondence: Mary Jane Cunningham, Incyte Pharmaceuticals, Incorporated, 3174 Porter Drive, Palo Alto, CA 94304. Voice: 650-855-0555; fax: 650-855-0572. maryjane@incyte.com

bind to methylated CpG sites in the p53 gene at sites where mutations are known to occur.[7] Mutations in this tumor suppressor gene have been discovered in over 50% of human cancers.[8]

APAP is a well-recognized and widely used analgesic. It is metabolized by cytochrome P450 (mainly 1A1, 1A2, 2E1, and 3A4) with the majority of the drug undergoing glucuronidation and sulfation.[9,10] A small portion is metabolized to an active intermediate, N-acetyl-p-benzoquinone imine (NAPQI), which is subsequently conjugated by glutathione (GSH). However, at large nontherapeutic doses, NAPQI is not detoxified, but (due to the depletion of GSH) covalently binds to hepatic proteins, causing cell damage and eventually hepatic failure.[11]

CLO is an antilipidemic drug whose function is to lower elevated levels of serum triglycerides. In rodents, chronic treatment produces hepatomegaly, an increase in hepatic peroxisomes, and has been shown to be a hepatocarcinogen, but not a mutagen.[12] CLO activates a peroxisome proliferator activated receptor (PPARα) and transcriptional activation of peroxisomal enzymes leading to peroxisomal proliferation.[13] In addition, CLO induces cytochrome P450, mainly the CYP4A isozymes, but also other CYP isozymes to a lesser extent.[14–16]

Several data analysis methods have been developed that can be applied to scoring gene expression profiles from microarray data. One such method is the Expectation Ratio Likelihood (ERL) [unpublished]. ERL is designed to detect genes that are differentially expressed in several hybridization experiments. The higher the ERL value, the lower the likelihood that the expression difference is due to measurement errors. ERL = Σ abs[log(R_t/R_c)], where R_t and R_c are the expression ratios in the treated and time-matched control experiments (assuming a common reference sample), respectively; abs(…) and log(…) are the absolute value and logarithm functions; and the sum is over pairs of treated/control experiments.

Another method is an information theoretic measure known as Shannon entropy.[17] This method is a measure of the information content of a series of events or dynamic pattern and is defined as $H = -\Sigma p_i \log_2 p_i$, where p_i is the probability (frequency) of a level of expression of a gene. The dynamic pattern, in this case, is a time series of gene expression where high entropy indicates that a gene expression pattern is very variable over time, while zero entropy indicates an unchanging pattern of expression. The greater the variation or change in a pattern, the higher the entropy. This concept should not be confused with disorder or randomness.

Change or variation in gene expression is also the criterion used to determine which genes are physiologically relevant to the biological process being studied. In this paper, ERL and Shannon entropy were applied to gene expression data from rat livers treated with known hepatotoxins to help analyze and visualize the resulting toxic responses.

MATERIALS AND METHODS

Animal Treatment

Male Sprague-Dawley rats (6–8 weeks old) were dosed ip with one of the following compounds: (a) BP at 10 mg/kg bw given 3 times per week for 2 weeks, (b) CLO at 250 mg/kg bw, (c) APAP at 1000 mg/kg bw, or (d) DMSO (control vehicle) at

<2 mL/kg bw. All chemicals were purchased from Acros (Geel, Belgium). Physical signs and body weights were monitored daily and prior to necropsy, and blood samples were drawn by cardiac puncture for determination of serum alanine transferase [ALT] and aspartate aminotransferase [AST] (diagnostic kits, Sigma Chemical Co., St. Louis, MO). At necropsy, observations of gross pathology and liver weights were recorded. The liver, kidney, brain, spleen, and pancreas from each rat were harvested, flash-frozen in liquid nitrogen, and stored at −80°C until RNA isolation.

mRNA Isolation

Total RNA was isolated by the Trizol procedure (Life Technologies, Gaithersburg, MD) following the modifications for liver RNA isolation. mRNA was selected and purified from total RNA by the OligoTex™ purification kit (Qiagen, Valencia, CA). The purified mRNA was treated with DNase 1 (Life Technologies), phenol/chloroform-extracted, and ethanol-precipitated. Quantification was performed by OD_{260} measurement.

Production of Cy3 and Cy5 Probes

The reverse transcription reaction was performed in a 25-µL volume containing 200 ng of polyA$^+$ RNA with GEMBright Kits (Incyte Pharmaceuticals, Fremont, CA) and incorporating the Cy3 and Cy5 fluorescent dyes (Amersham Pharmacia Biotech, Piscataway, NJ). Four specific control polyA$^+$ RNAs (YCFR06, YCFR45, YCFR67, YCFR85, YCFR43, YCFR22, YCFR23, YCFR25, YCFR44, and YCFR26) were synthesized by *in vitro* transcription from noncoding yeast genomic DNA. As quantitative controls, the control mRNAs (YCFR06, YCFR45, YCFR67, and YCFR85) of 0.002 ng, 0.02 ng, 0.2 ng, and 2 ng were diluted into the reverse transcription reaction at ratios of 1:100,000, 1:10,000, 1:1000, and 1:100 (w/w), respectively, to sample mRNA. The control mRNAs (YCFR43, YCFR22, YCFR23, YCFR25, YCFR44, and YCFR26) were diluted into the reverse transcription reaction at ratios of 1:3, 3:1, 1:10, 10:1, 1:25, and 25:1 (w/w), respectively, to sample mRNA differential expression patterns. After incubation at 37°C for 2 h, each reaction sample (one with Cy3 and another with Cy5 labeling) was treated with 2.5 µL of 0.5 M sodium hydroxide and incubated for 20 min at 85°C to stop the reaction and degrade the RNA. Probes were purified using two successive Chroma Spin™ 30 columns (Clontech, Palo Alto, CA), combined, and precipitated using 1 µL of glycogen (1 mg/mL), 60 µL of sodium acetate, and 300 µL of 100% ethanol.

Hybridization onto GEMs

The probes were resuspended in 1 µL of hybridization buffer (5× SSC plus 0.2% SDS) and were applied to the 4-cm^2 hybridization area of microarrays as described previously.[18] Hybridized microarrays were scanned at two separate channels for Cy3 and Cy5 emission signals, respectively, and analyzed.[19]

Production of GEMs

Incyte proprietary clones from cDNA rat liver and kidney libraries in the ZooSeq™ database (Incyte Pharmaceuticals, Palo Alto, CA) were clustered and a list containing a representative EST correlating to each gene was compiled. Approximately 500 ESTs corresponding to known genes involved in toxicity were added to the list. The vector used for cDNA library construction of each clone resulting in an EST was pINCY (Incyte Pharmaceuticals, Palo Alto, CA). Inserts of cDNA clones were amplified by PCR using primers that were complementary to vector sequences flanking both sides of the cDNA insert. Plasmid template (1–2 ng) was added to the 100 μL PCR mixture containing 0.2 mM of each nucleotide, 1 μM of each primer (SK853, GCTCGTATGTTGTGTGGAA, and SK536, GCGAAAGGGGGATGT-GCTG), 1.5 mM of Mg^{+2}, and 10 units of Taq polymerase. Inserts were amplified using 30 cycles (94°C for 30 s, 56°C for 30 s, 72°C for 90 s) with an initial denaturation at 95°C for 3 min and a final extension at 72°C for 5 min. Five μL of each finished reaction was electrophoresed on a 1.5% agarose gel to confirm amplification quality and quantity. PCR products were purified using Sephacryl™-400 columns (Amersham Pharmacia Biotech) and lyophilized dry for subsequent preparation for microarray fabrication. In general, the total quantity of each PCR product was greater than 5 μg. The average size of inserts was around 1000 bp.

PCR products were suspended in 10 μL of 2× SSC buffer and arrayed from 96-well microtiter plates onto silylated microscope slides using high-speed robotics as described.[19] A total of 7404 cDNA sequences, representing 7404 rat liver and kidney genes, and a variety of control elements, including 14 synthetic DNA control sequences, human genomic DNA, and yeast genomic DNA, were arrayed in a 1.8-cm^2 area of silylated microscope slides. Each DNA preparation was enough to make 500 copies of microarray.

Data Analysis

To assure that the data analysis is based only on the most reliable measurements, the data were subjected to stringent filtering. A microarray signal (GEMtools™ software, Incyte Pharmaceuticals) is deemed reliable if the intensity is ≥250, the signal-to-background ratio is ≥2.5, and the signal from the spotted area is ≥40%. To allow for comparative analysis, genes were selected only if all signals for all time points and drug treatments pass the quality-control thresholds. Out of 7680 clones on the array, 1714 passed these stringent criteria. For the entropy method, the highest entropy genes of $H = 1$ were selected, resulting in a total of 283. In order to be able to compare all three methods, the thresholds for the ERL and X-fold methods were set to 2.65 and 2.5, respectively, resulting in the same number of 283 genes for each.

The values used in the X-fold method are ratios of P1 signal (Cy3 channel) to P2 signal (Cy5 channel) after the P2 signal is adjusted with a balance coefficient. The balance coefficient corrects for signal differences in the two channels using the yeast genomic standards described above. A significant differential expression value is generally considered to be ±2-fold, while a threshold of ±2.5-fold is being used here in the comparison of the three analysis methods.

ERL values for the 1714 genes were calculated using the aforementioned formula $ERL = \Sigma \; abs[log(R_t/R_c)]$, where R_t and R_c are the expression ratios in the experiments using hepatotoxin-treated and time-matched DMSO-treated control rat livers. The summation is carried out over all time points for each gene. This formula is based on an analysis of error probability for clones on the GEM that correspond to the same gene. The ERL score is proportional to minus the logarithm of the error probability; thus, the larger the score, the more unlikely it is that the difference in expression is caused by measurement error.

To calculate Shannon entropy[17] for the 1714 genes, expression data for each gene were first normalized to the maximal expression for that gene (i.e., the maximum expression for each gene equals 1.0 for the time series) and then separated into one of two expression categories: <0.5 or ≥0.5. Shannon entropy was then calculated according to the formula $H = -\Sigma p_i \log_2 p_i$, where H is Shannon entropy and p_i is the probability (frequency) of a level of gene expression (<0.5 or ≥0.5) in the time series.

RESULTS

The male Sprague-Dawley rats dosed with BP showed increased liver weight to body weight ratios from day 3 to day 28 compared to rats dosed only with the control vehicle, DMSO. Increased liver to body weight ratios were also observed with the APAP- and CLO-dosed rats from the day 3 time point. Serum concentrations of ALT were increased in APAP-dosed rats at 12 h, 24 h, and day 14 and in CLO-dosed rats at 12 h. Increased serum concentrations of AST were also observed with APAP- and CLO-dosed rats at 12 and 24 h and with BP-dosed rats at day 7. There was no increase in ALT serum concentrations with the BP-dosed rats. At necropsy, cloudy spleens for most of the BP-dosed rats were observed, while only one cloudy spleen was observed with the CLO-treated rats at the day 28 time point. Approximately half of the APAP-treated rats presented with fused or adhered liver lobes.

Three different analysis methods were applied to the microarray data and compared. The first method is the X-fold differential gene expression. FIGURE 1 shows the log-log graph of the fluorescent signal intensities from the competitive hybridization of cDNA from a rat liver treated with the control vehicle (DMSO) in the Cy3 channel and cDNA from a rat liver treated with BP at 12 h post-last-dose in the Cy5 channel. The majority of the expression values are within ±2-fold differential expression. For the 12 h time point of the BP treatment, 229 genes were upregulated and 113 genes were downregulated (using a within ±2-fold threshold, not the ±2.5-fold threshold). In addition, 5.8% of the total expressed genes were not observed in the public domain databases. In FIGURE 1, three clones are noted that annotated to CYP1A2 and two clones that annotated to sulfotransferase (ST2A1).

The second method of analysis is ERL. ERL provides an indication of the difference between a treated and a control times series or a measure of deviation of one time series from another, both in the shapes of patterns and in absolute expression levels. An example of the comparison of the results for APAP and BP are shown in FIGURE 2. The same three clones of CYP1A2 and two clones of ST2A1, which were noted in FIGURE 1, are marked in this figure.

Finally, the third method is Shannon entropy, a measure of the information content of a series of events. High entropy indicates that a gene expression pattern is highly variable over time, while zero entropy indicates an unchanging pattern of expression. FIGURE 3 shows histograms of the entropy values for all three treatments: APAP, BP, and CLO. In each case, most of the expressed genes have zero or midrange entropy. Only a select few have the highest entropy value of $H = 1$.

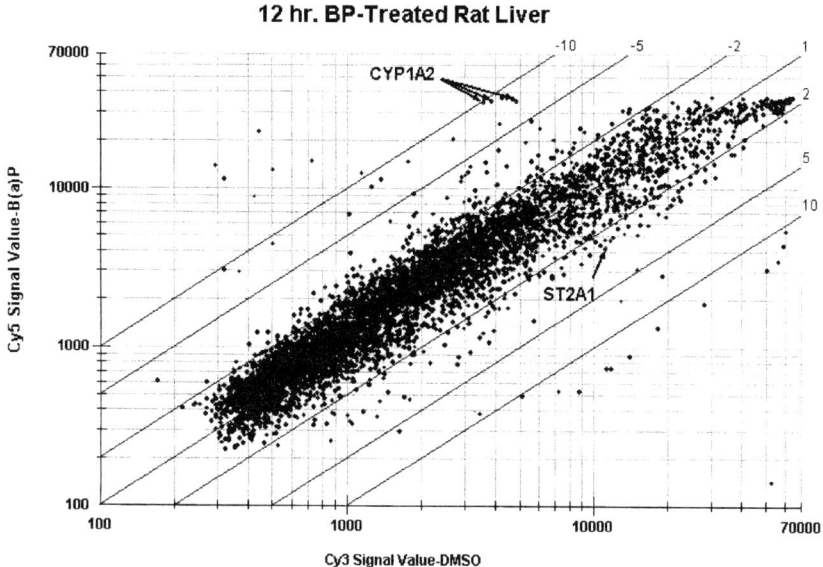

FIGURE 1. A log-log graph showing the signal values from a comparison of BP-treated rat liver at 12 h post-last-dose and DMSO-treated rat liver. The Cy3 channel is the cDNA from the control liver and the Cy5 channel is the cDNA from the BP-treated liver. The arrows note three clones representing CYP1A2 and two clones representing ST2A1.

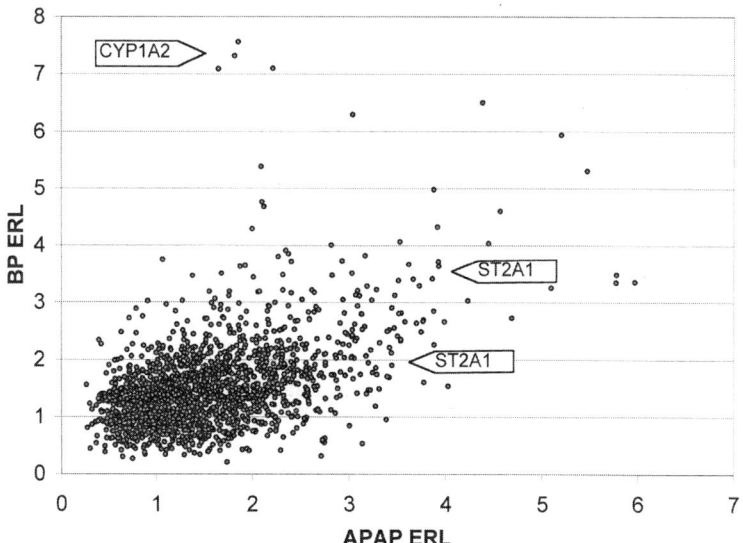

FIGURE 2. A graph depicting ERL values for APAP (x-axis) and BP (y-axis). The same CYP1A2 and ST2A1 clones that were noted in FIGURE 1 are noted here.

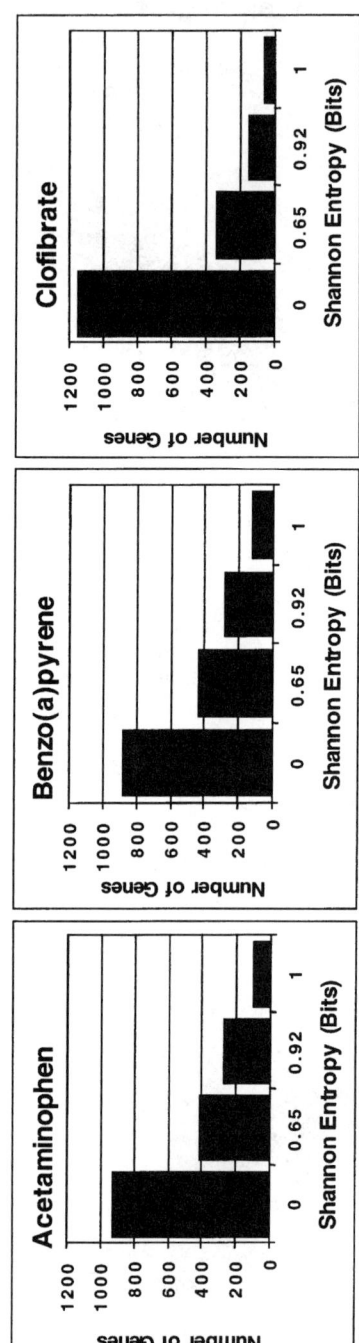

FIGURE 3. Shannon entropy for APAP, BP, and CLO experiments. The calculation of entropy for each of these three treatments results in four entropy values in each case. Histograms appear to show an exponential distribution of entropy values, with most genes having low entropy.

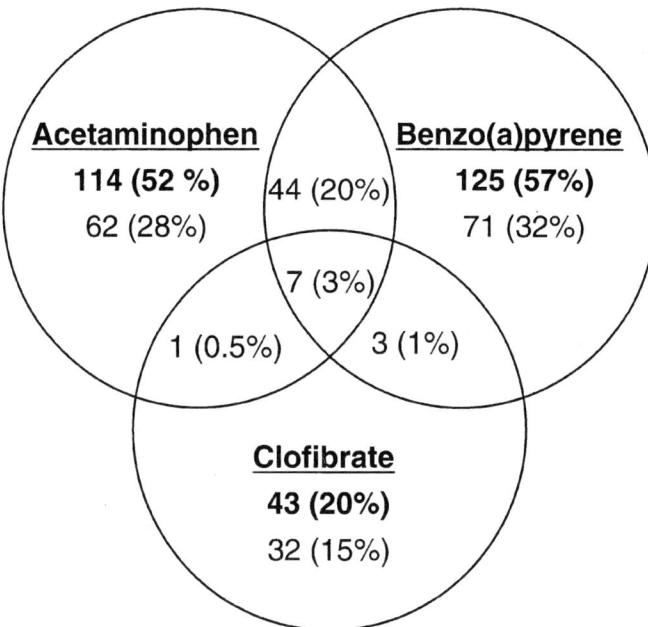

FIGURE 4A. Venn diagram comparing drug treatments according to the X-fold scoring method. The number of genes identified using this particular scoring method for a drug is shown in bold; the number solely identified by this method is shown immediately below. The intersections reflect which genes are affected by more than one treatment. Percentages are with respect to a total of 283 genes identified. (**A**) Genes exhibiting a ≥2.5-fold change.

For each method, the number of genes that showed the highest level of differential expression (283 genes total) was compared for each compound treatment (see FIGURES 4A–C). The number of genes in common between all three treatment groups is 0.4% for Shannon entropy, 3% for X-fold, and 6% for ERL, respectively. While all three methods detect a similar number of genes for APAP and BP, entropy clearly highlights the most genes for CLO (62), followed by X-fold (43) and ERL (29). For each method, the highest percentage of similarity is seen between APAP and BP (20% for X-fold, 18% for ERL, and 6% for entropy). Overall, entropy gives the best separation between drugs, that is, minimal overlap between genes identified in different treatments.

A Venn diagram showing the overlap of all three methods is shown in FIGURE 5. As already suggested by FIGURES 4A–C, the number of genes uniquely identified by a method is highest for entropy, followed by X-fold and then ERL. The highest overlap is between X-fold and ERL, followed by entropy versus ERL and entropy versus X-fold. Only 4% of genes are identified by all three methods. This demonstrates that each method independently captures meaningful relationships and suggests that all three methods should be included in a well-rounded analysis of expression profiles for toxicology analysis.

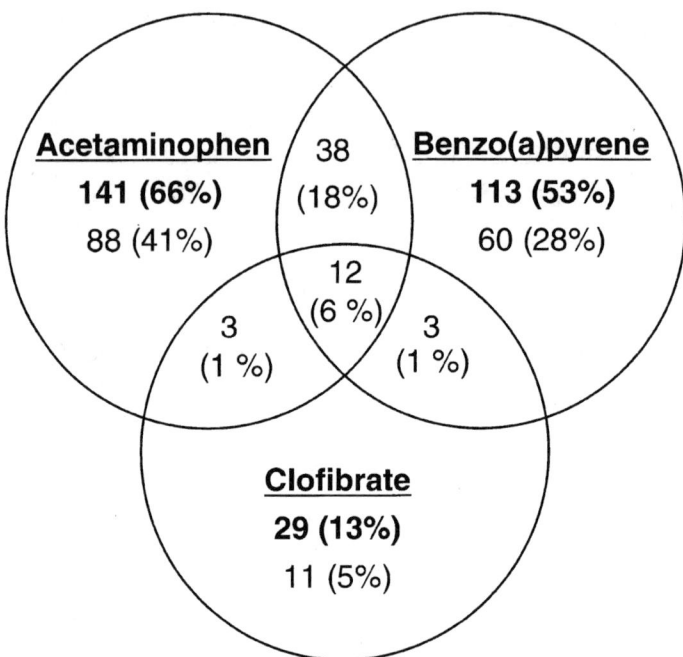

FIGURE 4B. Venn diagram comparing drug treatments according to the ERL scoring method. The number of genes identified using this particular scoring method for a drug is shown in bold; the number solely identified by this method is shown immediately below. The intersections reflect which genes are affected by more than one treatment. Percentages are with respect to a total of 283 genes identified. **(B)** Genes exhibiting an ERL ≥ 2.65.

Examination of individual expression profiles confirms the fidelity of the measurement technology and provides further detail on the behavior of different isozymes. FIGURE 6 shows several clones that are annotated to the same description and show the same pattern across all three time courses. In the top part of the figure, three clones (ZooSeq™ clone 700483145, 70013747, and 700606570) annotate to the gene CYP1A2 (g205938 and g203762, rat cytochrome P450d under the old nomenclature system) and show a similar expression pattern across the APAP, BP, and CLO time courses. The values for CLO are high throughout the time course, reaching even higher values at day 7. The values for APAP peak at day 7 and those for BP peak at 12 h. The values for BP were found to be significant using both the X-fold and ERL methods, whereas the values for APAP were significant with entropy.

The same pattern across all three time courses is also seen for two clones designated as cytochrome P4504A3 (g204989), three clones designated as fatty-acid transport protein 5 (FATP5, g3341461 and g3335570, same TrEMBL accession number of O88694), and two clones designated as sulfotransferase ST2A1 (g204670).

In another comparison depicted in FIGURE 7, clones annotating to CYP1A2 show a different pattern than a ZooSeq™ clone 700138667, annotating to CYP2B1. High values are seen for APAP, BP, and CLO with CYP2B1, but the peaks are seen at dif-

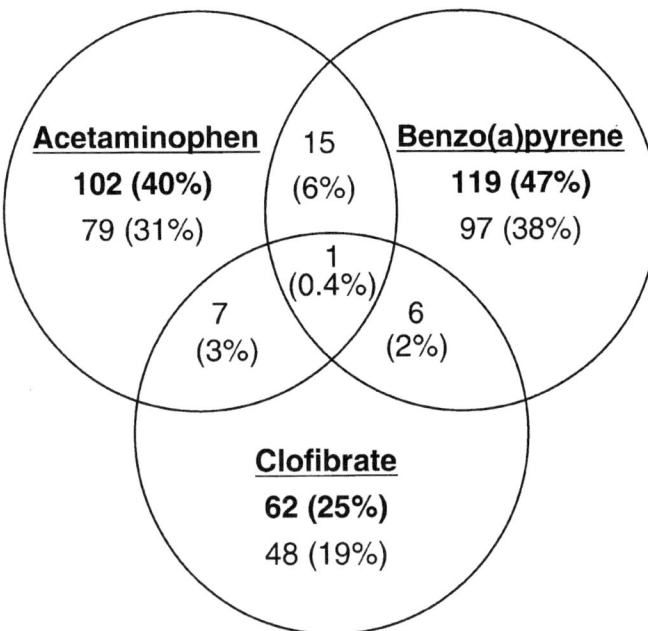

FIGURE 4C. Venn diagram comparing drug treatments according to the entropy scoring method. The number of genes identified using this particular scoring method for a drug is shown in bold; the number solely identified by this method is shown immediately below. The intersections reflect which genes are affected by more than one treatment. Percentages are with respect to a total of 283 genes identified. (C) Genes showing entropy values of $H = 1.0$.

ferent times than with CYP1A2. For example, the peak of expression for BP with CYP1A2 is at 12 h, while the peak is at day 7 with CYP2B1. Dissimilar expression patterns are also seen between isozymes of a detoxification family of enzymes, glutathione S-transferases (GST). Clones from the GST-α isozyme family show high expression patterns for APAP, peaking at 12 h with a later peak occurring from day 3 to day 28, and for BP, peaking at 12 h and from day 3 to day 7. In the case of CLO, the expression values remain high throughout the time course, with a slight decrease at day 7. The expression values for the GST-θ class of isozymes show a different pattern in the APAP and CLO time courses, but a similar pattern in the BP time course. The peak for APAP does not occur until day 3 and the peak for CLO occurs with one clone at 12 h with a later peak at day 3. The peak in values for BP occurs at 12 h and then from day 3 to day 7, as was seen with the GST-α isozyme clones.

DISCUSSION

Genes whose expression levels change in response to a disease or perturbation are logical candidates for putative drug or toxicity targets since a subset of these genes may actively participate in adverse effects. It is for this reason that we have com-

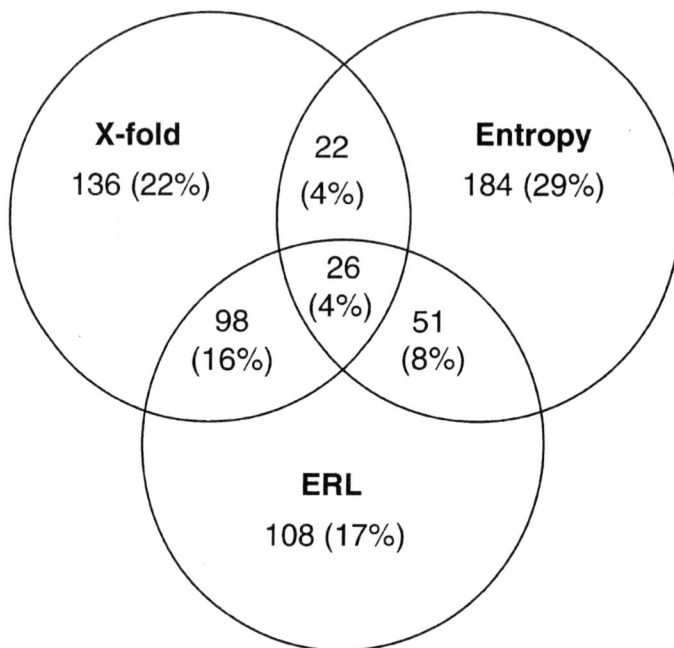

FIGURE 5. Venn diagram comparing scoring methods. Thresholds were adjusted such that each method detected exactly 283 genes. The entropy measure has the highest number of unique hits not identified by the other methods. Conversely, the highest overlap is between X-fold and ERL scoring (16%).

pared Shannon entropy, ERL, and X-fold change data analysis methods for the selection of interesting genes. An initial data analysis using Shannon entropy was discussed in Fuhrman et al.[20] Although entropy reveals nothing about the shape of the temporal expression pattern, it provides a measure of a gene's expression activity during a process. Ranking hundreds or thousands of genes using Shannon entropy permits the selection of the most "active" genes for further use as candidate toxicity markers or drug targets.

In each of the three methods, a high score selects a different set of genes, although there is some overlap with genes selected by the other two methods (as seen in FIGURES 4A–C and 5). The percentage of common genes varies with each method and may correlate with the fact that these three compounds are unrelated hepatotoxins. However, these common genes may be general markers of toxicity. The percentage of genes shared between treatments is most similar for X-fold and ERL. This is not surprising since both X-fold and ERL scoring depend on the degree of differential expression, as opposed to expression pattern diversity measured by entropy.

In all three methods, there was more overlap of common up- and downregulated genes from the APAP and BP treatments than the common genes from the APAP and CLO treatments or from the CLO and BP treatments. This result is surprising because APAP and CLO are both nongenotoxic compounds, while BP is a genotoxic

Gene	APAP0hr	APAP12hr	APAP24hr	APAP3d	APAP7d	APAP28d	BP0hr	BP12hr	BP24hr	BP3d	BP7d	BP28	Clo0hr	Clo12hr	Clo24hr	Clo3d	Clo7d	Clo28d
CYP1A2	0.6	0.5	0.5	1.0	1.0	0.9	0.1	1.0	1.0	0.6	0.5	0.2	0.6	0.6	0.7	0.6	1.0	0.8
CYP1A2	0.5	0.4	0.3	0.6	1.0	0.5	0.1	1.0	0.6	0.4	0.4	0.1	0.6	0.7	0.5	0.6	1.0	0.6
CYP1A2	0.7	0.4	0.3	0.7	1.0	0.9	0.1	1.0	0.7	0.5	0.5	0.1	0.6	0.6	0.6	0.5	1.0	0.6
CYP4A3	0.3	1.0	0.7	0.3	0.7	0.6	0.3	0.9	0.5	0.1	1.0	0.8	0.8	0.9	0.9	1.0	0.5	0.6
CYP4A3	0.2	1.0	0.6	0.2	0.5	0.5	0.2	0.8	0.5	0.1	1.0	0.6	0.8	0.9	0.9	1.0	0.5	0.6
FATP5	0.3	0.2	1.0	0.5	0.5	0.5	0.5	0.5	0.8	0.5	0.9	1.0	0.7	0.8	1.0	1.0	1.0	0.9
FATP5	0.4	0.2	1.0	0.7	0.4	0.5	0.6	0.7	1.0	0.6	1.0	0.9	0.6	0.7	1.0	0.8	1.0	0.8
FATP5	0.3	0.2	1.0	0.6	0.6	0.4	0.5	0.6	0.9	0.5	1.0	1.0	0.6	0.5	0.9	0.8	1.0	0.8
ST2A1	0.3	0.1	0.4	0.5	0.3	1.0	0.3	0.2	0.8	0.4	0.2	0.6	0.4	0.4	1.0	0.3	0.3	0.5
ST2A1	0.4	0.1	0.5	0.6	0.4	1.0	0.4	0.2	0.8	0.5	0.3	0.6	0.5	0.6	1.0	0.4	0.4	0.6

FIGURE 6. Similar gene expression patterns are shown for clones that are annotated to the same gene. Examples are noted for clones of CYP1A2, CYP4A3, FATP5, and sulfotransferase 2A1.

compound (i.e., acts by a DNA-damaging mechanism). The closer similarity between genes perturbed by APAP and BP may be due to the main mechanism of action involving the cytochrome P450 pathway. While cytochrome P450 is also involved in CLO metabolism, it has been suggested that long-chain dicarboxylic acids metabolized by the CYP4A family of P450 isozymes actually mediate the more active peroxisomal β-oxidation pathway.[21–23]

By looking at genes with highly significant expression values, pathways of their action can be observed. For example, some of the CYP genes are highly expressed with APAP, BP, and CLO. CYP1A2 shows significant high expression with APAP and BP (FIGURE 6) and high expression over the entire time course with CLO. CYP1A2 is induced by both APAP and BP,[2,9] but there is no published association with CLO. All three compounds induce CYP2B1,[4,5,10,15,16] but the pattern of expression is different (FIGURE 7).

Another example is the expression pattern for CLO. High expression values are observed with CYP1A2, CYP2B1, and CYP4A3 (FIGURES 6 and 7). CYP4A3 is also lauric acid omega hydroxylase and one of the major isozymes in the CYP4A family that metabolizes CLO. In addition, the fatty-acid pathway is seen by the high expression of FATP5 (FIGURE 6). The suggestion by Kaikaus *et al.*[22] and Waxman[23] implies that CYP4A3 would be expressed before the enzymes from the peroxisomal β-oxidation pathway. FIGURE 6 shows that the expression of CYP4A3 is highest from 0 h to day 3, whereas the expression of FATP5 peaks from 12 to 24 h and remains high until day 28. This observation is consistent with the conclusions put forth by both authors.[22,23]

Gene	CYP1A2	CYP1A2	CYP1A2	CYP2B1	GST-α	GST-α	GST-α	GST-θ	GST-θ
Clo28d	0.8	0.6	0.6	1.0	1.0	1.0	1.0	0.3	0.4
Clo7d	1.0	1.0	1.0	1.0	0.5	0.6	0.5	0.6	0.7
Clo3d	0.6	0.6	0.5	0.5	0.9	0.7	0.9	1.0	1.0
Clo24hr	0.7	0.5	0.6	1.0	0.8	0.7	0.8	0.2	0.2
Clo12hr	0.6	0.7	0.6	0.8	0.8	0.9	0.9	0.6	0.8
Clo0hr	0.6	0.6	0.6	0.7	0.8	0.9	0.8	0.4	0.5
BP28	0.2	0.1	0.1	0.1	0.4	0.3	0.3	0.1	0.1
BP7d	0.5	0.4	0.5	1.0	0.8	0.8	0.8	1.0	1.0
BP3d	0.6	0.4	0.5	0.3	1.0	1.0	0.8	1.0	0.7
BP24hr	1.0	0.6	0.7	0.2	0.5	0.6	0.5	0.2	0.2
BP12hr	1.0	1.0	1.0	0.1	1.0	1.0	1.0	0.8	0.8
BP0hr	0.1	0.1	0.1	0.2	0.7	0.7	0.5	0.4	0.3
APAP28d	0.9	0.5	0.9	0.8	0.9	0.6	0.7	0.2	0.2
APAP7d	1.0	1.0	1.0	1.0	0.7	0.9	1.0	0.7	0.6
APAP3d	1.0	0.6	0.7	0.5	0.7	1.0	0.8	1.0	1.0
APAP24hr	0.5	0.3	0.3	0.4	0.6	0.4	0.5	0.5	0.4
APAP12hr	0.5	0.4	0.4	0.3	0.6	0.7	0.6	0.6	0.5
APAP0hr	0.6	0.5	0.7	0.7	0.9	1.0	0.7	0.7	0.6

FIGURE 7. Different expression patterns resulted from different isozymes of cytochrome P450 and glutathione S-transferase (GST). The comparison shows CYP1A2 and CYP2B1 isozymes as well as isozymes from the alpha and theta families of GSTs.

The use of a time series allows for the observation of an entire physiological process and requires data analysis techniques more sophisticated than X-fold change. In that context, Shannon entropy is well suited to time course experiments since it requires a series of data points. Unlike ERL, entropy ignores X-fold change entirely and provides a measure of the complexity of a time series. With fewer than eight time points and only two expression level categories (as in the present study), the statistical variance may be substituted for entropy; however, entropy distinguishes itself as a measure of complexity with eight or more time points and more than two expression level categories.[20]

In all three treatments (APAP, BP, and CLO), the number of highly expressed genes decreases sharply as entropy increases, with less than 10% of genes having the highest entropy value. These highest entropy genes may serve as the focus for future studies of toxicity. Further research will be needed to determine if a bias toward low entropy is a general characteristic of liver and other tissues. Tissues with the majority of their genes in low entropy may be stabilized against perturbations caused by pharmaceutical compounds or toxic agents.

The use of ERL as a data analysis measure complements Shannon entropy in two ways. First, the change in gene expression may be a part of the normal developmental process and not induced specifically by the NCEs. ERL deals with this by comparing the changes in NCE-induced expression patterns with those of normal development. Second, significant changes in gene expression need to be differentiated from measurement noise. In that context, ERL is proportional to minus the logarithm of probability that the measured expression difference is due to the measurement error; therefore, the higher the score, the more unlikely that the expression difference from two hybridizations is due to a measurement error.

ERL may prove useful in temporal gene expression studies that involve significant changes in the control time series. For example, studies of subchronic toxicity models should take into account the normal aging process. In this case, genes exhibiting significant changes in expression caused by aging must be separated from those that are affected by toxicity. Once this has been accomplished, other methods, such as Shannon entropy, can be applied to the toxicity-specific genes selected by ERL. Future developments in the sorting of gene expression data may depend on the application of complementary computational techniques such as ERL and entropy.

In summary, when dealing with thousands of genes, all potentially interesting, it is desirable to rank the genes according to their degree of participation in a physiological process. Therefore, genes with the highest Shannon entropy and ERL can be selected as the best toxicity target candidates, permitting preclinical scientists to focus their research and resources on those genes.

ACKNOWLEDGMENTS

We would like to thank Glenn Fu, Irene Ni, Laura Kamagaki, and the cDNA library production group, and Warren Lei and the Microarray Division for their technical help. We would also like to thank Gary Zweiger and Scott Panzer for their technical help in designing the rat GEM 1.0 microarray.

REFERENCES

1. BENZO[A]PYRENE. 1983. IARC Monogr. Eval. Carcinog. Risk Chem. Hum. **32:** 211–224.
2. DEGAWA, M. et al. 1994. Metabolic activation and carcinogen-DNA adduct detection in human larynx. Cancer Res. **54:** 4915–4919.
3. KADLUBAR, F.F. & A.F. BADAWI. 1995. Genetic susceptibility and carcinogen-DNA adduct formation in human urinary bladder carcinogenesis. Toxicol. Lett. **82/83:** 627–632.
4. PARK, S.H. & R.A. SCHATZ. 1999. Effect of low-level short-term o-xylene inhalation of benzo(a)pyrene (BaP) metabolism and BaP-DNA adduct formation in rat liver and lung microsomes. J. Toxicol. Environ. Health **58:** 299–312.
5. CHRISTOU, M. et al. 1992. Selective suppression of the catalytic activity of cDNA-expressed cytochrome P4502B1 toward polycyclic hydrocarbons in the microsomal membrane: modification of this effect by specific amino acid substitutions. Biochemistry **31:** 2835–2841.
6. QU, S.X. & N.H. STACEY. 1996. Formation and persistence of DNA adducts in different target tissues of rats after multiple administration of benzo(a)pyrene. Carcinogenesis **17:** 53–59.
7. CHEN, J.X. et al. 1998. Carcinogens preferentially bind at methylated CpG in the p53 mutational hot spots. Cancer Res. **58:** 2070–2075.
8. GREENBLATT, M.S. et al. 1994. Mutations in the p53 tumor suppressor gene: clues to cancer etiology and molecular pathogenesis. Cancer Res. **54:** 4855–4878.
9. COHEN, S.D. & E.A. KHAIRALLAH. 1977. Selective protein arylation and acetaminophen-induced hepatotoxicity. Drug Metab. Rev. **29:** 59–77.
10. MYERS, T.G. et al. 1994. Preferred orientations in the binding of 4′-hydroxyacetanilide (acetaminophen) to cytochrome P450 1A1 and 2B1 isoforms as determined by ^{13}C- and ^{15}N-NMR relaxation studies. J. Med. Chem. **37:** 860–867.
11. KROGER, H. et al. 1997. Protection from acetaminophen-induced liver damage by the synergistic action of low doses of the poly(ADP-ribose) polymerase-inhibitor nicotinamide and the antioxidant N-acetylcysteine or the amino acid L-methionine. Gen. Pharmacol. **28:** 257–263.
12. NAKANISHI, Y. et al. 1989. Effects of chronic administration of the peroxisome proliferator, clofibrate, on cytosolic acetyl-CoA hydrolase in rat liver. Biochem. Pharmacol. **45:** 1403–1407.
13. TUGWOOD, J.D. et al. 1998. Peroxisome proliferator–activated receptors: structures and function. Ann. N.Y. Acad. Sci. **804:** 252–265.
14. SIMPSON, A.E. 1997. The cytochrome P450 4 (CYP4) family. Gen. Pharmacol. **28:** 351–359.
15. SUNDSETH, S.S. & D.J. WAXMAN. 1992. Sex-dependent expression and clofibrate inducibility of cytochrome P450 4A fatty acid omega-hydroxylases: male specificity of liver and kidney CYP4A2 mRNA and tissue-specific regulation by growth hormone and testosterone. J. Biol. Chem. **267:** 3915–3921.
16. CUMMINGS, B.S. et al. 1999. Cellular distribution of cytochromes P-450 in the rat kidney. Drug Metab. Dispos. **27:** 542–548.
17. SHANNON, C.E. & W. WEAVER. 1963. The Mathematical Theory of Communication. University of Illinois Press. Champaign, Illinois.
18. SCHENA, M. et al. 1996. Parallel human genome analysis: microarray-based expression monitoring of 1000 genes. Proc. Natl. Acad. Sci. U.S.A. **93:** 10614–10619.
19. SHALON, D. et al. 1996. A DNA microarray system for analyzing complex DNA samples using two-color fluorescent probe hybridization. Genome Res. **6:** 639–645.
20. FUHRMAN, S. et al. 1999. The application of Shannon entropy in the identification of putative drug targets. In BioSystems: Proceedings of the International Workshop on Information Processing in Cells and Tissues. In press.
21. AMACHER, D.E. et al. 1997. Hepatic microsomal enzyme induction, β-oxidation, and cell proliferation following administration of clofibrate, gemfibrozil, or bezafibrate in the CD rat. Toxicol. Appl. Pharmacol. **142:** 143–150.

22. KAIKAUS, R.M. et al. 1993. Induction of peroxisomal fatty acid beta-oxidation and liver fatty acid–binding protein by peroxisome proliferators: mediators via the cytochrome P-450IVA1 omega-hydroxylase pathway. J. Biol. Chem. **268:** 9593–9603.
23. WAXMAN, D.J. 1999. P450 gene induction by structurally diverse xenochemicals: central role of nuclear receptors CAR, PXR, and PPAR. Arch. Biochem. Biophys. **369:** 11–23.

In Silico Toxicology

SAMUEL HOLTZMAN[a]

Entelos, Incorporated, Menlo Park, California, USA

> ABSTRACT: It is toxicology's job to discover a new substance's harmful effects and suggest ways to prevent or mitigate those harmful effects. This paper offers a new possibility—*in silico* toxicology—to help address this multifaceted challenge.

We are living in extraordinary times. Scientific advances in molecular biology and chemistry coupled with breakthroughs in information, communication, and automation technologies have opened doors to exciting new medicines, agricultural products, foods, industrial and household materials, and many other novel substances that promise to improve the lives of billions of people. Yet every one of these new substances has the potential to do harm. While extensive industrial and regulatory safeguards shield us from many potentially harmful effects from new products, seemingly benign substances too frequently lead to significant adverse events, even death. Moreover, the challenge is getting tougher.

It is toxicology's job to discover each new substance's harmful effects and suggest ways to prevent or mitigate those harmful effects. However, as science and technology advance, so does toxicology's challenge. The challenge is as much economic and ethical as it is scientific and technical. We cannot simply impose further and stricter regulations based on traditional concepts without straining moral sensibilities (e.g., by conducting more *in vivo* tests) and unduly restricting or delaying the timely availability of valuable new products.

This paper offers a new possibility—*in silico* toxicology—to help address this multifaceted challenge.

CHALLENGES AND OPPORTUNITIES

Toxicology is a well-established field. The wide array of established test formats (from *in vitro* acute-toxicity assays and *in vivo* teratology studies to Ames mutagenicity tests and multiyear animal-carcinogenicity studies) is evidence of the field's long and successful history. Many mainstream toxicology tests have become seamlessly integrated into the regulatory structure of most industrialized countries. However, these mainstream tests may no longer address key toxicology challenges. For example, they do not address the unique characteristics of a recombinant hemoglo-

---

[a]Address for correspondence: Entelos, Incorporated, 4040 Campbell Avenue, Suite 200, Menlo Park, CA 94025-1007. Voice: 650-330-5200; fax: 650-330-5201.
holtzman@entelos.com

bin product, which is neither a drug nor a food. Similarly, we do not have established methods to measure the safety of a gene-repair vaccine that changes the patient's genetic makeup for life. How should we study the enormous number of potential drug combinations against HIV to determine each one's long-term safety profile? How should we compellingly evaluate the safety of genetically engineered fruits and vegetables? Will the milk from an interspecies clone be safe to drink in the long term?

Many of the key effects we want to measure may be very significant, but may occur in only a few among hundreds, thousands, and even millions of possible substance combinations, all or most of which must somehow be tested to identify those rare cases in which severe effects can occur. On the same vein, many important effects may require that we study phenomena spanning many years and even decades across very large populations. Testing for these effects can be prohibitively expensive and time-consuming. We may even want to test substances *before* a final form has been synthesized and we may want to test for specific effects before a corresponding assay is available.

In silico toxicology—the application of *in silico* (computer-based) simulation to toxicology—can greatly contribute to meeting such challenges. *In silico* toxicology studies can help focus *in vitro* and *in vivo* experiments to make the latter highly efficient. In some cases, *in silico* studies might even replace particularly expensive, lengthy, uninformative, or offensive *in vitro* or *in vivo* experiments. Moreover, by virtue of being computer-based and, hence, inexpensively replicable, *in silico* toxicology can vastly expand the applicability and availability of toxicologic analysis.

IN SILICO SIMULATION SYSTEMS

In silico simulation systems are commonly used in engineering. Companies that develop such highly complex devices as telephone switching systems, airplanes, and integrated circuits have for decades relied on *in silico* simulation as a core R&D activity. It would be engineering and economic folly to embark in the production of any of these devices and systems without first simulating them to test their operability and optimize their design. Similarly, oil exploration would be far less reliable without *in silico* simulation of geologic phenomena based on data from seismic and other tests of the target terrain.

In biology, *in silico* simulation has primarily focused on exploring the physiologic effects of intended interventions against disease.[1–5] Developments in this area have led to such commercial products as Entelos® Asthma PhysioLab™ and Entelos Obesity PhysioLab, which are being used by some of the world's leading pharmaceutical companies to increase the probability of R&D success and reduce the time it takes to bring a drug from discovery to the pharmacy shelves. [Note that Entelos is a registered trademark of Entelos, Incorporated. PhysioLab and ToxLab are trademarks and service marks of Entelos, Incorporated. All rights reserved.] FIGURE 1 illustrates the key facets of an Entelos PhysioLab.

In silico simulation systems allow researchers to explore the biologic effects of actual and hypothetical interventions quickly, inexpensively, and reliably. A well-designed *in silico* simulation system makes any set of parameters (among many

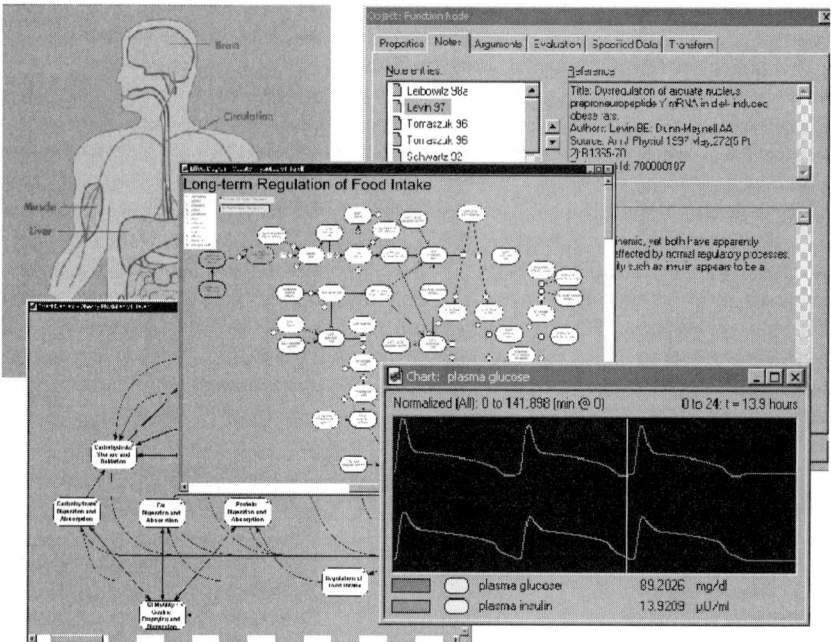

FIGURE 1. An Entelos® PhysioLab™ has four key facets: (i) a map of the physiology and pathophysiology of the disease at various levels of detail, (ii) extensive documentation supporting and explaining the disease map, (iii) a powerful simulation engine and corresponding experimental displays, and (iv) a collection of reference virtual patients, interventions, and experiments (not shown) [see www.entelos.com].

thousands represented) available for intervention and observation. A researcher could intervene anywhere in the body (e.g., by competitively binding to a target receptor with an inert ligand) and then observe any desired biologic parameter over time for the duration of the simulated experiment without concern for harming the subject or disturbing the course of the underlying biology.

For example, the clinical implications of a novel intervention pathway can be explored in detail before a compound that targets that pathway is identified. Clinical trials that would take months to execute can be represented *in silico* in a matter of hours and simulated in a matter of minutes. The behavior of any biologic factor represented in the simulation system can be tested against available data, and researchers can make adjustments to the PhysioLab (or, sometimes, to their knowledge!) wherever necessary. Such flexibility and speed are changing the nature of pharmaceutical research.

Like any other scientific endeavor, exploration using *in silico* simulation requires well-trained individuals working with an efficient experimental process. The process should be iterative and converge toward reliable scientific insights by coupling and mutually challenging simulation results with laboratory and clinical experimental data. In an ideal process, scientists would formulate their hypotheses in terms of the *in silico* system's parameters, evaluate the hypotheses through simulation, interpret the simulation results in meaningful scientific terms, and refine the formulation by incorporating any lessons learned from the interpreted results into a refined hypothesis and corresponding formulation, which are subsequently evaluated and the evaluation results reinterpreted. The iterative process continues as long as it keeps yielding valuable insights. Let us review these simulation steps in more detail.

To pose meaningful *in silico* questions, researchers must formulate their scientific questions in terms of a set of parameters selected from those available in the *in silico* system (a virtual experiment). The quality and thoughtfulness of this formulation is critical to obtaining insightful answers. For example, the administration of different pharmaceutical interventions must be represented in terms of the corresponding physiologic parameters in the *in silico* system. Exercise, environmental, dietary, and other lifestyle changes can also be parametrically represented in the *in silico* system. Virtual interventions can thus be defined in terms of their pharmaceutical and lifestyle components.

In addition, questions about an intervention's potential effectiveness should be asked from the perspectives of one or several specific disease etiologies. The common assumption that a common underlying etiology underlies similar clinical presentations can be a major source of confusion. Two clinically similar patients may have very different underlying dysfunctions and may require very different treatments for what is apparently the same condition. Patient variability to drug response can result in great frustration and expense during the pharmaceutical development process. *In silico* simulation studies can help prevent this frustration by allowing researchers to reflect in their study designs such factors as genetic predisposition, concurrent illnesses and treatments, different lifestyles, compliance patterns, variations in diet, and surgical interventions. Armed with insights about the key sources of patient variability, scientists can optimize study designs to increase their likelihood of yielding conclusive and actionable results.

Once the scientific question has been parametrically formulated, a wide range of corresponding *in silico* experiments can be designed and carried out. The following issues should be considered in designing *in silico* experiments. How many and what kinds of virtual patients should be tested? What dose regimens or exposure levels should be represented? What compliance (adherence) patterns should be studied? What time horizon should the experiment cover? What concurrent treatments should be included in the simulated experiments? A very large number of possible experimental variations can be efficiently and inexpensively tested *in silico*. Computational power is very economical in comparison with comparable *in vitro* or *in vivo* experiments.

Just as the original scientific question required translation into the *in silico* simulation system's parameters, *in silico* simulation results must be properly interpreted in scientifically meaningful terms. Knowledgeable individuals must translate the simulation results into actionable knowledge that reflects the scientific and human context in which experiments are being carried out. This translation highlights any simulation results that challenge prevailing knowledge and considers whether the behavior observed in simulation may reveal unseen biological phenomena or whether the simulation parameters need to be adjusted to more accurately reflect the scientific question being studied.

Researchers can then reformulate the desired scientific question to reflect the insights from the simulation and the ensuing discussion. Revised simulations yield further insights, and the iterative process continues until the scientific question being asked is sufficiently well addressed by the simulation. This process usually converges after only a few iterations.

IN SILICO TOXICOLOGY

In silico simulation systems can play an important role in enabling toxicology to better identify and help reduce or mitigate the potential harm of novel drugs, foods, agricultural products, and other potentially revolutionary substances.

In silico toxicology systems can reveal the complex physiologic pathways that underlie toxicity. Unlike more traditional animal, culture, and expression-array experimental models, organ-, tissue-, and cell-specific *in silico* simulation systems can allow researchers to observe harmful effects in detail early in the life of a new substance. *In silico* systems also enable researchers to observe many otherwise unobservable aspects of the process by which harmful effects occur. By studying harmful processes, it may be possible for scientists and engineers to identify biological, chemical, mechanical, and other means by which undesired effects might be mitigated. Moreover, *in silico* experiments are not subject to the biological or ethical limits that commonly apply to the use of *in vitro* and *in vivo* experimental models.

In silico simulation systems also can guide the use of and can help interpret the results of high-throughput *in vitro* assays. Such assays are attractive to pharmaceutical and other industrial developers of novel substances because assays can rapidly and inexpensively provide large quantities of biologic data. However, the data they provide tend to be narrowly focused. *In silico* systems complement high-throughput assay technology by placing assay results into the fuller pathophysiologic context that translates basic biologic activity into clinically important events.

An *in silico* toxicology system can itself be used in high-throughput mode. A large set of virtual substances can be tested against a correspondingly large set of virtual patients under a wide range of simulated circumstances. Combinatoric variety that would be unthinkable with *in vitro* or *in vivo* models can be well within the reach of *in silico* experimentation. Moreover, *in silico* experiments can dramatically compress time and reduce costs. Experiments that in the laboratory or the clinic could cost millions of dollars and take months to design and years to carry out could be designed in hours and carried out in minutes in an *in silico* platform, all of this at a small fraction of their cost using more traditional methods. Very large batches of these experiments, which would be unthinkable with traditional methods, could be economically run overnight.

When toxic processes become well understood, it becomes possible to identify biologic means by which their harmful effects can be mitigated. Researchers can run *in silico* experiments to simulate and optimize their proposed mitigation strategies. Such strategies can be systematically refined before valuable (and often scarce) experimental resources are committed to verify the *in silico* prediction. Targeted and efficient studies can then confirm and update a compound's *in silico* toxicologic profile.

Once a compound is deemed to be safe enough to be tested in humans, it becomes critical that experimental subjects be selected to maximize the amount of information resulting from each trial and to minimize the potential harm that could be inflicted on the subjects. *In silico* simulation can help identify criteria for selecting or rejecting experimental subjects. Moreover, as individual data are obtained for each subject, the *in silico* toxicology system can provide an early warning of potential toxicologic problems. It could also suggest mitigation approaches in the event that they are needed.

In silico toxicology opens the door to much more efficient and economic toxicology. *In silico* simulation can become a primary means for toxicologic exploration. *In vitro* and, in particular, *in vivo* methods would then be better thought of as means to confirm a compound's toxicologic profile predicted *in silico*. Such confirmatory studies would be much more targeted, fast, and efficient than the more traditional exploratory studies.

INDIVIDUALIZED TOXICOLOGY

In silico simulation can make individualized toxicology readily available to clinicians, their patients, and any other interested individual with access to networked computing equipment. Consider an individual evaluating the personal advantages and disadvantages of alternative antihistamine therapies to treat atopic allergic reactions. Like many other people in this situation, such an individual may already be taking several medicines for other conditions. Moreover, it would not be uncommon for such an individual to suffer from moderate asthma. *In silico* toxicology makes it possible for that individual to, for example, log on to an Internet site at which, with the help of her clinician, she could characterize her physiotype to quickly create a custom personalized virtual patient. The medicines that she and her clinician are considering may have already been characterized in the *in silico* system. Therefore, with little effort, she would be able to test on her own simulated physiology each of the contemplated medicines or combinations thereof. She could also study the long-term effects on herself—both desired (efficacy) and undesired (toxicity)—of each alternative therapy being considered.

By combining *in silico* physiology simulation systems such as Entelos Asthma PhysioLab[6] with *in silico* toxicology systems, clinicians, patients, and other individuals could explore the potential consequences of medical treatments before embarking on a medical course of action. More broadly, these systems can be an integral part of automated decision systems, which can help individuals identify the best course of action in a broader personal and social context.[7,8] Such an automated decision system can help the individual decision maker understand key trade-offs among such uncertain factors as treatment efficacy, potential toxicity, and lifestyle and business consequences of the treatment and the underlying illness(es).

In silico toxicology systems are part of an exciting revolution that is changing the timing, economics, and success rate of the pharmaceutical industry and improving the development and availability of safe new foods, agricultural products, and other promising substances that can greatly benefit humanity.

REFERENCES

1. ZIPKIN, I. 1998 (October 5). Entelos: simulating disease. BioCentury.
2. STRAUSS, E. 1998. New ways to probe the molecules of life. Science **282:** 1406–1407.
3. KOO, M. 1999. E-R&D in a virtual lab. Helix **1**(no. 4): 18–20.
4. THIEL, K. 1999 (November 4). Virtual drug development: start-ups put biology in motion. Biospace feature (www.biospace.com).
5. WELLS, W. 2000 (February). Virtual cures, chemistry, and biology. See www.biomednet.com/hmsbeagle.
6. STOKES, C.L. 2000. Biological systems modeling: powerful discipline for biomedicine. AIChE J. **46**(issue 3): 430–433.
7. HOLTZMAN, S. 1989. Intelligent Decision Systems. Addison–Wesley. Reading, MA.
8. HOLTZMAN, S. et al. 1999. Decision analysis and Alzheimer disease: three case studies. Genet. Testing **3**(no. 1).

Toxicity Testing: The FDA Perspective

JANE E. HENNEY[a]

Food and Drug Administration, Rockville, Maryland, USA

It is abundantly evident that modern science and technology are providing new breakthrough products every day. These new developments present opportunities and challenges for a science-based regulatory agency like the Food and Drug Administration (FDA) that must be continually met with the greatest scientific expertise, cutting-edge knowledge, and an open mind.

As is well known, toxicity test results are a pivotal part of the decision process at the FDA. In this paper, I would like to focus my remarks on two areas regarding toxicity testing: (i) looking back on how we have progressed in this area and (ii) looking ahead—where we believe that we will need to be positioned to meet the needs and challenges of the future.

First, reflections and musing about the past and present. Unfortunately, where we thought we would be 15 years ago and where we are today are two very different things. Why is that? For one thing, the underlying science is much more complex than we had anticipated 15 years ago. The 1970s were a time of unbounded excitement—new methods of detecting genotoxic carcinogens had been promising, Our enthusiasm diminished when we realized in subsequent years that there are many mechanisms by which chemicals cause cancer. Carcinogens seen by the agency today are, for the most part, not genotoxic, but cause cancer by some other mechanism. Because of the diversity of "secondary" mechanisms of cancer and remaining unanswered questions about relevance to humans, these chemicals pose a larger challenge today than genotoxic carcinogens did in the past.

Another reason why we are not as far along as we originally thought is that some forms of toxicity have been refractory to better understanding. Interpretation of the results of reproductive and developmental toxicity tests is still largely an empirical process. Despite decades of research, mechanistic understanding of the causes of birth defects is limited to a very small number of chemicals and, even then, our understanding is at best incomplete.

Another factor that must be taken into consideration when reflecting on where we are today is that the number of issues and questions that warrant further testing or research increases continuously as we better understand toxicity in animals and humans. Such new concerns include the potential of chemicals to adversely affect children and the potential of chemicals to cause harm because of endocrine disrupter activity. Thus, instead of depending on a few standard tests, protocols have become more complicated and interpretation of the data has increased in complexity.

---

[a]Address for correspondence: Jane E. Henney, Commissioner of Food and Drugs, Food and Drug Administration, 5600 Fishers Lane, Room 14-71, Rockville, MD 20857. Voice: 301-827-2410; fax: 301-443-3100.

As a result, understanding of the mechanistic basis of chemical-induced toxicities has been slow to unravel. During past years, we hoped, believed, and maybe even prayed that mechanism-based toxicology tests would be the answer.

Unfortunately, we failed to understand the diversity of mechanisms by which chemicals cause damage to cells. Now that we have a clearer understanding of the diversity, it is evident that it would take hundreds of mechanism-based tests to predict the toxicity of chemicals previously untested if screened mechanism by mechanism, endpoint by endpoint—an approach that is neither pragmatic or practical.

Therefore, while the profile of data to support regulatory decisions is more comprehensive today than in years past, mechanistic understanding has been slow to accumulate. Thus, the expectation of a few years ago that tests would be faster, better, and cheaper has not been realized.

Even in the wake of these realities, I believe that we have every reason to be optimistic about the future. The application of knowledge gained from understanding of the genome of animals and humans will, without a doubt, aid our efforts exponentially. There may be a time in the not too distant future when DNA chip technology and other high-throughput systems will enable us to do short-term studies and predict outcomes based on effects on DNA, gene expression products, or protein synthesis. As we better understand the genome, we should be able to construct animal models that more closely resemble healthy and diseased humans.

How rapidly the science unfolds and evolves will determine much of what we are able to do and how we will be able to do it. Some of the many questions that we, as a regulatory agency, will need to ask and consider are as follows: Can data derived from areas such as gene expression and proteomics be used to support decisions about safety and efficacy of a product? How will we validate this information and what information will be sufficient to replace the old studies? What would we ask for in lieu of other data? Also, very importantly, is the FDA ready to receive these other data?

There are two underlying problems behind this series of questions: (i) our ability to generate more data than we know how to interpret and (ii) the fact that the sheer volume of data available will be potentially overwhelming. Let me expand on both of these challenges. Regarding the first problem, new technology will allow us to determine if thousands of genes are upregulated, downregulated, or unaffected by exposure to a chemical. The impact of such changes will be understood for some genes, but not for others. Simultaneous or sequential changes in large numbers of genes are more likely to be important than changes in a single gene. As with more traditional endpoints of toxicology, the temporal and dose-response aspects will be important, as well as the impact of repeated exposure versus single exposure to chemicals. The questions about species-specific responses and extrapolation from laboratory animals to humans will still exist. The data derived from new high-throughput technologies will eventually allow us to determine subtle changes in homeostasis that are predictive of toxicity in whole animal models, but we are not there yet today.

Now the second problem—the volume of data. As presented by contributors to these proceedings, the area of bioinformatics is essential for development of strategies and systems for handling large volumes of information, including the systems to integrate and model data to facilitate interpretation of data for decisions. Thus, improvements in toxicology testing through the use of totally new technologies will depend on convergence of several different developments over the same time course: better understanding of the biology that underlies the new molecular-level data to permit its use in predicting toxicity; validation of the new test methodologies to permit their use for regulatory decisions; and development and application of bioinformatics technology to permit effective use of the large volume of data that will be derived from high-throughput technologies.

Let me now address a critical question—what is the FDA doing to make itself prepared for this new era? Since my confirmation as commissioner, I have stressed the importance of having a strong, science-based regulatory agency. We cannot afford to not have the best science underpinning all of our decisions. Often, when I mention this issue, a "scientist" in a lab coat doing bench research comes to mind. However, my vision of where the agency should be headed goes far beyond that. From the researcher in our food labs to the reviewer in our drug divisions, from the inspectors out in the field to any employee articulating a new policy, all decisions should be based on the most recent scientific developments and knowledge. A certain confidence comes from knowing that the correct decision has been made because it was grounded in scientific data.

Within the past year, we have awarded new research and risk assessment grants, particularly in the food safety area, and established new procedures to better plan and coordinate research among federal partners. We have also funded seven cooperative agreements totaling $1 million, including ones with Washington State University, New England Medical Center, the University of Georgia, and the University of Wisconsin, to study the microbiological hazards associated with the food animal production environment, which includes animal feeds.

One example of the type of collaborative work that we are doing at our National Center for Toxicological Research (NCTR) involves cancer bioassays on chemicals of considerable public health concern such as fumonisin B1, a mycotoxin found in corn and corn-based food products. In addition to FDA scientists, these studies involved collaborators from the National Institute of Environmental Health Sciences and the U.S. Department of Agriculture. The research agenda included basic and applied research studies designed to facilitate the interpretation of the 2-year bioassays. These results, along with data from other studies and other laboratories within and outside of the FDA, will now form the basis for setting standards for exposure based on risk assessments. These studies are an excellent example of FDA scientists working with experts from several different sectors to protect the health of the public.

Other studies being done include evaluations of the carcinogenicity of chloral hydrate, primarily because of its use as a sedative in children; malachite green because of its use as an antifungal agent in the aquaculture industry; and the combination of ethanol and urethane because of the presence of small amounts of urethane in alcoholic beverages. Several compounds with hormonal properties, including genistein, nonylphenol, and ethinyl estradiol, are being evaluated for adverse reproductive effects and other toxicities over multiple generations as part of a larger study of endocrine disrupters.

Through the use of these types of agreements and collaborations with scientists outside of the FDA, we are effectively leveraging the resources and expertise of other outside entities. This not only enables our limited resources to go further, but also harnesses a greater breadth of experience within the scientific community. By working in cooperation with those outside the agency, we are able to attain a wide range of perspectives, while still being able to have all of our decisions grounded in good science.

One last area that needs to be touched upon involves how we lure the top scientists in the country to our agency—and keep them with us. It is critical that we invest wisely in those that we recruit and retain for these tasks that are so fundamental to effective protection of the public health. Since I have come back to the agency, I have been constantly searching for new opportunities for our scientific staff. This includes measures such as ensuring that more training opportunities and fellowships, as well as participation in research grants and cooperative agreements, are available to our employees.

Training and retraining of our scientists to have state-of-the-art knowledge of new scientific developments and new product technology are essential for us to remain a credible, science-based agency. Through use of our own facilities, such as NCTR, and by reaching out to institutions outside the FDA, our regulatory scientists need to go on sabbaticals to other federal research agencies, academia, and (given the right circumstances) industry, where they spend time shoulder to shoulder with laboratory scientists. The enhancement of the science base at the agency depends upon our ability to keep up with knowledge that is state of the art, including areas of new product technology and new science. By having these kinds of educational opportunities open to our scientists, we ultimately enable them to bring back to the agency deeper knowledge that translates into better and more efficient performance of regulatory tasks.

By enhancing our scientific infrastructure in the many ways that I have mentioned, we will bring the agency into the twenty-first century with the expertise we need to make science-based decisions. We must effectively provide the FDA with the tools that it needs to ensure that the agency is equipped to understand and access new breakthrough technology as it emerges. I am steadfastly committed to achieving this. However, it will take our working together, sharing information, and building collaborative partnerships to ensure that we will be as ready as possible for the challenges of tomorrow.

While development in the area of toxicity testing has not always gone according to plan, I am confident that we will be facing a future filled with great promise.

ACKNOWLEDGMENT

This paper was presented by Bernard A. Schwetz (Acting Deputy Commissioner and Senior Advisor for Science, FDA) at the conference.

p53 Tumor Suppressor Gene

At the Crossroads of Molecular Carcinogenesis, Molecular Epidemiology, and Human Risk Assessment

S. PERWEZ HUSSAIN,[a] MONICA H. HOLLSTEIN,[b] AND CURTIS C. HARRIS[a,c]

[a]*Laboratory of Human Carcinogenesis, National Cancer Institute, Bethesda, Maryland 20892, USA*

[b]*Division of Toxicology, German Cancer Research Center, D-69120 Heidelberg, Germany*

ABSTRACT: The molecular archaeology of the mutation spectra of tumor suppressor genes generates hypotheses concerning the etiology and molecular pathogenesis of human cancer. The spectrum of somatic mutations in the p53 gene implicates environmental carcinogens and both endogenous agents and processes in the etiology of human cancer.

Environmental, occupational, and recreational exposures to carcinogens contribute to cancer risk in humans. Cancer formation is a multistage process involving the activation of proto-oncogenes and the inactivation of tumor suppressor genes (see FIGURE 1).[1] Carcinogens can affect any of these stages through genetic and epigenetic mechanisms.

MOLECULAR ARCHAEOLOGY OF CANCER-RELATED GENES

Mutational spectra of cancer-related genes, for example, p53, ATM, and p16^{INK4}, may provide a molecular link between etiological agents and human cancer. Mutations in the evolutionarily conserved codons of the p53 tumor suppressor gene are common in diverse types of human cancer,[2–5] and the p53 mutational spectrum differs among cancers of the colon, lung, esophagus, breast, liver, brain, reticuloendothelial tissues, and hemopoietic tissues. Analysis of these mutations can provide clues to the mutagenic mechanisms and the function of specific regions of p53, and can generate hypotheses for investigation.[5] Most transversions in lung, breast, and esophageal carcinomas are dispersed among numerous evolutionarily conserved codons within the p53 domain responsible for sequence-specific DNA binding and transcriptional activity. Transitions predominate in colon, brain, and lymphoid ma-

---

[c]Corresponding author: Curtis C. Harris, Chief, Laboratory of Human Carcinogenesis, National Cancer Institute, NIH, Building 37, Room 2C01, 37 Convent Drive, MSC 4255, Bethesda, MD 20892-4255. Voice: 301-496-2048; fax: 301-496-0497.
Curtis_Harris@nih.gov

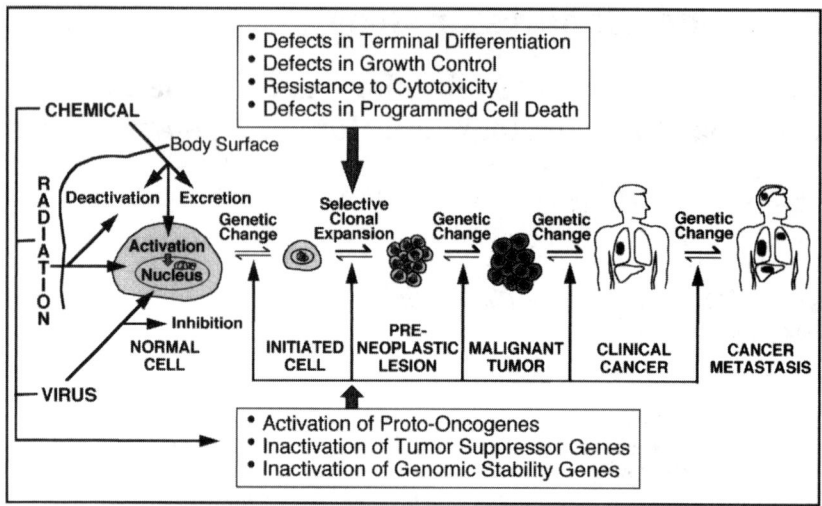

FIGURE 1. Molecular pathogenesis of human cancer.

lignancies. Mutational hot spots at CpG dinucleotides in codons 175, 248, 273, and 282 may reflect an endogenous mutagenic mechanism, for example, the deamination of 5-methylcytosine to thymidine. Oxyradicals may enhance the rate of deamination. For example, we have observed that (a) an increased production of nitric oxide (NO) by nitric oxide synthase-2 (NOS2) is associated with p53 C to T transitions during colon carcinogenesis;[6] (b) p53 transrepresses basal and cytokine-induced NOS2 expression *in vitro*[7] and *in vivo*;[8] and (c) NO increases the expression of the vascular endothelial growth factor, angiogenesis, and tumor growth.[9] p53 G:C to T:A transversions are the most frequent substitutions observed in cancers of the lung and liver, and are more likely to be due to bulky carcinogen-DNA adducts. G:C to T:A transversions also are more common in lung cancers from smokers when compared with never-smokers[5,10] and more frequent in lung cancers from women when compared with men.[11] The high frequency of G:C to T:A p53 transversions in the nontranscribed DNA strand is a reflection of strand-specific repair.[12] p53 also may contribute to DNA repair and apoptosis by protein-protein interactions with the transcription-repair factors, XPB and XPD, in TFIIH.[13–15] p53 mutation, allelic deletions, and/or posttranslationally modified protein can be early events in bronchial, mammary, or esophageal carcinogenesis[16–22] and may prove useful in the early diagnosis of cancer.

In liver tumors from persons living in geographic areas where aflatoxin B_1 and hepatitis B virus (HBV) are cancer-risk factors, most p53 mutations are at the third nucleotide pair of codon 249 (TABLE 1).[23–27] A dose-dependent relationship between dietary aflatoxin B_1 intake and codon 249^{ser} p53 mutations is observed in hepatocellular carcinoma. Exposure of aflatoxin B_1 to human liver cells *in vitro* produces 249^{ser} (AGG to AGT) p53 mutants.[28,29] The mutation load of 249^{ser} mutant cells in nontumorous liver also is positively correlated with dietary aflatoxin B_1 exposure.[30]

TABLE 1. Hypothesis: Dietary aflatoxin B_1 exposure can cause 249^{ser} (AGG→AGT) p53 mutations during human liver carcinogenesis—assessment of causation by the Bradford-Hill criteria[5,57]

- Strength of Association
  - Consistency
    - Positive dose-response correlation between estimated dietary aflatoxin B_1 exposure and frequency of 249^{ser} p53 mutations in three different ethnic populations on three continents
  - Specificity
    - 249^{ser} p53 mutant cells are observed in nontumorous liver in high HCC incidence geographic areas
- Biological Plausibility
  - AFB_1 is a potent mutagen and carcinogen in laboratory studies
  - AFB_1 is enzymatically activated by human hepatocytes, and the 8,9-AFB_1 oxide binds to the third base (G) in codon 249
  - AFB_1 exposure to human liver cells *in vitro* produces codon 249^{ser} p53 mutations
  - 249^{ser} p53 expression inhibits apoptosis and p53-mediated transcription, and enhances liver cell growth *in vitro*

These results indicate that the expression of the 249^{ser} mutant p53 protein provides a specific growth and/or survival advantage to liver cells. Because cellular context may influence the pathobiological effects of specific mutants of p53, the 249^{ser} mutant may be especially potent in hepatocytes due to the enhanced growth rate of p53-null HEP-3B cells by transfected 249^{ser} mutant p53, indicating a gain of oncogenic function.[31] The 249^{ser} mutant p53 is more effective than other p53 mutants (143^{ala}, 175^{his}, 248^{trp}, and 282^{his}) in inhibiting wild-type p53 transcriptional activity in human liver cells.[32] An alternative model is that rare, oxyradical-induced heterozygotic codon 249^{ser} p53 mutant hepatocytes are highly sensitive to the genotoxicity of aflatoxin B_1 that either leads to loss of the wild-type p53 allele or mutates other cancer-related genes.

HBV also has important pathobiological effects. For example, the HBVX gene is frequently integrated and expressed in human hepatocellular carcinomas from high-risk geographic areas.[33,34] Hepatitis B viral gene products may form complexes with cellular transcription factors (e.g., ATF2),[35] upregulate transcription of cellular and viral genes[36-40] (including NOS2[41]), or activate the ras-raf-MAP kinase signaling cascade.[42] The inactivation of the p53 tumor suppressor gene functions, including DNA repair and apoptosis, may be another consequence of the cellular protein–HBV oncoprotein complex formation. The HBVX protein binds to p53,[13,43,44] sequesters it in the cytoplasm,[41] and inhibits its sequence-specific DNA binding and transcriptional activity.[13] The HBVX protein also inhibits p53-dependent apoptosis.[45] In nucleotide excision DNA repair, the HBVX protein may modulate p53 function,[14,46] including the repair of AFB_1-DNA adducts. HBV integration also could increase genomic instability, including abnormal chromosomal segregation, and increase the rates of DNA recombination.[47,48]

TABLE 2. Hypothesis: Sunlight exposure can cause a characteristic CC to TT tandem double mutation in p53 in human skin cancer—assessment of causation by the Bradford-Hill criteria[5,57]

- Strength of Association
  - Consistency
    - Prevalence of CC to TT tandem double mutation in squamous and basal cell skin carcinoma
  - Specificity
    - Tandem dipyrimidine CC to TT mutations are uncommon in other types of cancer
  - Temporality
    - CC to TT mutations are found in normal and precancerous skin
- Biological Plausibility
  - UV is a mutagen and carcinogen in laboratory studies
  - Cyclobutane pyrimidine dimers and pyrimidine photoproducts are the two major DNA base modifications produced by UV irradiation and induce C to T, at non-CpG sites, and CC to TT mutations
  - Skin cancer in xeroderma pigmentosum patients, with defective nucleotide excision repair, contains a high frequency of CC to TT mutations
  - UV exposure produces CC to TT mutations in studies using phage, bacteria, and mice

Three other associations between the p53 mutational spectra and carcinogen exposure have been observed. The induction of skin carcinoma by ultraviolet light is indicated by the occurrence of p53 mutations at dipyrimidine sites, including CC to TT double-base changes (TABLE 2).[49,50] The p53 mutational spectrum in radon-associated lung cancer from uranium miners also differs from lung cancer caused by tobacco smoking alone.[16] Hepatic angiosarcoma induced by occupational exposure to vinyl chloride has a high frequency of A:T to T:A p53 mutations when compared with sporadic angiosarcoma[51] (unpublished results). In summary, these differences in mutational frequency and spectra among human cancer types indicate the following: (a) the etiological contributions of both exogenous and endogenous factors to human carcinogenesis; (b) specific proliferative effects conferred by different mutant p53 genes in different human cell types; and (c) hypotheses for investigation.[5] These genetic changes in the tumor suppressor genes also have implications for cancer diagnosis, prognosis, and therapy.[4,52]

MOLECULAR EPIDEMIOLOGY OF HUMAN CANCER RISK

The association of a suspected carcinogenic exposure and cancer risk can be studied in populations with classic epidemiologic techniques. However, these techniques are not applicable to the assessment of risk in individuals. A goal of molecular epidemiology is to integrate molecular biology, *in vitro* and *in vivo* laboratory models, biochemistry, and epidemiology to infer individual cancer risk.[1,53–56] Carcinogen-macromolecular adduct levels and somatic cell mutations can be measured to determine the biologically effective dose of a carcinogen. Molecular epidemiology also explores host cancer susceptibilities, such as carcinogen metabolic activation, DNA repair, endogenous mutation rates, and inheritance of mutated tumor suppressor genes. Substantial interindividual variation for each of these biologic endpoints has been shown[1] and, therefore, highlights the need for assessing cancer risk on an individual basis. Given the pace of the last decade, it is feasible that future advances will allow molecular epidemiologists to develop a cancer-risk profile for an individual that includes assessment of a number of exposure and host factors. This will help focus preventive strategies and strengthen quantitative risk assessments.

ACKNOWLEDGMENTS

We thank Dorothea Dudek for her editorial and graphic assistance.

REFERENCES

1. HARRIS, C.C. 1991. Chemical and physical carcinogenesis: advances and perspectives. Cancer Res. **51:** 5023s–5044s.
2. HOLLSTEIN, M., D. SIDRANSKY, B. VOGELSTEIN et al. 1991. p53 mutations in human cancers. Science **253:** 49–53.
3. GREENBLATT, M.S., W.P. BENNETT, M. HOLLSTEIN et al. 1994. Mutations in the p53 tumor suppressor gene: clues to cancer etiology and molecular pathogenesis. Cancer Res. **54:** 4855–4878.
4. HARRIS, C.C. 1996. Structure and function of the p53 tumor suppressor gene: clues for rational cancer therapeutic strategies. J. Natl. Cancer Inst. **88:** 1442–1455.
5. HUSSAIN, S.P. & C.C. HARRIS. 1998. Molecular epidemiology of human cancer: contribution of mutation spectra studies of tumor suppressor genes. Cancer Res. **58:** 4023–4037.
6. AMBS, S., W.P. BENNETT, W.G. MERRIAM et al. 1999. Characteristic p53 mutations correlate with inducible NO synthase expression in human colorectal cancer. J. Natl. Cancer Inst. **91:** 86–88.
7. FORRESTER, K., S. AMBS, S.E. LUPOLD et al. 1996. Nitric oxide–induced p53 accumulation and regulation of inducible nitric oxide synthase (NOS2) expression by wild-type p53. Proc. Natl. Acad. Sci. U.S.A. **93:** 2442–2447.
8. AMBS, S., M.O. OGUNFUSIKA, W.G. MERRIAM et al. 1998. Upregulation of NOS2 expression in cancer-prone p53 knockout mice. Proc. Natl. Acad. Sci. U.S.A. **95:** 8823–8828.
9. AMBS, S., W.G. MERRIAM, M.O. OGUNFUSIKA et al. 1998. p53 and vascular endothelial growth factor regulate tumour growth of NOS2-expressing human carcinoma cells. Nat. Med. **4:** 1371–1376.
10. TAKESHIMA, Y., T. SEYAMA, W.P. BENNETT et al. 1993. p53 mutations in lung cancers from non-smoking atomic-bomb survivors. Lancet **342:** 1520–1521.
11. GUINEE, D.G., W.D. TRAVIS, G.E. TRIVERS et al. 1995. Gender comparisons in human lung cancer: analysis of p53 mutations, anti-p53 serum antibodies, and C-erbB-2 expression. Carcinogenesis **16:** 993–1002.
12. EVANS, M.K., B.G. TAFFE, C.C. HARRIS et al. 1993. DNA strand bias in the repair of the p53 gene in normal human and xeroderma pigmentosum group C fibroblasts. Cancer Res. **53:** 5377–5381.
13. WANG, X.W., K. FORRESTER, H. YEH et al. 1994. Hepatitis B virus X protein inhibits p53 sequence-specific DNA binding, transcriptional activity, and association with transcription factor ERCC3. Proc. Natl. Acad. Sci. U.S.A. **91:** 2230–2234.
14. WANG, X.W., H. YEH, L. SCHAEFFER et al. 1995. p53 modulation of TFIIH-associated nucleotide excision repair activity. Nat. Genet. **10:** 188–195.

15. WANG, X.W., W. VERMEULEN, J.D. COURSEN *et al.* 1996. The XPB and XPD helicases are components of the p53-mediated apoptosis pathway. Genes Dev. **10:** 1219–1232.
16. VAHAKANGAS, K.H., J.M. SAMET, R.A. METCALF *et al.* 1992. Mutations of p53 and ras genes in radon-associated lung cancer from uranium miners. Lancet **339:** 576–580.
17. BENNETT, W.P., M.C. HOLLSTEIN, R.A. METCALF *et al.* 1992. p53 mutation and protein accumulation during multistage human esophageal carcinogenesis. Cancer Res. **52:** 6092–6097.
18. BARTEK, J., J. BARTKOVA, B. VOJTESEK *et al.* 1990. Patterns of expression of the p53 tumour suppressor in human breast tissues and tumours *in situ* and *in vitro*. Int. J. Cancer **46:** 839–844.
19. DAVIDOFF, A.M., P.A. HUMPHREY, J.D. IGLEHART *et al.* 1991. Genetic basis for p53 overexpression in human breast cancer. Proc. Natl. Acad. Sci. U.S.A. **88:** 5006–5010.
20. SUNDARESAN, V., P. GANLY, P. HASLETON *et al.* 1992. p53 and chromosome 3 abnormalities, characteristic of malignant lung tumours, are detectable in preinvasive lesions of the bronchus. Oncogene **7:** 1989–1997.
21. NUORVA, K., Y. SOINI, D. KAMEL *et al.* 1993. Concurrent p53 expression in bronchial dysplasias and squamous cell lung carcinomas. Am. J. Pathol. **142:** 725–732.
22. SOZZI, G., M. MIOZZO, R. DONGHI *et al.* 1992. Deletions of 17p and p53 mutations in preneoplastic lesions of the lung. Cancer Res. **52:** 6079–6082.
23. HSU, I.C., R.A. METCALF, T. SUN *et al.* 1991. Mutational hot spot in the p53 gene in human hepatocellular carcinomas. Nature **350:** 427–428.
24. BRESSAC, B., M. KEW, J. WANDS *et al.* 1991. Selective G to T mutations of p53 gene in hepatocellular carcinoma from southern Africa. Nature **350:** 429–431.
25. SCORSONE, K.A., Y.Z. ZHOU, J.S. BUTEL *et al.* 1992. p53 mutations cluster at codon 249 in hepatitis B virus–positive hepatocellular carcinomas from China. Cancer Res. **52:** 1635–1638.
26. LI, D., Y. CAO, L. HE *et al.* 1993. Aberrations of p53 gene in human hepatocellular carcinoma from China. Carcinogenesis **14:** 169–173.
27. SOINI, Y., S.C. CHIA, W.P. BENNETT *et al.* 1996. An aflatoxin-associated mutational hot spot at codon 249 in the p53 tumor suppressor gene occurs in hepatocellular carcinomas from Mexico. Carcinogenesis **17:** 1007–1012.
28. AGUILAR, F., S.P. HUSSAIN & P. CERUTTI. 1993. Aflatoxin B1 induces the transversion of G→T in codon 249 of the p53 tumor suppressor gene in human hepatocytes. Proc. Natl. Acad. Sci. U.S.A. **90:** 8586–8590.
29. MACE, K., F. AGUILAR, J.S. WANG *et al.* 1997. Aflatoxin B1 induced DNA adduct formation and p53 mutations in CYP450-expressing human liver cell lines. Carcinogenesis **18:** 1291–1297.
30. AGUILAR, F., C.C. HARRIS, T. SUN *et al.* 1994. Geographic variation of p53 mutational profile in nonmalignant human liver. Science **264:** 1317–1319.
31. PONCHEL, F., A. PUISIEUX, E. TABONE *et al.* 1994. Hepatocarcinoma-specific mutant p53-249ser induces mitotic activity, but has no effect on transforming growth factor beta 1–mediated apoptosis. Cancer Res. **54:** 2064–2068.
32. FORRESTER, K., S.E. LUPOLD, V.L. OTT *et al.* 1995. Effects of p53 mutants on wild-type p53-mediated transactivation are cell type dependent. Oncogene **10:** 2103–2111.
33. UNSAL, H., C. YAKICIER, C. MARCAIS *et al.* 1994. Genetic heterogeneity of hepatocellular carcinoma. Proc. Natl. Acad. Sci. U.S.A. **91:** 822–826.
34. PATERLINI, P., K. POUSSIN, M. KEW *et al.* 1995. Selective accumulation of the X transcript of hepatitis B virus in patients negative for hepatitis B surface antigen with hepatocellular carcinoma. Hepatology **21:** 313–321.
35. MAGUIRE, H.F., J.P. HOEFFLER & A. SIDDIQUI. 1991. HBV X protein alters the DNA binding specificity of CREB and ATF-2 by protein-protein interactions. Science **252:** 842–844.
36. SHIRAKATA, Y., M. KAWADA, Y. FUJIKI *et al.* 1989. The X gene of hepatitis B virus induced growth stimulation and tumorigenic transformation of mouse NIH3T3 cells. Jpn. J. Cancer Res. **80:** 617–621.
37. KEKULË, A.S., U. LAUER, M. MEYER *et al.* 1990. The preS2/S region of integrated hepatitis B virus DNA encodes a transcriptional transactivator. Nature **343:** 457–461.

38. TWU, J.S. & R.H. SCHLOEMER. 1987. Transcriptional trans-activating function of hepatitis B virus. J. Virol. **61:** 3448–3453.
39. SPANDAU, D.F. & C.H. LEE. 1988. Trans-activation of viral enhancers by the hepatitis B virus X protein. J. Virol. **62:** 427–434.
40. CASELMANN, W.H., M. MEYER, A.S. KEKULË et al. 1990. A trans-activator function is generated by integration of hepatitis B virus preS/S sequences in human hepatocellular carcinoma DNA. Proc. Natl. Acad. Sci. U.S.A. **87:** 2970–2974.
41. ELMORE, L.W., A.R. HANCOCK, S.F. CHANG et al. 1997. Hepatitis B virus X protein and p53 tumor suppressor interactions in the modulation of apoptosis. Proc. Natl. Acad. Sci. U.S.A. **94:** 14707–14712.
42. BENN, J. & R.J. SCHNEIDER. 1994. Hepatitis B virus HBx protein activates Ras-GTP complex formation and establishes a Ras, Raf, MAP kinase signaling cascade. Proc. Natl. Acad. Sci. U.S.A. **91:** 10350–10354.
43. PIRISI, L., S. YASUMOTO, M. FELLER et al. 1987. Transformation of human fibroblasts and keratinocytes with human papillomavirus type 16 DNA. J. Virol. **61:** 1061–1066.
44. UEDA, H., S.J. ULLRICH, J.D. GANGEMI et al. 1995. Functional inactivation, but not structural mutation of p53 causes liver cancer. Nat. Genet. **9:** 41–47.
45. WANG, X.W., M.K. GIBSON, W. VERMEULEN et al. 1995. Abrogation of p53-induced apoptosis by the hepatitis B virus X gene. Cancer Res. **55:** 6012–6016.
46. JIA, L., X.W. WANG & C.C. HARRIS. 1999. Hepatitis B virus X protein inhibits nucleotide excision repair. Int. J. Cancer **80:** 875–879.
47. HINO, O., K. NOMURA, K. OHTAKE et al. 1989. Instability of integrated hepatitis B virus DNA with inverted repeat structure in a transgenic mouse. Cancer Genet. Cytogenet. **37:** 273–278.
48. HINO, O., S. TABATA & Y. HOTTA. 1991. Evidence for increased *in vitro* recombination with insertion of human hepatitis B virus DNA. Proc. Natl. Acad. Sci. U.S.A. **88:** 9248–9252.
49. BRASH, D.E., J.A. RUDOLPH, J.A. SIMON et al. 1991. A role for sunlight in skin cancer: UV-induced p53 mutations in squamous cell carcinoma. Proc. Natl. Acad. Sci. U.S.A. **88:** 10124–10128.
50. ZIEGLER, A., A.S. JONASON, D.J. LEFFELL et al. 1994. Sunburn and p53 in the onset of skin cancer. Nature **372:** 773–776.
51. HOLLSTEIN, M., M.J. MARION, T. LEHMAN et al. 1994. p53 mutations at A:T base pairs in angiosarcomas of vinyl chloride–exposed factory workers. Carcinogenesis **15:** 1–3.
52. HARRIS, C.C. & M. HOLLSTEIN. 1993. Clinical implications of the p53 tumor-suppressor gene. N. Engl. J. Med. **329:** 1318–1327.
53. SHIELDS, P.G. & C.C. HARRIS. 1991. Molecular epidemiology and the genetics of environmental cancer. JAMA **266:** 681–687.
54. PERERA, F.P. & R. SANTELLA. 1993. Carcinogenesis. *In* Molecular Epidemiology: Principles and Practices, pp. 277–300. Academic Press. New York.
55. PERERA, F.P. 1997. Environment and cancer: who are susceptible? Science **278:** 1068–1073.
56. PONDER, B. 1997. Genetic testing for cancer risk. Science **278:** 1050–1054.
57. HILL, A.B. 1965. The environment and disease: association or causation. Proc. R. Soc. Med. **58:** 295–300.

Mechanisms of Cell Transformation in the Syrian Hamster Embryo (SHE) Cell Transformation System

ROBERT J. ISFORT[a]

Research Division, Procter & Gamble Pharmaceuticals, Cincinnati, Ohio, USA

ABSTRACT: The Syrian hamster embryo (SHE) cell transformation system has been used for investigational studies of basic mechanisms of neoplastic transformation, as well as determining the carcinogenic potential of chemical, physical, and biological agents. Many of these investigations utilize an intermediate step in the SHE cell neoplastic transformation process, known as morphological transformation, as an indicator that the cells have acquired an increased potential to progress to malignancy. While the nature of the morphologically transformed phenotype is not completely understood, it is believed to result from a block in the cellular differentiation of stem cells present within the SHE cell population. In terms of determination of the transforming potential of biological/chemical/physical agents, more than 500 agents have been tested in the SHE cell transformation assay with an 80–90% correlation between MT and carcinogenic potential. As such, the SHE cell transformation assay has utility as a test to provide short-term information on the carcinogenic potential of chemicals. One class of agents of current interest with regard to SHE cell transformation assay utilization consists of growth and differentiation factors (GDFs). Analysis of the SHE cell transformation potential of the GDFs, epidermal growth factor (EGF), fibroblast growth factor 4 (FGF-4), platelet-derived growth factor AA (PDGF AA), PDGF AB, PDGF BB, and the antimitogenic GDF, transforming growth factor beta one (TGF-β1), was performed. All GDFs, with the exception of TGF-β1, induced SHE cell transformation. However, an interesting difference between the GDFs was observed—PDGF A/B and PDGF B/B, but not PDGF A/A, EGF, or FGF-4, induced transformation after both a transient 1-day exposure and a continuous 7-day exposure, while continuous 7-day exposure was required for transformation by PDGF A/A, EGF, and FGF-4. Interestingly, both transient 1-day and continuous 7-day TGF-β1 exposure resulted in suppression of transformation induced by a variety of transforming agents including growth factors, Ames assay–positive carcinogens, Ames assay–negative carcinogens, and spontaneous transformation. Interestingly TGF-β1 was not able to suppress transformation by the tumor promoter, TPA. Together, these data demonstrate the utility of the Syrian hamster embryo cell transformation system for analyzing the transforming potential of GDFs and for characterizing differences in transforming mechanisms between different GDFs.

[a]Address for correspondence: Research Division, Procter & Gamble Pharmaceuticals, Health Care Research Center, 8700 Mason-Montgomery Road, Mason, OH 45040-9317. Voice: 513-622-2899; fax: 513-622-1195.
isfortrj@pg.com

INTRODUCTION

The Syrian hamster embryo (SHE) cell transformation system has been useful for investigational studies of basic mechanisms of neoplastic transformation, as well as determining the carcinogenic potential of chemical, physical, and biological agents.[1-6] Many of these investigations utilize an intermediate step in the SHE cell neoplastic transformation process, known as morphological transformation, as an indicator that the cells have acquired an increased potential to progress to malignancy.[1,4] While the nature of the morphologically transformed phenotype is not completely understood, it is believed to result from a block in the cellular differentiation of stem cells, at multiple stages in the differentiation process with the potential to differentiate into epithelial and mesenchymal cells, present within the SHE cell population.[1,7-9] Analysis of agents that increase the number of MT colonies indicates that carcinogenic agents can induce MT by either a transient (24-hour) or continuous (7-day) exposure to the transforming agent.[10-12] For example, genotoxic carcinogens, which are believed to act by mutation of DNA, induce MT following transient exposure, while tumor promoters, which act through a variety of mechanisms, require continuous exposure for MT induction.[10-12] In terms of determination of the transforming potential of biological/chemical/physical agents, more than 500 agents have been tested in the SHE cell transformation assay with an 80–90% correlation between MT and carcinogenic potential.[10] As such, the SHE cell transformation has utility as a test to provide short-term information on the carcinogenic potential of chemicals.

With the advent of the use of recombinant GDFs as therapeutic agents, analysis of the carcinogenic potential of GDFs is essential for the safe clinical use of these drugs. Currently, only long-term rodent bioassays are being utilized for the tumorigenic assessment of GDFs. A short-term reliable assay would greatly aid in the carcinogenic analysis of GDFs. Therefore, we have tested GDFs in the SHE cell transformation assay in order to determine their transforming potential.

MATERIALS AND METHODS

SHE Cell Transformation Assays

A comprehensive protocol for the conduct of the SHE cell transformation assay has been published.[12] Briefly, reconstituted SHE feeder cells were X ray–irradiated (5000 rad) and seeded into 60-mm culture dishes at a density of 4×10^4 cells/dish. Twenty-four hours later, reconstituted SHE target cells were seeded at a clonal density (80–100 cells/60-mm culture dish) onto the feeder cells. Following 24 hours of growth, target cells were treated with TGF-β1, EGF, FGF-4, PDGF AA, PDGF AB, PDGF BB (all from R&D Systems, Inc.), benzo[a]pyrene (B[a]P), lead acetate (PbAc), diethylhexylphthalate (DEHP), or 12-*O*-tetradecanoylphorbol-13-acetate (TPA) (all from Sigma) and then returned to incubation at 37°C and 10% CO_2 in 90% humidified air for 7 days of clonal growth (continuous exposure protocol). For the 24-hour exposure phenotype stability SHE cell transformation assay, test agents were removed at 24 hours after dosing and the cultures were refed with culture medium, lacking the test materials. At the end of the 7-day clonal growth period, SHE colonies were fixed with methanol, stained with Giemsa, and examined for morphological transformation (MT). Growth factor MT data were tested pairwise with the solvent control MT for statistical significance. A test chemical is considered to be SHE assay–positive if it causes a statistically significant ($p < 0.05$) increase in MT relative to the solvent control in at least two dose groups, or it causes a statistically significant increase in MT in one dose with a statistically significant ($p < 0.05$) positive dose-response trend test. Test doses for the GDFs were chosen based upon the mitogenic assay so as to encompass several mitogenic doses and nonmitogenic doses to ensure full coverage of potential biological activity. Top dose was selected based on maximal mitogenic effect so that at least two doses were at full mitogenic activity. Importantly, all the GDFs tested in the SHE assay are present in fetal bovine serum at subnanogram/milliliter concentrations, that is, concentrations well below the ED_{50} needed for mitogenic and transformation activity in SHE cells.

Mitogenesis Analysis

Mitogenesis analysis of the GDFs was performed as previously described.[13] Briefly, 2000 cells were plated/well in a 96-well Falcon microtiter plate with 200 µL of 10% FBS/DMEM and allowed to sit down overnight. The cells were then serum-starved in 50 µL/well of serum-free DMEM for 8 hours followed by the addition of the growth and differentiation factor (GDF) of interest in 50 µL/well of serum-free DMEM. Following an overnight incubation, 10 µL/well of 2 Ci/mmol [3H]-thymidine (Amersham) was added; the cells were incubated for an additional 6 hours, after which the cells were harvested; and the amount of incorporated [3H]-thymidine was quantitated by scintillation counting. All mitogenesis assays were performed in triplicate with an SEM < 3% for any specific experimental set of three assays. A positive mitogenic response is defined as a mitogen-induced [3H]-thymidine incorporation response that is 1.5 times the background [3H]-thymidine incorporation rate. Inhibition of mitogenesis is the [3H]-thymidine incorporation response, which is 0.7 times the background rate.

RESULTS

SHE Cell Transformation with GDFs

The mitogenic effects of the six GDFs—EGF, FGF-4, PDGF AA, PDGF AB, TGF-β1, and PDGF BB—on wild-type SHE cells are presented in TABLE 1. EGF, FGF-4, PDGF AA, PDGF AB, and PDGF BB were mitogenic for SHE cells in a dose-dependent manner, whereas TGF-β1 inhibited SHE cell mitogenesis in a dose-dependent manner. Importantly, the levels of the GDFs needed for either mitogenic stimulation or mitogenic inhibition in serum-free conditions (5–100 ng/mL) are greater than 50-fold above the levels of the GDFs present in 20% FBS, indicating that saturation of the GDF receptors by GDFs present in FBS has not occurred. From the above mitogenic data, doses for the SHE cell morphological transformation (MT) assay were selected, with the top dose selected being the maximal mitogenic stimulated dose, the bottom dose being a no-effect dose in the mitogenic assay, and the middle two doses selected to be evenly spaced between the bottom dose and the

TABLE 1. SHE cell mitogenic stimulation by GDFs

Growth factor	Fold stimulation over background
Media	1.0
10% FBS	9.5
0.01 ng/mL TGF-β1	0.8
0.1 ng/mL TGF-β1	0.7
1.0 ng/mL TGF-β1	0.7
10.0 ng/mL TGF-β1	0.6
0.05 ng/mL EGF	1.2
0.5 ng/mL EGF	2.6
5.0 ng/mL EGF	2.8
50.0 ng/mL EGF	2.3
0.035 ng/mL FGF-4	1.0
0.35 ng/mL FGF-4	1.7
3.5 ng/mL FGF-4	2.7
35.0 ng/mL FGF-4	2.1
0.05 ng/mL PDGF AA	0.8
0.5 ng/mL PDGF AA	1.1
5.0 ng/mL PDGF AA	0.9
50.0 ng/mL PDGF AA	2.1
0.05 ng/mL PDGF AB	0.8
0.5 ng/mL PDGF AB	1.0
5.0 ng/mL PDGF AB	1.3
50.0 ng/mL PDGF AB	2.3
0.05 ng/mL PDGF BB	0.8
0.5 ng/mL PDGF BB	1.2
5.0 ng/mL PDGF BB	1.7
50.0 ng/mL PDGF BB	2.2

top dose. The results of the SHE cell MT assays of the six GDFs tested are given in TABLE 2. TGF-β1, in a 7-day exposure SHE transformation assay, did not result in significant MT induction at any of the doses tested, although TGF-β1 did demonstrate a positive inverse dose versus MT response trend test result ($p = 0.0145$). Interestingly, TGF-β1 at the 1 and 10 ng/mL level suppressed the background MT frequency. In contrast, EGF induced a significant MT response with a positive trend test compared to controls in the 7-day exposure SHE cell transformation assay. Treatment of SHE cells with FGF-4 at the 3.5 and 35 ng/mL dose levels demonstrated a statistically significant induction of MT with a positive trend test compared to controls in the 7-day exposure SHE cell transformation assay. Finally, PDGF AB and BB at doses of 5 and 50 ng/mL and PDGF AA at a dose of 50 ng/mL resulted in a

TABLE 2. GDF SHE cell morphological transformation assay results

GDF exposure	Dose (ng/mL)	RPE (%)[a]	Number of MT[b]/ total colonies	MTF (%)[c]	Fisher's exact p value
TGF-β1					
24-hour	Control	100 (48)[d]	2/1746	0.12	0.1596[g]
	0.01	90	4/1564	0.26	0.2935
	0.1	75	2/1313	0.15	0.5747
	1.0	46	2/1728	0.12	0.6837
	10.0	34	0/1284	0.00	0.3320
7-day	Control	100 (38)[d]	5/1536	0.33	0.0145[f]
	0.01	93	5/1429	0.35	0.5781
	0.1	70	4/1067	0.38	0.5423
	1.0	66	0/1021	0.00	0.0780
	10.0	69	0/1054	0.00	0.0732
EGF					
24-hour	Control	100 (38)[d]	3/1340	0.22	0.0392[f]
	0.05	89	1/1222	0.08	0.3477
	0.5	92	4/1266	0.32	0.4689
	5.0	96	3/1321	0.23	0.6497
	50.0	101	8/1385	0.58	0.1238
7-day	Control	100 (38)[d]	5/1536	0.33	0.0042[f]
	0.05	99	7/1529	0.46	0.3839
	0.5	98	8/1501	0.53	0.2758
	5.0	103	24/1575	1.52	0.0003[e]
	50.0	96	10/1470	0.68	0.1310
FGF-4					
24-hour	Control	100 (47)[d]	2/1687	0.12	0.1140[g]
	0.035	89	0/1462	0.00	0.2869
	0.35	94	3/1581	0.19	0.4696
	3.5	97	5/1632	0.31	0.2129
	35.0	99	3/1676	0.18	0.4969
7-day	Control	100 (41)[d]	3/1491	0.20	0.0058[f]
	0.035	102	8/1482	0.54	0.1109
	0.35	102	9/1519	0.59	0.0772
	3.5	103	11/1534	0.72	0.0320[e]
	35.0	103	14/1531	0.91	0.0073[e]
PDGF AA					
24-hour	Control	100 (46)[d]	3/1658	0.18	0.3020[g]
	0.05	96	3/1594	0.19	0.6378
	0.5	100	4/1657	0.24	0.4997
	5.0	101	2/1682	0.12	0.4933
	50.0	102	2/1695	0.12	0.4896

—continued

TABLE 2. GDF SHE cell morphological transformation assay results

GDF exposure	Dose (ng/mL)	RPE (%)[a]	Number of MT[b]/ total colonies	MTF (%)[c]	Fisher's exact p value
7-day	Control	100 (46)[d]	4/1605	0.25	0.0007[f]
	0.05	96	2/1578	0.13	0.3517
	0.5	99	2/1623	0.12	0.3384
	5.0	93	2/1531	0.13	0.3660
	50.0	92	15/1510	0.99	0.0066[e]
PDGF AB					
24-hour	Control	100 (38)[d]	3/1340	0.22	0.0000[f]
	0.05	92	5/1270	0.39	0.3341
	0.5	86	8/1178	0.68	0.0765
	5.0	84	8/1151	0.70	0.0710
	50.0	84	22/1158	1.90	0.0000[e]
7-day	Control	100 (37)[d]	7/1476	0.47	0.0000[f]
	0.05	98	2/1446	0.14	0.0947
	0.5	88	8/1293	0.62	0.3970
	5.0	95	23/1403	1.64	0.0016[e]
	50.0	86	63/1270	4.96	0.0000[e]
PDGF BB					
24-hour	Control	100 (44)[d]	3/1589	0.19	0.0000[f]
	0.05	97	3/1535	0.20	0.6400
	0.5	100	5/1596	0.31	0.2655
	5.0	97	5/1532	0.33	0.3433
	50.0	97	20/1540	1.30	0.0002[e]
7-day	Control	100 (44)[d]	3/1589	0.19	0.0000[f]
	0.05	100	4/1593	0.25	0.5014
	0.5	92	5/1461	0.34	0.3182
	5.0	88	21/1389	1.51	0.0000[e]
	50.0	90	49/1434	3.42	0.0000[e]

[a]Relative plating efficiency (RPE) = (test group plating efficiency/solvent control plating efficiency) × 100.

[b]Morphologically transformed colony.

[c]Morphological transformation frequency (MTF) = (number of MT colonies/total number of colonies) × 100.

[d]Actual target cell plating efficiency in parentheses = (number of colonies per dish/number of cells seeded) × 100.

[e]MTF values are significantly greater than control MTF values at $p < 0.05$ as determined by Fisher's exact test.

[f]MTF values are trend test positive at $p < 0.05$ as determined by an unstratified binomial exact permutation trend test (Cytel Software).

[g]MTF values are *not* trend test positive at $p < 0.05$ as determined by an unstratified binomial exact permutation trend test (Cytel Software).

statistically significant increase in MT with a positive trend test compared to controls in the 7-day exposure SHE cell transformation assay.

To determine the stability of the GDF-induced transformed phenotypes, SHE cell transformation assays were performed employing the 24-hour exposure protocol. Neither EGF, FGF-4, nor PDGF AA resulted in significant MT in the 24-hour exposure SHE cell transformation assay. In contrast, the 24-hour exposure SHE cell transformation assay of PDGF AB and PDGF BB yielded significant MT ($p < 0.05$) at the 50 ng/mL dose level along with a positive dose versus MT response trend test ($p < 0.05$). A 24-hour exposure SHE cell transformation assay of TGF-β1 at the 10 ng/mL dose level resulted in the stable suppression of MT.

Inhibition of SHE Cell Transformation by TGF-β1

Experiments were performed designed to evaluate the TGF-β1-induced suppression of SHE cell transformation utilizing several different classes of transforming agents acting by different mechanisms. This entailed treating SHE cells with the following transforming agents—GDFs (PDGF AB and EGF), an Ames assay–positive genotoxic carcinogen (B[a]P), two Ames assay–negative carcinogens (PbAc and DEHP), and a tumor promoter (TPA)—and comparing transformation either with or without TGF-β1 present. The results presented in TABLE 3 demonstrate that TGF-β1 is able to significantly reduce SHE cell transformation induced by PDGF AB, EGF, B[a]P, PbAc, and DEHP. Transformation with PDGF AB was performed with multiple doses of TGF-β1 in the 7-day continuous and 24-hour intermittent dosing regimens in order to characterize the TGF-β1 dose-response curve and to investigate whether the reduction in transformation was a reversible effect. As can be seen in TABLE 3, TGF-β1 reduction of PDGF AB transformation was an irreversible effect and occurred at TGF-β1 doses higher than 0.1 ng/mL in the continuous (7-day) exposure SHE cell transformation assay and at TGF-β1 doses of 0.75 ng/mL and higher in the transient (24-hour) exposure SHE cell transformation assay. Significantly, TGF-β1 reduction of transformation in the 24-hour transient exposure SHE cell assay was observed at doses where toxicity was not observed. In contrast to the above agents, TGF-β1 was not able to significantly reduce transformation caused by TPA, even though the toxicity caused by exposure to TGF-β1 was not altered with the concomitant exposure to TPA.

DISCUSSION

The Syrian hamster embryo cell transformation assay has been utilized to evaluate the transformation potential of over 500 chemical, physical, and biological agents with an 80–90% correlation between morphological transformation and rodent tumorigenicity. One class of biological agents that has not been thoroughly evaluated in the SHE cell transformation assay consists of growth and differentiation factors (GDFs). We tested a variety of GDFs in the SHE cell transformation assay and demonstrated that multiple GDFs can induce morphological transformation in SHE cells and that PDGF AB and PDGF BB, but not EGF, FGF-4, and PDGF AA, are able to induce morphological transformation in SHE cells in an irreversible man-

TABLE 3. Morphological transformation of SHE cells by transforming agents PDGF AB, EGF, B[a]P, PbAc, TPA, and DEHP with and without added TGF-β1

Chemical	Dose (ng/mL)	RPE (%)[a]	Number of MT[b]/ total colonies	MTF (%)[c]	Fisher's exact p value control vs. test chem	Fisher's exact test chem vs. TGF-β1 + test chem
PDGF AB + TGF-β1						
24-hour						
50 ng/mL PDGF AB	Control	100 (45)[d]	2/810	0.25		
50 ng/mL PDGF AB + 0.1 ng/mL TGF-β1		96	9/776	1.16	0.0274[e]	
50 ng/mL PDGF AB + 0.25 ng/mL TGF-β1		76	4/612	0.65	0.2233	0.2474
50 ng/mL PDGF AB + 0.5 ng/mL TGF-β1		84	4/682	0.59	0.2667	0.1896
50 ng/mL PDGF AB + 0.75 ng/mL TGF-β1		70	4/570	0.70	0.1972	0.2898
50 ng/mL PDGF AB + 1.0 ng/mL TGF-β1		86	1/700	0.14	0.5546	0.0159[e]
		76	0/615	0.00	0.3229	0.0051[e]
7-day						
50 ng/mL PDGF AB	Control	100 (42)[d]	1/750	0.13		
50 ng/mL PDGF AB + 0.1 ng/mL TGF-β1		90	20/677	5.31	0.0000[e]	
50 ng/mL PDGF AB + 0.25 ng/mL TGF-β1		55	6/412	1.46	0.0095[e]	0.0831
50 ng/mL PDGF AB + 0.5 ng/mL TGF-β1		51	1/362	0.28	0.5453	0.0014[e]
50 ng/mL PDGF AB + 0.75 ng/mL TGF-β1		35	0/265	0.00	0.7389	0.0012[e]
50 ng/mL PDGF AB + 1.0 ng/mL TGF-β1		30	0/221	0.00	0.7724	0.0033[e]
		32	0/238	0.00	0.7591	0.0022[e]

—*continued*

[a]Relative plating efficiency (RPE) = (test group plating efficiency/solvent control plating efficiency) × 100.
[b]Morphologically transformed colony.
[c]Morphological transformation frequency (MTF) = (number of MT colonies/total number of colonies) × 100.
[d]Actual target cell plating efficiency in parentheses = (number of colonies per dish/number of cells seeded) × 100.
[e]MTF values are significantly greater than control MTF values at $p < 0.05$ as determined by Fisher's exact test.

TABLE 3. *Continued*

EGF + TGF-β1				
7-day	Control	100 (38)[d]	2/1360	0.15	
5.0 ng/mL EGF		98	10/1296	0.77	0.0155[e]
0.5 ng/mL TGF-β1		56	1/766	0.13	0.7042
5.0 ng/mL EGF + 0.25 ng/mL TGF-β1		62	0/846	0.00	0.3800	0.0065[e]
B[a]P + TGF-β1					
7-day	Control	100 (29)[d]	3/1172	0.26	
10.0 μg/mL B[a]P		87	17/1014	1.68	0.0004[e]
0.25 ng/mL TGF-β1		45	0/1054	0	
10.0 μg/mL B[a]P + 0.25 ng/mL TGF-β1		65	7/1518	0.46	0.2969	0.0021[e]
PbAc + TGF-β1					
7-day	Control	100 (29)[d]	3/1172	0.26	
50.0 μg/mL PbAc		89	35/1043	3.36	0.0000[e]
0.25 ng/mL TGF-β1		45	0/1054	0	
50.0 μg/mL PbAc + 0.25 ng/mL TGF-β1		64	10/1484	0.67	0.1033	0.0000[e]
TPA + TGF-β1					
7-day	Control	100 (26)[d]	1/1035	0.10	
1.0 μg/mL TPA		101	25/1047	2.39	0.0000[e]
0.25 ng/mL TGF-β1		53	0/1104	0	
1.0 μg/mL TPA + 0.25 ng/mL TGF-β1		53	21/1103	1.90	0.0000[e]	0.2657
DEHP + TGF-β1					
7-day control		100 (25)[d]	1/1400	0.07	
0.625 μg/mL DEHP		91	8/1240	0.65	0.0123[e]
0.25 ng/mL TGF-β1		46	0/1300	0	
0.625 μg/mL DEHP + 0.25 ng/mL TGF-β1		55	2/1509	0.13	0.5281	0.0276[e]

ner, while the mitogenic inhibitor TGF-β1 is able to suppress morphological transformation in an irreversible manner.

SHE cells, which are a mixture of cell types including progenitor and differentiated cells of mesenchymal and epithelial origin, respond mitogenically in the absence of fetal bovine serum to PDGF family members, EGF family members, and FGF family members and are mitogenically inhibited in the absence of fetal bovine serum by TGF-β family members. With regard to morphological transformation, treatment of SHE cells continuously for 7 days with the mitogens, EGF, FGF-4, and PDGF AA, resulted in statistically significant morphological transformation, although transient 24-hour exposure of SHE cells did not result in morphological transformation. These results demonstrate the need for continuous stimulation by these GDFs for maintenance of the morphologically transformed phenotype. We have observed this type of SHE cell transformation assay result (the need for continuous exposure to the transforming agent) with tumor promoters and agents that modulate mitogenic signal transduction pathways.[11] Others have demonstrated that EGF and FGF act in a tumor promoter–like manner *in vitro* and *in vivo*.[14–17] In contrast, treatment of SHE cells either continuously for 7 days or intermittently for 24 hours with the mitogens PDGF AB and PDGF BB resulted in statistically significant morphological transformation. We have observed this type of SHE cell transformation assay response (positive transformation with both intermittent and continuous treatment) with complete carcinogens.[11] Interestingly, the 7-day exposure SHE cell MT response at the 50 ng/mL PDGF AB and PDGF BB dose was ~2.5 times the 24-hour exposure SHE cell MT response at the 50 ng/mL PDGF AB and PDGF BB dose, indicating that additional target cells are transformed with continuous exposure and that a majority of these cells revert to normal upon removal of PDGF AB and PDGF BB. These data support a dual "initiator-like" and "promoter-like" role for PDGF AB and PDGF BB in comparison to the "promoter-like"-only effect observed with EGF, FGF-4, and PDGF AA. PDGF BB has been shown to modulate differentiation and enhance proliferation in a number of normal cell types, as well as function as a complete carcinogen when transduced by retroviruses as the v-sis oncogene.[17]

In contrast to the mitogens listed above, treatment of SHE cells, either continuously or intermittently with the antimitogenic agent, TGF-β1, resulted in an inhibition of the spontaneous transformation rate. In addition, TGF-β1 suppressed the morphological transformation induced by a variety of transforming agents including the GDFs, PDGF AB and EGF; the Ames assay–positive carcinogen, B[a]P; and the Ames assay–negative carcinogens, PbAc and DEHP. Interestingly, TGF-β1 did not suppress MT induced by the tumor promoter, TPA. The transformation inhibitory effect of TGF-β1 on SHE cells is not due to toxicity since inhibition of PDGF AB–induced MT in the transient transformation assay was observed without toxicity and TGF-β1 did not inhibit TPA-induced MT even though toxicity was observed. Finally, TGF-β1 could not completely suppress the morphological transforming ability of B[a]P, PbAc, and DEHP, but was able to completely suppress EGF, PDGF AB, and spontaneous morphological transformation. These data suggest that multiple morphological transformation pathways exist, including pathways that are sensitive to TGF-β-induced suppression and reversible and irreversible pathways.

REFERENCES

1. ISFORT, R.J. & R.A. LEBOEUF. 1996. The Syrian hamster embryo (SHE) cell transformation system: a biologically relevant *in vitro* model—with carcinogen predicting capabilities—of *in vivo* neoplastic transformation. Crit. Rev. Oncog. **6:** 251–260.
2. ISFORT, R.J. & R.A. LEBOEUF. 1996. Application of *in vitro* cell transformation assays to predict the carcinogenic potential of chemicals. Mutat. Res. **365:** 161–173.
3. BERWALD, Y. & L. SACHS. 1963. In vitro transformation with chemical carcinogens. Nature **200:** 1182–1184.
4. BARRETT, J.C. 1979. The progressive nature of neoplastic transformation of Syrian hamster embryo cells in culture. Prog. Exp. Tumor Res. **24:** 17–27.
5. BARRETT, J.C. *et al.* 1984. Use of cell transformation systems for carcinogenicity testing and mechanistic studies of carcinogenesis. Pharmacol. Rev. **36:** 53s–70s.
6. DIPAOLO, J.A. & B.C. CASTO. 1978. *In vitro* carcinogenesis with cells in early passage. Natl. Cancer Inst. Monogr. **48:** 245–257.
7. KERCKAERT, G.A. *et al.* 1996. pH effects on the lifespan and transformation frequency of Syrian hamster embryo (SHE) cells. Carcinogenesis **17:** 1819–1824.
8. ISFORT, R.J. *et al.* 1996. Isolation and biological characterization of morphological transformation-sensitive Syrian hamster embryo cells. Carcinogenesis **17:** 997–1005.
9. ISFORT, R.J. *et al.* 1997. Role of the H19 gene in Syrian hamster embryo cell tumorigenicity. Mol. Carcinog. **20:** 189–193.
10. ISFORT, R.J. *et al.* 1996. Comparison of the standard and reduced pH Syrian hamster embryo (SHE) cell *in vitro* transformation assays in predicting the carcinogenic potential of chemicals. Mutat. Res. **356:** 11–64.
11. LEBOEUF, R.A. *et al.* 1996. The pH 6.7 Syrian hamster embryo cell transformation assay for assessing the carcinogenic potential of chemicals. Mutat. Res. **356:** 85–127.
12. KERCKAERT, G.A. *et al.* 1996. A comprehensive protocol for conducting the Syrian hamster embryo cell transformation assay at pH 6.7. Mutat. Res. **356:** 65–84.
13. ISFORT, R.J. *et al.* 1994. Growth factor responsiveness and alterations in growth factor homeostasis in Syrian hamster embryo cells during *in vitro* transformation. Carcinogenesis **15:** 1203–1209.
14. STERN, D.F. *et al.* 1986. Differential responsiveness of myc- and ras-transfected cells to growth factors: selective stimulation of myc-transfected cells by EGF. Mol. Cell. Biol. **6:** 870–877.
15. GOSPODAROWICZ, D. *et al.* 1986. Fibroblast growth factor. Mol. Cell. Endocrinol. **46:** 187–204.
16. HUANG, S. *et al.* 1986. Transforming growth factor activity of bovine brain-derived growth factor. Biochem. Biophys. Res. Commun. **139:** 619–625.
17. SPORN, M.B. & A.B. ROBERTS. 1990. The multifunctional nature of peptide growth factors. *In* Peptide Growth Factors and Their Receptors, pp. 3–15. Springer-Verlag. New York/Berlin.

Neurochemical Effects of Environmental Chemicals

In Vitro and *In Vivo* Correlations on Second Messenger Pathways[a]

PRASADA RAO S. KODAVANTI[b] AND HUGH A. TILSON

Cellular and Molecular Toxicology Branch, Neurotoxicology Division, National Health and Environmental Effects Research Laboratory, United States Environmental Protection Agency, Research Triangle Park, North Carolina 27711, USA

ABSTRACT: Polychlorinated biphenyls (PCBs) are persistent, bioaccumulative, toxic, and widely distributed environmental chemicals. There is now both epidemiological and experimental evidence that PCBs cause cognitive deficits; however, the underlying cellular or molecular mechanism(s) is not known. We have hypothesized that altered signal transduction/second messenger homeostasis by PCBs may be associated with these effects since second messengers in signal transduction pathways, such as calcium, inositol phosphates (IP), and protein kinase C (PKC), play key roles in neuronal development and their function. *In vitro* studies using cerebellar granule neurons and isolated organelle preparations indicate that *ortho*-PCBs increase intracellular free Ca^{2+} levels by inhibiting microsomal and mitochondrial Ca^{2+} buffering and the Ca^{2+} extrusion process. *Ortho*-PCBs also increase agonist-stimulated IP accumulation and cause PKC translocation at low micromolar concentrations where no cytotoxicity is observed. On the other hand, non-*ortho*-PCBs are not effective in altering these events. Further SAR studies indicate that congeners with chlorine substitutions favoring non-coplanarity are active *in vitro*, while congeners favoring coplanarity are relatively inactive. Subsequent *in vivo* studies have shown that repeated exposure to a PCB mixture, Aroclor 1254, increases PKC translocation and decreases Ca^{2+} buffering in the brain, similar to *in vitro* studies. These changes *in vivo* are associated with elevated levels of non-coplanar *ortho*-PCB congeners at levels equivalent to 40–50 µM in brain, the concentrations that significantly inhibited second messenger systems in neuronal cultures *in vitro*. Current research is focusing on PCB-induced alterations in second messenger systems following developmental exposure.

---

[a]The research described in this article has been reviewed by the National Health and Environmental Effects Research Laboratory, U.S. Environmental Protection Agency, and approved for publication. Approval does not signify that the contents necessarily reflect the views and policies of the Agency nor does mention of trade names or commercial products constitute endorsement or recommendation for use.

[b]Address for correspondence: Prasada Rao S. Kodavanti, Neurotoxicology Division, MD 74B, National Health and Environmental Effects Research Laboratory, U.S. Environmental Protection Agency, Research Triangle Park, NC 27711. Voice: 919-541-7584; fax: 919-541-4849.
kodavanti.prasada@epamail.epa.gov

INTRODUCTION

Humans are exposed to a number of chemicals in their day-to-day life. Although many chemicals can enhance and even save lives by ensuring food security and protecting health, several other chemicals are not beneficial. The United Nations Environment Programme (UNEP) has identified a dozen chemicals as significant threats to human and wildlife health on a global basis. These chemicals are highly persistent, travel thousands of miles, accumulate in food chain, and persist in the environment, taking up to centuries to fully degrade. These chemicals are categorized as "persistent organic pollutants" (POPs) or "persistent bioaccumulative toxicants" (PBTs), and polychlorinated biphenyls (PCBs) belong to this category of environmental pollutants.[1–3] POPs or PBTs are the chemicals of concern for the next millennium in terms of human health and environmental damage.

PCBs exist as mixtures containing up to 209 possible congeners and are ubiquitous environmental contaminants resulting from intensive industrial use and inadequate disposal over past decades.[4] PCB mixtures as well as congeners possess a surprising array of biological activity leading to toxicity.[5] It is known that some PCBs and other halogenated hydrocarbons such as 2,3,7,8-tetrachlorodibenzo-*p*-dioxin (TCDD) produce their biological effects through a receptor-mediated response by binding to the cytosolic aryl hydrocarbon (Ah) receptor followed by induction of a number of genes.[6,7] It has been proposed that non-*ortho* substitutions on the biphenyl ring (lateral substitutions at the *meta-* and *para-*positions) promote coplanarity and are associated with the TCDD-like toxic effects of certain PCB congeners.[8] Ah receptor involvement is associated with reproductive, immunologic, teratogenic, and carcinogenic effects of PCBs;[6,9] however, recent studies indicate that neurotoxic effects of PCBs might not be mediated through the Ah receptor.[10,11]

There is now both epidemiological and experimental evidence that developmental exposure to PCBs causes cognitive deficits in humans[12,13] and animals;[14,15] however, the underlying cellular or molecular mechanism(s) is not known.[16,17] We have hypothesized that altered signal transduction/second messenger homeostasis by PCBs may be associated with these effects. This hypothesis is based on the following reasons: (a) the most significant neurotoxic effects of PCBs seen in humans are learning and memory deficits;[12,13] (b) laboratory studies indicate that PCBs inhibit long-term potentiation (LTP, a form of synaptic plasticity) and impair learning/memory *in vivo*;[14,15] (c) LTP is often described as a physiological model for neuronal development, learning, and memory;[18] (d) second messengers such as calcium, inositol phosphates, protein kinase C (PKC), arachidonic acid (AA), and nitric oxide synthase (NOS) have been shown to modulate LTP and play key roles in neuronal development;[18] and (e) epidemiological studies indicate that infants born to mothers who consumed contaminated cooking oil in Yusho, Japan, showed abnormal calcification of the skull, indicating that PCBs might interfere with calcium metabolism.[19] Based on this reasoning, we have conducted both *in vitro* and *in vivo* studies to understand the effects of PCBs on second messenger systems. *In vitro* experiments were conducted using cerebellar granule cell cultures as well as brain homogenate preparations, while *in vivo* studies were conducted by the repeated exposure of adult rats to a PCB mixture, Aroclor 1254.

IN VITRO EFFECTS OF PCBs

In vitro studies were conducted with prototypic *ortho* (2,2′-dichlorobiphenyl, DCB) and non-*ortho* (3,3′,4,4′,5-pentachlorobiphenyl, PeCB; or 4,4′-DCB) PCBs. Granule cells from rat cerebellum were isolated from 6- to 8-day-old pups of Long-Evans hooded rats following the enzymatic disruption method.[20,21] These cells at 7 days in culture were utilized for the measurements of % lactate dehydrogenase (LDH) leakage from the exposed cells to indicate cytotoxicity,[22] alterations in intracellular free Ca^{2+} with fluorescent dyes (Fluo-3AM and Fura-2AM),[23] [^{3}H]-arachidonic acid release,[24] PKC translocation,[25] and PKC activity.[26] Cerebellar fractions were obtained from cerebella of adult male rats by the sucrose-gradient centrifugation method[21,27] and were utilized for the measurements of $^{45}Ca^{2+}$ uptake by mitochondria and microsomes,[28] synaptosomal Ca^{2+}-ATPase,[21] and nitric oxide synthase activity.[29]

Calcium homeostasis: Ours is the first report showing that PCB congeners increase cerebellar granule cell $[Ca^{2+}]_i$. The *ortho*-substituted 2,2′-DCB was more effective than the non-*ortho*-substituted 3,3′,4,4′,5-PeCB. The increase in $[Ca^{2+}]_i$ was slow and a steady rise was observed with time.[21] Further literature reports also indicated similar increases in $[Ca^{2+}]_i$ in cerebellar granule neurons[30] as well as in human granulocytes.[31] Results characterizing the mechanisms of $[Ca^{2+}]_i$ increase indicated that 2,2′-DCB was a potent inhibitor of $^{45}Ca^{2+}$ uptake by mitochondria and microsomes, with IC_{50} (concentration that inhibits control activity by 50%) values of 6–8 μM. 3,3′,4,4′,5-PeCB inhibited Ca^{2+} sequestration, but the effects were much less than those produced by equivalent concentrations of 2,2′-DCB. Synaptosomal Ca^{2+}-ATPase, involved in the Ca^{2+} extrusion process, was only inhibited by 2,2′-DCB, but not by 3,3′,4,4′,5-PeCB[21] (TABLE 1). Further structure-activity relationship (SAR) studies indicated that congeners that are non-coplanar inhibited $^{45}Ca^{2+}$ uptake by microsomes and mitochondria, while coplanar congeners did not.[32]

Inositol phosphates (IP): The disruption of Ca^{2+} homeostasis may have a significant effect on signal transduction pathways (IP second messengers) regulated or modulated by Ca^{2+}. 2,2′-DCB (but not 3,3′,4,4′,5-PeCB) affected basal IP accumulation in cerebellar granule cells. Concentrations of 2,2′-DCB up to 50 μM increased carbachol (CB)–stimulated IP accumulation. At concentration of 100 μM 2,2′-DCB, CB-stimulated IP accumulation was decreased. 3,3′,4,4′,5-PeCB, on the other hand, had no effect on CB-stimulated IP accumulation at concentrations up to 100 μM.[33] Further studies indicated that any modulation of CB-stimulated IP accumulation is due to Ca^{2+} overload and not due to activation of PKC activity[34] (TABLE 1).

Arachidonic acid (AA) release: AA is released intracellularly following activation of membrane phospholipases and this is an important second messenger in releasing Ca^{2+} from endoplasmic reticulum.[35] We have characterized the effects of PCBs on second messengers that contribute to the perturbations in Ca^{2+} homeostasis and the possible mechanism by which PCBs activate phospholipases. Aroclor 1254 and 2,2′-DCB increased [^{3}H]-AA release in cerebellar granule cells, while 4,4′-DCB did not, and this is in agreement with previous SAR studies on Ca^{2+} buffering and PKC translocation.[16,32] The release caused by PCBs was linear with time of exposure and a significant release was seen as early as 2 min. Phospholipase A_2 (PLA_2) inhibitor completely blocked the release. Removal of extracellular Ca^{2+} or inhibition

TABLE 1. *In vitro* effects of prototypic *ortho*-substituted non-coplanar (2,2'-DCB) and non-*ortho*-substituted coplanar (3,3',4,4',5-PeCB) congeners on signal transduction mechanisms in neuronal cultures and brain homogenate preparations

		Significant effect	
		Ortho-PCB	Non-*ortho*-PCB
Cytotoxicity:	LDH leakage	100–200 µM	Not toxic at 200 µM
Ca^{2+} homeostasis:	$[Ca^{2+}]$ levels—fluorescent probe	25 µM	25–50 µM
	Ca^{2+} buffering by mitochondria and microsomes	5 µM	50–75 µM
	Ca^{2+} extrusion by Ca^{2+}-ATPase	10 µM	NOE[a]
Inositol phosphates:	Basal PI metabolism	100 µM	NOE
	Carb-stimulated PI metabolism	↑ at 30–50 µM; ↓ at 100 µM	NOE
Arachidonic acid release:	Basal release	3 µM	50 µM
	Characterizing DCB-increased arachidonic acid release	Seen as early as 2 min after exposure	
		Blocked by PLA_2 inhibitor	
		External Ca^{2+} partially necessary	
		$[Ca^{2+}]_i$ release partially necessary	
PKC translocation:	[^{3}H]-Phorbol ester binding		
	Without preincubation	30 µM	NOE
	With preincubation	30 µM	NOE
	Characterizing DCB-increased [^{3}H]-PDBu binding	External Ca^{2+} necessary	
		Additive with glutamate	
		No effect with verapamil	
		No effect with tetradotoxin	
		No effect with MK-801, CPP, or CNQX	
		Sphingosine blocked PCB effect	
Nitric oxide synthase (NOS):	Cytosolic NOS	10 µM	NOE
	Membrane NOS	10 µM	NOE

[a]No effect up to 100 µM.

of intracellular Ca^{2+} release only partially blocked the [^{3}H]-AA release,[36] suggesting that PCB-induced [^{3}H]-AA release could be due to activation of both Ca^{2+}-dependent and Ca^{2+}-independent PLA_2.

PKC translocation: One of the downstream effects of perturbed Ca^{2+} homeostasis is translocation of PKC from cytosol to the membrane where it gets activated.[37] [^{3}H]-Phorbol ester ([^{3}H]-PDBu) binding was used as an indicator of PKC translocation. 2,2′-DCB increased [^{3}H]-PDBu binding in a concentration-dependent manner in cerebellar granule cells. 3,3′,4,4′,5-PeCB had no effect at concentrations up to 100 μM (TABLE 1). The effect of 2,2′-DCB was time-dependent and also dependent on the presence of external Ca^{2+} in the medium. Sphingosine, a PKC translocation blocker, prevented 2,2′-DCB-induced increases in [^{3}H]-PDBu binding (TABLE 1). Experiments with several pharmacologic agents revealed that the effects are additive with glutamate, and none of the channel (glutamate, calcium, and sodium) antagonists blocked the response of 2,2′-DCB.[33] Subsequent SAR studies indicated that congeners that are non-coplanar increased PKC translocation, while coplanar congeners did not (for review, see reference 16).

Nitric oxide synthase (NOS): Nitric oxide produced by NOS is a first gaseous neurotransmitter that has an important role as a retrograde messenger in LTP, learning, and memory processes, and endocrine function.[38,39] 2,2′-DCB (but not 4,4′-DCB) inhibited both cytosolic (nNOS) and membrane (eNOS) forms of NOS (see TABLE 1).

Cytotoxicity: To understand whether changes in second messengers following exposure to PCBs are a result of cell death or can lead to cell death, we determined cytotoxicity by measuring LDH leakage. 2,2′-DCB was cytotoxic at >100 μM after 4 hours of exposure in cerebellar granule cells. 3,3′,4,4′,5-PeCB, on the other hand, was not cytotoxic even at 200 μM during 4 hours of exposure[21] (TABLE 1).

These *in vitro* studies clearly demonstrate that second messenger systems, involved in neuronal function and development of the nervous system, are sensitive targets for the *ortho*-substituted PCBs. *Ortho*-PCBs increased intracellular free Ca^{2+}, inhibited Ca^{2+} buffering mechanisms, stimulated phospholipases, inhibited NOS, and caused PKC translocation at low micromolar concentrations and shorter exposure periods where cytotoxicity is not evident. On the other hand, non-*ortho*-PCBs had marginal effects on intracellular free Ca^{2+}, Ca^{2+} buffering, and phospholipases, and no effect on NOS and PKC translocation. These *in vitro* studies demonstrate direct effects of both *ortho*- and non-*ortho*-PCBs on signal transduction pathways involved in LTP, learning, and memory. Such effects might be a mode of action for PCB effects on the nervous system.

IN VIVO EFFECTS OF PCBs

In vivo effects of PCBs were investigated by dosing Long-Evans hooded rats (adult male; 200–250 g) orally by gavage with Aroclor 1254 (Lot no. 6024, AccuStandard, New Haven, CT) in corn oil (2 mL/kg). The selected dosages were 0, 10, or 30 mg/kg/day. The rats were dosed once a day, 5 times a week, for 4 weeks. At 24 h after the last dosage, rats were sacrificed and brains removed and dissected into frontal cortex, cerebellum, and striatum for neurochemical and PCB analyses.

TABLE 2. *In vivo* effects of a commercial PCB mixture (Aroclor 1254) on signal transduction mechanisms in different brain regions

Parameter	Cerebellum	Frontal cortex	Striatum
Ca^{2+} buffering			
Microsomes	Inhibited	Inhibited	Inhibited
Mitochondria	Inhibited	No effect	No effect
Total PKC	Inhibited	No effect	No effect
Membrane PKC (% total)	Increased	No effect	No effect
Total PCBs	13 ppm	15 ppm	8 ppm

NOTE: Adult male rats were repeatedly dosed with Aroclor 1254 (10 or 30 mg/kg/day) for 4 weeks. Ca^{2+} buffering, PKC activity, and total PCBs were determined in different brain regions.

Ca^{2+} buffering,[28] PKC activity,[26] and congener-specific analysis of PCBs were performed.[40] The reasons for these adult studies are twofold. The first one is to determine whether changes in Ca^{2+} homeostasis and PKC translocation observed after *in vitro* exposure also occur after exposure *in vivo*. The second one is to examine whether concentrations of PCBs that altered second messenger systems *in vitro* are achievable *in vivo*.

Following Aroclor 1254 treatment, body weight gain in the high-dose group was significantly lower than in the control and low-dose groups. Ca^{2+} buffering by microsomes was significantly lower in all three brain regions from the 30-mg/kg group. In the same dose group, mitochondrial Ca^{2+} buffering was affected in cerebellum, but not in cortex or striatum. Similarly, total cerebellar PKC activity was decreased significantly, while the % of PKC activity associated with the membrane was significantly elevated at 10 and 30 mg/kg. PKC activity was not altered in either cortex or the striatum[41] (TABLE 2). These results indicate that *in vivo* exposure to a PCB mixture can produce changes in second messenger systems that are similar to those observed after *in vitro* exposure of neuronal cell cultures and brain homogenate preparations.

Total PCBs accumulated in some brain regions were equivalent to 40–50 µM (13–15 ppm) and most of the PCBs accumulated in brain are *ortho*-substituted, noncoplanar congeners[42] (TABLE 2). At these concentrations, intracellular second messengers were significantly affected in neuronal cultures and brain homogenate preparations. Currently, we are focusing on the PCB-induced alterations in intracellular second messengers following developmental exposure.

Although we have demonstrated direct effects of PCBs on several intracellular second messengers and accumulation of PCBs, especially *ortho*-PCBs, in brain at concentrations where *in vitro* effects are observed, it is very difficult to extrapolate these neurochemical changes to the neurotoxic effects of PCBs. Apart from having effects on second messengers, PCBs have been shown to decrease circulating thyroid hormones,[43] decrease brain dopamine concentrations,[44] and alter the cholinergic system.[45] Additional studies are needed to test whether one or more of these mechanisms are responsible for the effects of PCBs in the nervous system. Since metabolites of PCBs have been detected in mammalian tissue and blood samples,[46] it is necessary to understand the role of metabolites in the final outcome of toxicity. It is also essential to understand the potential interactive effects among PCB congeners and with other environmental contaminants.

ACKNOWLEDGMENTS

We thank James D. McKinney and Jae-Ho Yang for their comments on an earlier version of this document. We also thank Ethel C. Derr-Yellin for excellent technical assistance.

REFERENCES

1. VALLACK, H.W. et al. 1998. Controlling persistent organic pollutants—what next? Environ. Toxicol. Pharmacol. **6**: 143–175.
2. SWEDISH ENVIRONMENTAL PROTECTION AGENCY. 1998. Persistent organic pollutants: a Swedish view of an international problem. Monitor 16.
3. FISHER, B.E. 1999. Most unwanted persistent organic pollutants. Environ. Health Perspect. **107**: A18–A23.
4. ERICKSON, M.D. 1986. Analytical Chemistry of PCBs. Butterworths. Boston/London.
5. WORLD HEALTH ORGANIZATION. 1993. Environmental Health Criteria 140: Polychlorinated Biphenyls and Terphenyls. Second edition. International Programme on Chemical Safety, Geneva, Switzerland.
6. SAFE, S. 1994. Polychlorinated biphenyls (PCBs): environmental impact, biochemical and toxic responses, and implications for risk assessment. CRC Crit. Rev. Toxicol. **24**: 87–149.
7. OKEY, A.B., D.S. RIDDICK & P.A. HARPER. 1994. The Ah receptor: mediator of the toxicity of 2,3,7,8-tetrachlorodibenzo-p-dioxin (TCDD) and related compounds. Toxicol. Lett. **70**: 1–22.
8. MCKINNEY, J.D. & C.L. WALLER. 1994. Polychlorinated biphenyls as hormonally active structural analogues. Environ. Health Perspect. **102**: 290–297.
9. KAFAFI, S.A., H.Y. AFEEFY, A.H. ALI, H.K. SAID & A.G. KAFAFI. 1993. Binding of polychlorinated biphenyls to the aryl hydrocarbon receptor. Environ. Health Perspect. **101**: 422–428.
10. SCHANTZ, S.L. 1996. Developmental neurotoxicity of PCBs in humans: what do we know and where do we go from here? Neurotoxicol. Teratol. **18**: 217–227.
11. SEEGAL, R.F. 1996. Epidemiological and laboratory evidence of PCB-induced neurotoxicity. CRC Crit. Rev. Toxicol. **26**: 709–737.
12. JACOBSON, J.L. & S.W. JACOBSON. 1996. Intellectual impairment in children exposed to polychlorinated biphenyls *in utero*. N. Engl. J. Med. **335**: 783–789.
13. PATANDIN, S., C.I. LANTING, P.G.H. MULDER, E.R. BOERSMA, P.J.J. SAUER & N. WEISGLAS-KUPERUS. 1999. Effects of environmental exposure to polychlorinated biphenyls and dioxins on cognitive abilities in Dutch children at 42 months of age. J. Pediatr. **134**: 33–41.
14. SCHANTZ, S.L., J. MOSHTAGHIAN & D.K. NESS. 1995. Spatial learning deficits in adult rats exposed to *ortho*-substituted PCB congeners during gestation and lactation. Fundam. Appl. Toxicol. **26**: 117–126.
15. NIEMI, W.D., J. AUDI, B. BUSH & D.O. CARPENTER. 1998. PCBs reduce long-term potentiation in the CA1 region of rat hippocampus. Exp. Neurol. **151**: 26–34.
16. KODAVANTI, P.R.S. & H.A. TILSON. 1997. Structure-activity relationships of potentially neurotoxic PCB congeners in the rat. Neurotoxicology **18**: 425–442.
17. TILSON, H.A. & P.R.S. KODAVANTI. 1997. Neurochemical effects of polychlorinated biphenyls: an overview and identification of research needs. Neurotoxicology **18**: 727–744.

18. LYNCH, M.A. 1998. Analysis of the mechanisms underlying the age-related impairment in long-term potentiation in the rat. Rev. Neurosci. **9:** 169–201.
19. YAMASHITA, F. & M. HAYASHI. 1985. Fetal PCB syndrome: clinical features, intrauterine growth retardation, and possible alteration in calcium metabolism. Environ. Health Perspect. **59:** 41–45.
20. GALLO, V., A. KINGSBURY, R. BALAZS & O.S. JERGENSEN. 1987. The role of depolarization in the survival and differentiation of cerebellar granule cells in culture. J. Neurosci. **7:** 2203–2213.
21. KODAVANTI, P.R.S., D. SHIN, H.A. TILSON & G.J. HARRY. 1993. Comparative effects of two polychlorinated biphenyl congeners on calcium homeostasis in rat cerebellar granule cells. Toxicol. Appl. Pharmacol. **123:** 97–106.
22. AMADOR, E., L.E. DORFMAN & W.E.C. WACKER. 1963. Serum lactic dehydrogenase: an analytical assessment of current assays. Clin. Chem. **9:** 391–399.
23. GRYNKIEWICZ, G., M. POENIE & R.Y. TSIEN. 1985. A new generation of Ca^{2+} indicators with greatly improved fluorescence properties. J. Biol. Chem. **260:** 3340–3350.
24. LAZAREWICZ, J.W., J.T. WROBLEWSKI & E. COSTA. 1990. N-Methyl-D-aspartate-sensitive glutamate receptors induce calcium-mediated arachidonic acid release in primary cultures of cerebellar granule cells. J. Neurochem. **55:** 1875–1881.
25. VECCARINO, F.M., S. LILJEQUIST & J.F. TALLMAN. 1991. Modulation of protein kinase C translocation by excitatory and inhibitory amino acids in primary cultures of neurons. J. Neurochem. **57:** 391–396.
26. CHEN, S-J., E. KLANN, M.C. GOWER, C.M. POWELL, J.S. SESSOMS & J.D. SWEATT. 1993. Studies with synthetic peptide substrates derived from the neuronal protein neurogranin reveal structural determinants of potency and selectivity for protein kinase C. Biochemistry **32:** 1032–1039.
27. DODD, P.R., J.A. HARDY, A.E. OAKLEY, J.A. EDWARDSON, E.K. PERRY & J.P. DELAUNOY. 1981. A rapid method for preparing synaptosomes: comparison with alternative procedures. Brain Res. **226:** 107–118.
28. MOORE, L., T. CHEN, H.R. KNAPP, JR. & E.L. LANDON. 1975. Energy dependent calcium sequestration activity in rat liver microsomes. J. Biol. Chem. **250:** 4562–4568.
29. BREDT, D. & S. SNYDER. 1990. Isolation of nitric oxide synthetase, a calmodulin-requiring enzyme. Proc. Natl. Acad. Sci. U.S.A. **87:** 682–685.
30. CARPENTER, D.O., C.R.T. STONER & D.A. LAWRENCE. 1997. Flow cytometric measurements of neuronal death triggered by PCBs. Neurotoxicology **18:** 507–514.
31. VOIE, O.A. & F. FONNUM. 1998. Ortho-substituted polychlorinated biphenyls elevate intracellular $[Ca^{2+}]$ in human granulocytes. Environ. Toxicol. Pharmacol. **5:** 105–112.
32. KODAVANTI, P.R.S., T.R. WARD, J.D. MCKINNEY & H.A. TILSON. 1996. Inhibition of microsomal and mitochondrial Ca^{2+} sequestration in rat cerebellum by polychlorinated biphenyl mixtures and congeners: structure-activity relationships. Arch. Toxicol. **70:** 150–157.
33. KODAVANTI, P.R.S. et al. 1994. Differential effects of polychlorinated biphenyl congeners on phosphoinositide hydrolysis and protein kinase C translocation in rat cerebellar granule cells. Brain Res. **662:** 75–82.
34. SHAFER, T.J., W.R. MUNDY, H.A. TILSON & P.R.S. KODAVANTI. 1996. Disruption of inositol phosphate accumulation in cerebellar granule cells by polychlorinated biphenyls: a consequence of altered Ca^{2+} homeostasis. Toxicol. Appl. Pharmacol. **141:** 448–455.
35. STRIGGOW, F. & B.E. EHRLICH. 1997. Regulation of intracellular calcium release channel function by arachidonic acid and leukotriene B4. Biochem. Biophys. Res. Commun. **237:** 413–418.
36. DERR-YELLIN, E.C. & P.R.S. KODAVANTI. 1999. Stimulation of [^{3}H]arachidonic acid release in rat cerebellar granule neurons by PCBs: structure-activity relationships and possible mechanism(s). Toxicologist **48:** 276.
37. TRILIVAS, I. & J.H. BROWN. 1989. Increases in intracellular Ca^{2+} regulate the binding of [^{3}H]phorbol 12,13-dibutyrate to intact 1321N1 astrocytoma cells. J. Biol. Chem. **264:** 3102–3107.
38. SCHUMAN, E.M. & D.V. MADISON. 1994. Nitric oxide and synaptic function. Annu. Rev. Neurosci. **17:** 153–183.

39. MCCANN, S.M., M. KIMURA, A. WALCZEWSKA, S. KARANTH, V. RETTORI & W.H. YU. 1998. Hypothalamic control of FSH and LH by FSH-RF, LHRH, cytokines, leptin, and nitric oxide. Neuroimmunomodulation **5:** 193–202.
40. BUSH, B., R.W. STREETER & R.J. SLOAN. 1989. Polychlorinate biphenyl (PCB) congeners in striped bass (*Morone saxatilis*) from marine and estuarine waters of New York State determined by capillary gas chromatography. Arch. Environ. Contam. Toxicol. **19:** 49–61.
41. KODAVANTI, P.R.S. *et al.* 1998. Repeated exposure of adult rats to Aroclor 1254 causes brain region–specific changes in intracellular Ca^{2+} buffering and protein kinase C activity in the absence of changes in tyrosine hydroxylase. Toxicol. Appl. Pharmacol. **153:** 186–198.
42. KODAVANTI, P.R.S. *et al.* 1998. Congener-specific distribution of PCBs in brain regions, blood, liver, and fat of adult rats following repeated exposure to Aroclor 1254. Toxicol. Appl. Pharmacol. **153:** 199–210.
43. MORSE, D.C. *et al.* 1993. Interference of PCBs in hepatic and brain thyroid hormone metabolism in fetal and neonatal rats. Toxicol. Appl. Pharmacol. **122:** 27–33.
44. SEEGAL, R.F., K.O. BROSCH & R.J. OKONIEWSKI. 1997. Effects of *in utero* and lactational exposure of the laboratory rat to 2,4,2′,4′- and 3,4,3′,4′-tetrachlorobiphenyl on dopamine function. Toxicol. Appl. Pharmacol. **146:** 95–103.
45. JUAREZ DE KU, L.M., M. SHARMA-STOKKERMANS & L.A. MESERVE. 1994. Thyroxine normalizes polychlorinated biphenyl (PCB) dose-related depression of choline acetyltransferase (ChAT) activity in hippocampus and basal forebrain of 15-day-old rats. Toxicology **94:** 19–30.
46. BERGMAN, A., E. KLASSON-WEHLER & H. KUROKI. 1994. Selective retention of hydroxylated PCB metabolites in blood. Environ. Health Perspect. **102:** 464–469.

Culture Models of Neurodegenerative Disease

D. A. FIGLEWICZ,[a] L. DONG, M. MLODZIENSKI, AND J. C. TURCOTTE

Departments of Neurology and Neurobiology/Anatomy, University of Rochester Medical Center, Rochester, New York 14642, USA

> ABSTRACT: In order to investigate how mutant SOD1 protein or environmental exogenous stressors lead to the death of motor neurons, we have established several *in vitro* model systems. We describe some features of the various models in order to demonstrate the advantages and shortcomings of each system.

Amyotrophic lateral sclerosis (ALS) is an adult-onset degenerative disorder involving loss of motor neurons in the cerebral cortex, brain stem, and ventral spinal cord. Approximately 10% of ALS cases are inherited (FALS), and mutations in the Cu/Zn superoxide dismutase gene (SOD1) have been identified in a subset of FALS kindreds.[1] In order to investigate how mutant SOD1 protein (mSOD) or environmental exogenous stressors lead to the death of motor neurons, we have established several *in vitro* model systems. Here, we describe some features of the various models in order to demonstrate the advantages and shortcomings of each system.

MATERIALS AND METHODS

Cell Culture Systems

Purified motor neurons were prepared from E14 ventral spinal cord of Sprague-Dawley rats using the panning method described by Camu and Henderson.[2] B27 media with or without antioxidant supplement (Gibco) were both tested. Growth factors, when included, were added during the panning stage: BDNF (4 ng/mL), GDNF (4 ng/mL), CNTF (200 ng/mL), and IGF-1 (5 ng/mL) (all from Sigma Chemical Company).

The RN46A cell line was obtained from Dr. Scott Whittemore. RN46A cells are serotonergic cells isolated from E13 rat medullary raphe and infected with a temperature-sensitive mutant retrovirus. Under permissive conditions, these cells differentiate into distinctive neuronal phenotypes.[3] Mutant or wild-type human SOD1 cDNAs were cloned into the expression vector pCEP4.[4,5] Mutant SODs used in these studies were Ala4 → Val (pC4), Gly37 → Arg (pC37), Leu38 → Val (pC38), Gly41 → Ser (pC41A), Gly93 → Ala (pC93A), Gly93 → Cys (pC93B), Ile113 → Thr (pC113), Asn139 → Lys (pC139), Ile149 → Thr (pC149), and wild-type SOD1

---

[a]Address for correspondence: Denise A. Figlewicz, Department of Neurology, University of Rochester Medical Center, 601 Elmwood Avenue, Box 673, Rochester, NY 14642. Voice: 716-275-4055; fax: 716-273-1255.

Denise_Figlewicz@urmc.rochester.edu

(pCN). Transfection and selection: 6×10^4 cells/well in a 24-well plate were transfected with 2 μL of lipofectamine (Gibco/BRL) and 0.2 μg of plasmid DNA, for 2 h at 33°C, without serum. After 2 h, an equal volume of media with 2× serum (20%) was added. Cells were incubated for 24 h, washed, and selected for stable transfection by adding 200 mg/mL of hygromycin (Sigma) in complete media with serum (CNS + 10% FBS). To differentiate, confluent cells were washed and incubated at 39°C with CNS media without serum. After ~4 days, the cells stopped dividing and started to differentiate.

Dissociated mouse spinal cord cultures were prepared from E13 CD1 mouse spinal cord. Details of the culture system, microinjection of constructs for the expression of mSOD or wild-type SOD1 (wtSOD) cDNAs, evaluation of viability, immunocytochemistry, and exposure to antioxidant agents, glutathione ethyl ester and PBN, have been previously described.[4,5]

Purified Motor Neuron Counting/Viability

Cover glasses were mounted on slides for viewing with an Olympus IX70 microscope. Pictures were taken with a Spot digital camera (Diagnostic Instruments, Inc.) for image analysis (Image-Pro Plus Software, Media Cybernetics, Inc.). Data were also collected using a Nikon microscope fitted with an MTI CCD72 camera (Dage MTI, Michigan City, MI) connected to a G3 Macintosh computer using Image (version 1.62), a program developed by the National Institutes of Health. The technique for image analysis was similar for both programs. Briefly, both microscopes were adjusted for Köhler illumination. The Nikon microscope was fitted with a Wratten filter (Eastman Kodak, Rochester, NY) in order to obtain the best image transfer. The microscopes and cameras were focused on a slide with a black dot. This black image was used to adjust the color scale to the darkest pixel and the lightest pixel for a range between approximately 5 and 250. Cells magnified at 20× were isolated for counting or for densitometry using a color segmentation method. Cells were isolated from the image background and counted or measured for size and density automatically. The cells imaged with the NIH program were isolated from the surrounding background tissue by four standard deviations from the mean density. All analysis was done with the experimenter blind to the day in culture and type of media. Cells were included for analysis if they had cell processes of at least two cell body diameters in length. This somewhat short dendrite length was chosen due to the short processes present on some cells at day 1.

Cell counts: Motor neurons were counted using the color segmentation methods described above. Using Image Pro, cells were counted from an area comprising 20% of the 12-mm cover glass, and the total number of cells was extrapolated from the sum of these counts from 3 cover glasses/experimental condition. Alternatively, cell counts were obtained by eye over the entire cover glass and counts from 3 cover glasses/condition averaged. These methods yielded similar cell counts.

Cell size: Color segmentation also provided a measure of cell body area. Cells were chosen in random order focusing from the top of the cover glass to the bottom until at least 15 cells were included for each cover glass, giving a total number of 30 cells/media condition. Some cell areas were sorted below or above 300 mm in order to obtain a general impression of the number of large motor neurons in each condition over time.

Immunocytochemistry

Motor neurons were stained for ChAT (Chemicon), Islet-1 (ATCC), GFAP (Chemicon), or antineurofilament antibody SMI 31 (Sternberger Monoclonals). Cultures were rinsed with Tris-buffered saline (TBS pH 7.2) and fixed in 3% paraformaldehyde for 20 min at room temperature. Following additional rinses (3× 5 min), cells were refrigerated in buffer containing 0.1% sodium azide until used for immunocytochemistry. Prior to immunostaining, cells were incubated in blocking serum containing TBS, 10% normal goat serum (Vector Laboratories, Burlingame, CA), 0.25% Triton X-100, 1% bovine serum albumin, and 1% hydrogen peroxide for 30 min. Primary antibodies were diluted in buffer containing TBS and 5% normal goat serum, and cells incubated overnight at 4°C. The following day, cells were rinsed three times with TBS and incubated in buffer containing 5% normal goat serum and either biotinylated goat anti-rabbit or goat anti-mouse IgGs for 90 min. Cells were rinsed again (3× TBS) and incubated in A and B reagents (Elite Kit, Vector Laboratories), 9 µL/mL, in TBS for 90 min. Following the second incubation, cells were rinsed (3× TBS) and incubated in DAB solution (Vector) until brown reaction product was observed (1–10 min). Fluorescent immunostaining for SOD1 has been previously described.[5]

SOD Activity

Total SOD activity was measured using the method of Misra and Fridovich,[6] based on the ability of SOD to inhibit the auto-oxidation of epinephrine at pH 10.2. Formation of adenochrome was followed spectrophotometrically at 480 nm. Total activity was calculated as the % inhibition of the reaction. Transfected RN46A cells (1×10^6) were lysed in 0.1 mM EDTA, 0.05 M Na_2CO_3, and 0.1% Nonidet NP-40; 5–40 µL of the lysate was used in the spectrophotometric assay, which was standardized using 1–100 ng of bovine SOD (Sigma). The contribution of Mn-SOD (SOD2) to the total activity was determined by the addition of NaCN to paired samples to be approximately 2 U/mg protein.

Western Blotting Protocol

RN46A cells (1×10^5) transfected with wild-type and mutant human SOD1 were lysed in SDS sample buffer (62.5 mM Tris-HCl, pH 6.8; 10% glycerol; 2% SDS; 5% β-mercaptoethanol), electrophoresed on a 15% polyacrylamide gel, and transferred to PVDF. After 1-h blocking with 5% nonfat dry milk/TBS, membranes were washed twice in 0.5% Tween-TBS. Human and murine SOD1 were identified using 1:1000 anti-SOD1 antibody (The Binding Site) followed by ECL (LumiGLO/KPL) according to the manufacturer's instructions. The blot was exposed to BioMax film for 30 s. Ratios of human SOD1 protein to native rodent SOD1 protein levels were quantitated from the blots by densitometry using ImageQuant software (Molecular Dynamics). Five separate determinations were made from harvested RN46A cell lines over the course of 2 years.

Apoptosis

Cells undergoing apoptosis were detected as follows: Cells were fixed in 2% buffered formalin, permeabilized with 0.2% Triton X-100, and labeled with Biotin-14-dCTP using 15 U of terminal deoxynucleotide transferase/100 mL reaction volume. TUNEL+ cells have dark nuclei and were quantitated by counting. Chromatin condensation and fragmentation were visualized by Hoechst staining.

Statistics

Student's t tests were calculated to determine significant differences in number, size, and intensity. One-way ANOVAs were also calculated to demonstrate significant differences and interactions between different media conditions, and time in culture.

RESULTS

In purified rat motor neuron cultures, cells were identified as motor neurons based upon morphology and immunostaining (FIG. 1). When cultures were double-labeled for the motor neuron marker, ChAT, and for glial fibrillary acidic protein (GFAP), a glial-specific marker, over 90% of the cells were immunoreactive for ChAT and not for GFAP, indicating a low percent of glial cell contamination. A subset of ChAT+ neurons were also labeled with the developmentally regulated marker Islet-1;[7] these were mostly larger motor neurons. Without media supplements, very

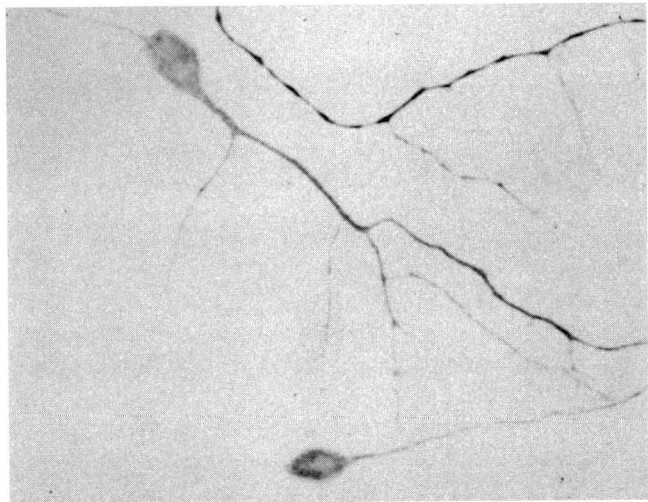

FIGURE 1. This photograph depicts a representative example of purified rat spinal motor neurons, fixed on day 6 in culture. Neurons are fixed and immunostained with antibody SMI 31 (Sternberger Monoclonals, Inc.), which characteristically stains highly phosphorylated neurofilaments in neuronal processes.

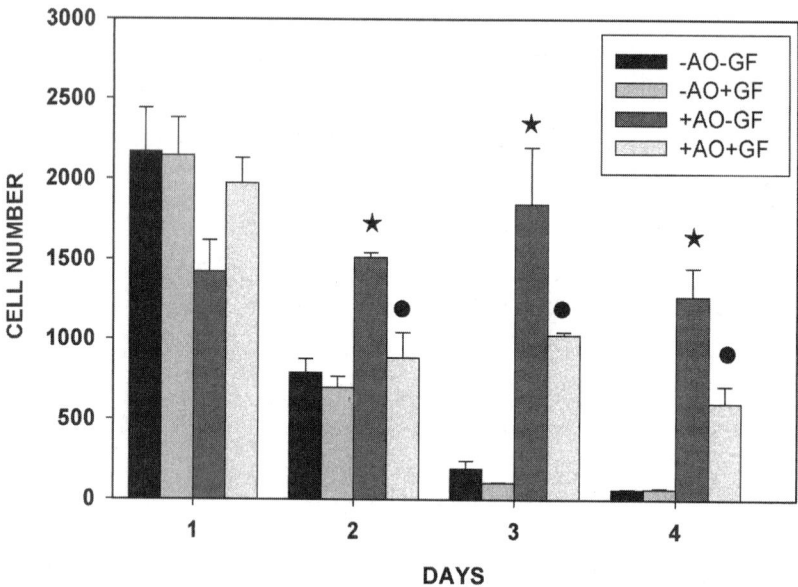

FIGURE 2. Total number of purified embryonic rat motor neurons surviving with and without growth factor and antioxidant media supplements during the first 4 days in culture. Addition of antioxidants to the media contributed to motor neuron survival ($p < 0.001$; one-way ANOVA and Scheffe F test). The contribution of growth factors to survival was not significant, and the combination of antioxidants plus growth factors proved to be less beneficial than addition of antioxidants alone.

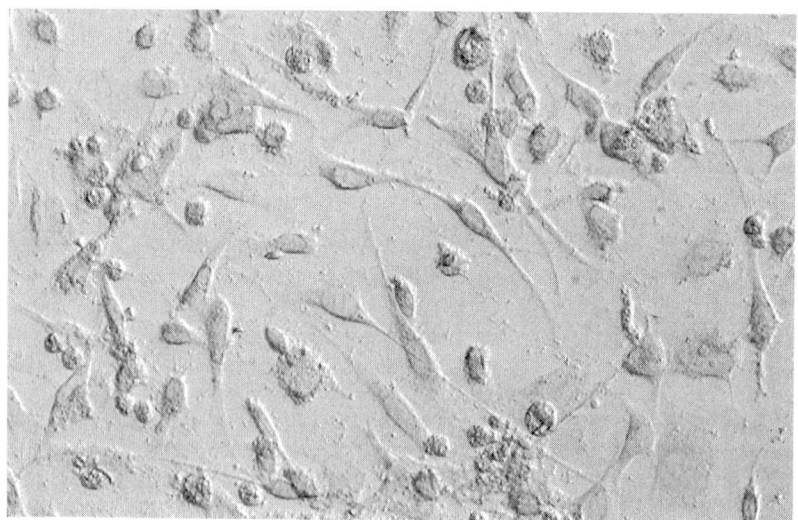

FIGURE 3. RN46A serotonergic cell line derived from E13 rat medullary raphe undergoing differentiation.

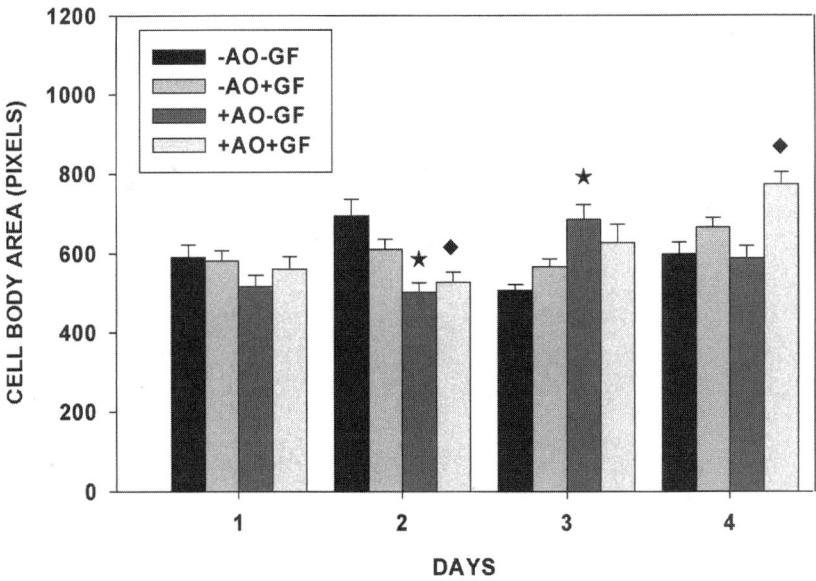

FIGURE 4. Cell body size of purified motor neurons in media with and without growth factors and antioxidant media supplements during the first 4 days in culture. Overall, cell body size did not appear to increase significantly over the course of 4 days; however, there was a highly significant contribution of growth factors to cell body size by day 4 ($p = 0.0001$; ANOVA and Scheffe F test).

few purified motor neurons survive beyond 6 days in culture (FIG. 2). In contrast, stably transfected RN46A cell lines grow confluent and survive for weeks when not challenged (FIG. 3). Murine dissociated spinal cord cultures survive 8–10 weeks;[8] motor neurons in these cultures survive an average of 6–12 days once they have been microinjected.[5]

When media in purified motor neuron cultures were supplemented with a cocktail of growth factors, there was a significant increase in cell body size (FIG. 4) and number of Islet+ motor neurons (FIG. 5) after 4 days in culture. Apoptosis, or programmed cell death, is an active process requiring protein synthesis and is characterized by morphological changes including chromatin condensation, cell shrinkage, and fragmentation of the cell with formation of apoptotic bodies.[9] Apoptosis plays an important role in developmental cell death and tissue morphogenesis; however, its contribution to cell death in adult-onset neurodegenerative disorders is still subject to debate.[10,11] The mode of cell death for >90% of purified motor neurons appeared to be apoptosis (FIGS. 6A and 6B). The most significant benefit to purified motor neuron cultures was provided by the antioxidant supplement to the media, which improved survival of motor neurons throughout the time in culture (FIG. 2). The antioxidant-mediated decrease in apoptosis (FIG. 6B) appeared to be independent of the addition of the growth factor cocktail.

The immortalized neuronal cell line, RN46A, was stably transfected with plasmid expression constructs bearing one of several mutant, or wild-type, human SOD1

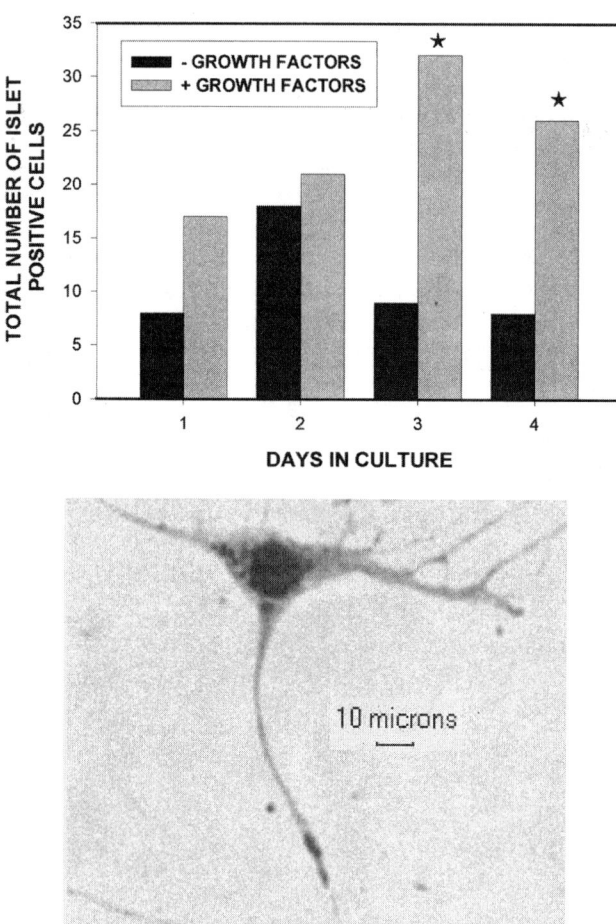

FIGURE 5. Islet-1, an intranuclear marker expressed at early stages of motor neuron differentiation, was identified in a subset of ChAT+ purified motor neurons that appeared to be primarily large motor neurons. **(Top)** The number of Islet+ neurons in 20% of 4 cover glasses was counted. Addition of neurotrophic factor cocktail (BDNF, GDNF, CNTF, and IGF-1) to the media led to an increase in the total number of Islet+ motor neurons at 3 and 4 days in culture ($p < 0.05$). **(Bottom)** An Islet+ neuron after 3 days in culture stained with Islet-1 and ChAT, both markers for motor neurons.

cDNAs. With transfection followed by hygromycin selection, and maintenance of the cultures in a low concentration of hygromycin, it was possible to obtain cell populations where virtually 100% of the cells expressed human SOD1 (FIG. 7). The stably transfected cell lines showed no significant differences in survival compared to controls. Sufficient numbers of mSOD- or wtSOD-expressing cells could be grown and isolated to measure SOD activity (FIG. 8A) and to determine how much human SOD

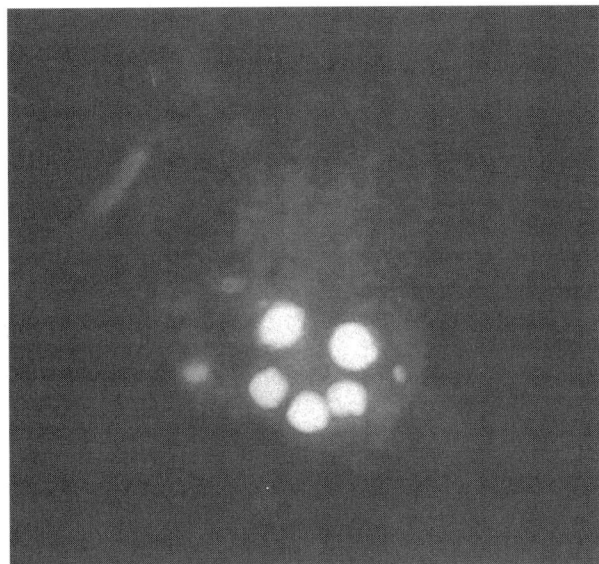

FIGURE 6A. The majority of purified motor neurons appeared to die by apoptosis: Hoechst staining of motor neuron nucleus displaying chromatin condensation and fragmentation.

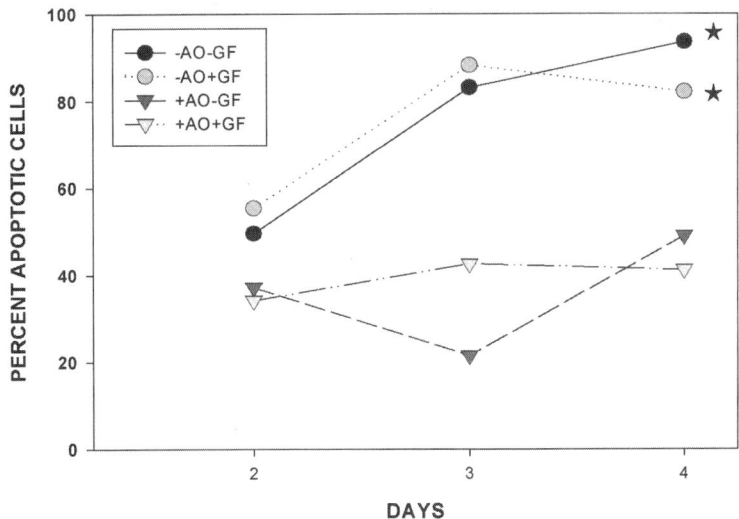

FIGURE 6B. The majority of purified motor neurons appeared to die by apoptosis: The fraction of *surviving* purified motor neurons undergoing apoptosis at any time in culture continued to increase over the course of 4 days. Apoptosis was significantly decreased by the addition of antioxidants to the culture media; addition of neurotrophic factor cocktail had no significant effect.

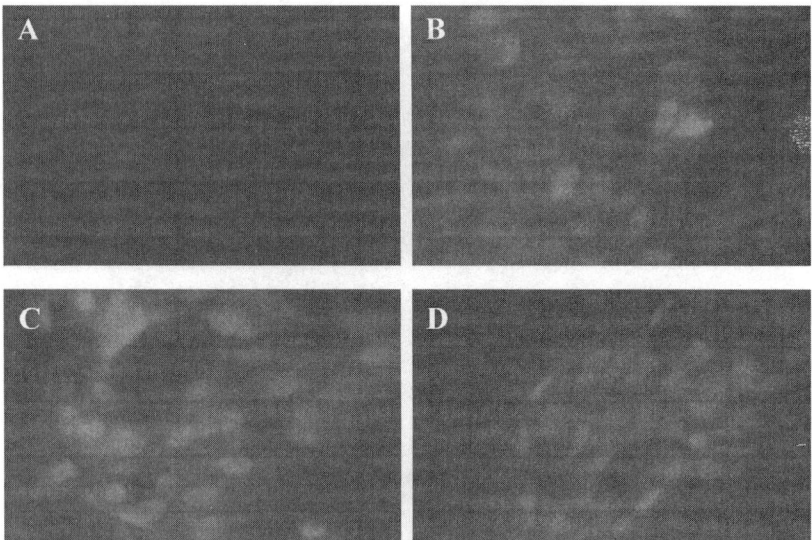

FIGURE 7. The RN46A serotonergic cell line was transfected with the plasmid pCEP4; mutant or wild-type human SOD1 cDNAs were cloned into this expression vector. After selection of stably transfected cell lines with hygromycin, expression of the human SOD1 protein (human-specific SOD1 antibody, Sigma) could be detected via Texas Red immunofluorescence in virtually 100% of cells: **(A)** pCEP4 empty vector alone; **(B)** pCN wild-type SOD1; **(C)** pC93B mutant SOD1; **(D)** pC149 mutant SOD1.

protein was being synthesized compared to native SOD1 (FIGS. 8B and 8C). Surprisingly, total SOD activity remained within a normal range of 4–8 U/mg protein in both control and mSOD cell lines. In fact, with the exception of cell line RN46A-pC37, levels of human SOD1 protein expressed did not vary significantly among the cell lines. Rapid turnover of the mutant protein in the cell lines combined with decreased catalytic activity of mSODs might account for the normal levels of SOD activity that were obtained. An original rationale for creating the stably transfected mSOD cell lines was to test how expression of mSOD might increase the vulnerability of neuronal cells to environmental toxins. Addition of Pb (70 µM), paraquat (0.5 mM), or styrene oxide (0.4–0.5 mM) to the culture media for 4 days led to variable onset of cell death that was predominantly apoptotic (FIG. 9A). Cell lines expressing mSOD were not always more vulnerable to the toxin than control cell lines (FIG. 9B), and no correlation could be established between vulnerability to an exogenous toxin and cellular SOD activity or SOD protein load in the various cell lines.

DISCUSSION

In addition to the *in vitro* models presented here, a third system involving primary culture of dissociated embryonic murine spinal cord has already been described.[5] In the dissociated spinal cord cultures, large motor neurons are able to fully differenti-

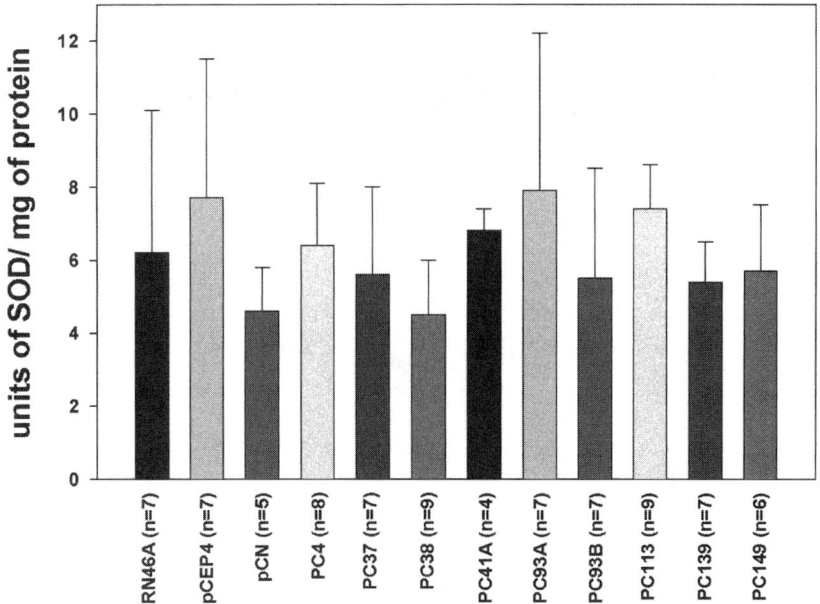

FIGURE 8A. SOD enzyme activity and protein levels in stably transfected RN46A cell lines: Units of SOD1 per mg total cellular protein in (left to right) native RN46A cells, pCEP4 only, pCN wild-type human SOD1, and 9 mutant SOD1 lines (pC4, pC37, pC38, pC41A, pC93A, pC93B, pC113, pC139, and pC149).

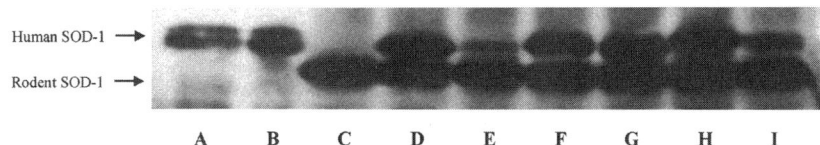

FIGURE 8B. SOD enzyme activity and protein levels in stably transfected RN46A cell lines: Western blot with immunodetection of human and rodent SOD1 (The Binding Site antibody). RN46A cells were transfected with wild-type or mutant human SOD1; 1×10^5 cells were lysed and electrophoresed on 15% polyacrylamide gel and transferred to PVDF. Human and/or rodent SOD1 could be detected (left to right): 100 ng human SOD1 standard; 50 ng human SOD1 standard; RN46A cell line; pCN wild-type human SOD1 transfected; mutant SOD1 transfected (pC37, pC93A, pC93B, pC113, and pC149).

ate and establish functional synapses; undisturbed, the cultures can survive for 2 months or longer. Motor neurons in the dissociated cultures express mSOD or wtSOD after nuclear microinjection of the plasmid constructs described above. In contrast to the purified motor neurons or the stably transfected neuronal lines, mature motor neurons die by necrotic mechanisms as often as by apoptotic mechanisms.[4,5] Moreover, antioxidants do not appear to be as effective a neuroprotective strategy for the motor neurons in dissociated cultures as they are in the purified

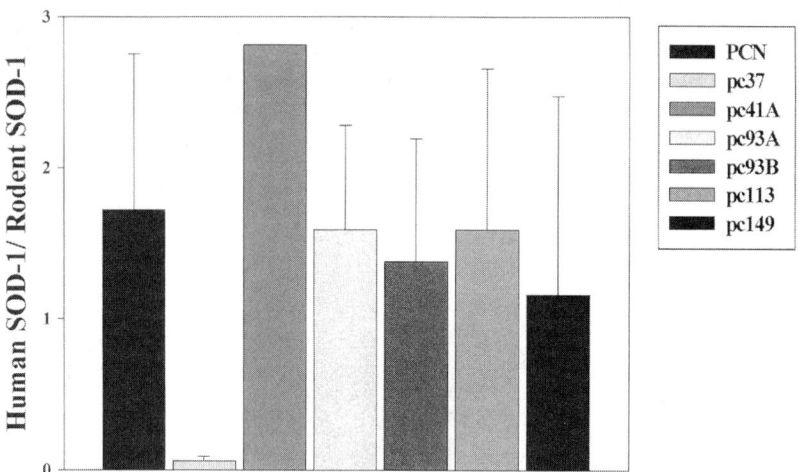

FIGURE 8C. SOD enzyme activity and protein levels in stably transfected RN46A cell lines: The ratio of human:rodent SOD1 protein was quantitated from Western blots by densitometry using Image Quant software (Molecular Dynamics) in five separate determinations per cell line. Left to right: pCN transfected wild-type human SOD1; transfected mutant SOD1 (pC37, pC41A, pC93A, pC93B, pC113, and pC149).

motor neuron cultures. For example, treatment of the dissociated cultures with glutathione ethyl ester provided complete protection against paraquat toxicity, partial protection against exogenous glutamate, and no protection against the expression of mSOD.[4] In comparison to mSOD-expressing neuronal cell lines, mature motor neurons in dissociated cultures were more vulnerable to exogenous environmental stressors. Tenfold or greater concentrations of paraquat or lead were needed before significant levels of cell death were seen in the transfected RN46A cells. The largest disadvantage of the microinjection/dissociated spinal cord culture system is that the small number of large motor neurons microinjected for a single time point (40–100 neurons) rules out the possibility of measuring transgene dosage, SOD enzymatic activity, or other biochemical parameters.

Although motor neurons in both primary culture systems originate from the equivalent embryonic stage of spinal cord, purified motor neurons do not thrive in the absence of glial or muscle-derived trophic support. Even addition of neurotrophic factor cocktail to these cultures does not appear to aid survival, but perhaps promotes differentiation. The purified motor neuron culture system may serve as a very useful model for understanding the apoptotic cell death process, which is a normal stage in development of the neuromuscular system.

Neuronal cell lines stably transfected and expressing mSOD appear to have adaptive survival ability, presumably a function of their immortalized status, which makes them more resistant than primary motor neurons to both expression of mSOD protein and addition of exogenous toxins. These cell lines might be employed in differential gene expression studies to identify genes that mediate their enhanced survival capabilities.

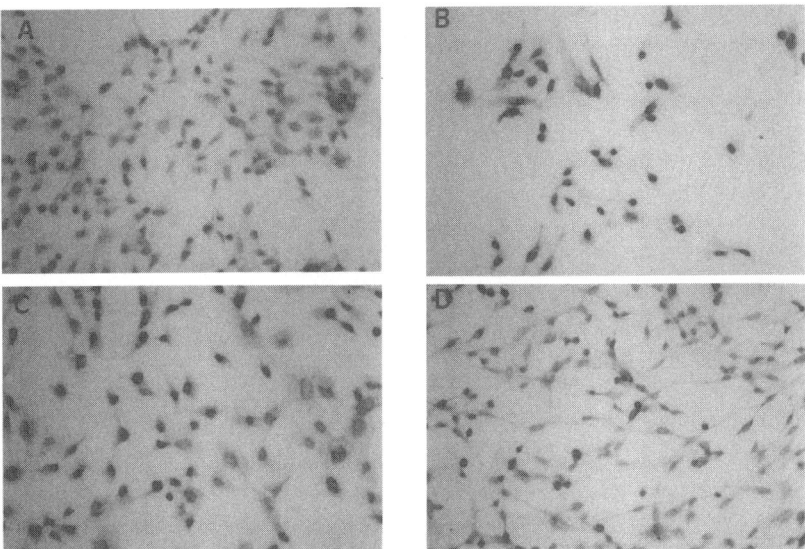

FIGURE 9A. Stably transfected RN46A cell lines were used to determine the relationship between expression of mutant SOD1 and vulnerability to environmental toxins: Apoptosis in the cell lines was measured after 4 days of exposure to the toxins using Biotin-14-dCTP labeling of DNA by terminal deoxynucleotide transferase enzyme. TUNEL+ cells have prominent darkly stained nuclei. Panels: (**A**) control media; (**B**) 70 μM Pb; (**C**) 0.5 mM paraquat; (**D**) 0.4 mM styrene oxide.

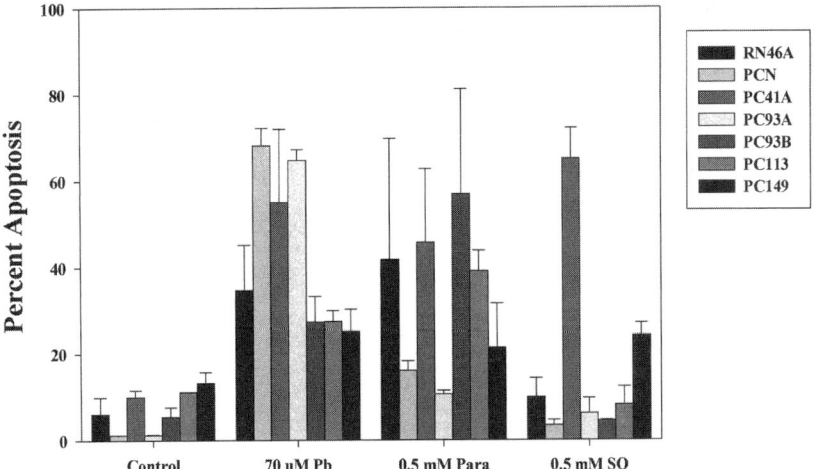

FIGURE 9B. Stably transfected RN46A cell lines were used to determine the relationship between expression of mutant SOD1 and vulnerability to environmental toxins: TUNEL+ cells were quantitated by counting and are shown as % of total cell number.

In conclusion, our studies with *in vitro* models of neurodegeneration have identified unique advantages and drawbacks of each system. Selection of an *in vitro* model system for investigation of neurodegeneration clearly requires consideration of some of the variable characteristics; assessment of these may render studies employing a particular model relatively meaningless. Likewise, care must be taken when comparing and interpreting data obtained from studies using different *in vitro* models of neurodegeneration.

ACKNOWLEDGMENTS

We would like to acknowledge the assistance of Dr. Martha Bohn, Dr. Heather Durham, and Rita Giuliano in these studies of *in vitro* models. The RN46A cell line was the generous gift of Dr. Scott Whittemore. Support for these studies was obtained from the following: ALS Association, MDA-USA, and NIHRO1 (to D. A. Figlewicz), and NIA/T32-AG00107 (to J. C. Turcotte).

REFERENCES

1. ROSEN, D.R., T. SIDDIQUE, D. PATTERSON *et al.* 1993. Mutations in Cu/Zn superoxide dismutase gene are associated with familial amyotrophic lateral sclerosis. Nature **362:** 59–62.
2. CAMU, W. & C.E. HENDERSON. 1992. Purification of embryonic rat motor neurons by panning on a monoclonal antibody to the low affinity NGF receptor. J. Neurosci. Methods **44:** 59–70.
3. WHITE, L.A., M.J. EATON, M.C. CASTRO *et al.* 1994. Distinct regulatory pathways control neurofilament expression and neurotransmitter synthesis in immortalized serotonergic neurons. J. Neurosci. **14:** 6744–6753.
4. ROY, J., S. MINOTTI, L. DONG *et al.* 1998. Glutamate potentiates the toxicity of mutant Cu/Zn superoxide dismutase in motor neurons by postsynaptic calcium-dependent mechanisms. J. Neurosci. **18:** 9673–9684.
5. DURHAM, H.D., J. ROY, L. DONG *et al.* 1997. Aggregation of mutant Cu/Zn superoxide dismutase proteins in a culture model of ALS. J. Neuropathol. Exp. Neurol. **56:** 523–530.
6. MISRA, H.P. & I. FRIDOVICH. 1972. The univalent reduction of oxygen by reduced flavins and quinones. J. Biol. Chem. **247:** 3170–3175.
7. ERICSON, J., S. THOR, T. EDLUND *et al.* 1992. Early stages of motor neuron differentiation revealed by expression of homeobox gene Islet-1. Science **256:** 1555–1560.
8. DOROUDCHI, M.M. & H.D. DURHAM. 1996. Activation of protein kinase C induces neurofilament fragmentation, hyperphosphorylation of perikaryal neurofilaments, and proximal dendritic swellings in cultured motor neurons. J. Neuropathol. Exp. Neurol. **55:** 246–256.
9. COLUMBANO, A. 1995. Cell death: current difficulties in discriminating apoptosis from necrosis in the context of pathological processes *in vivo*. Cell Biochem. **58:** 181–190.
10. MARTIN, L.J. 1999. Neuronal death in amyotrophic lateral sclerosis is apoptosis: possible contribution of a programmed cell death mechanism. J. Neuropathol. Exp. Neurol. **58:** 459–471.
11. MIGHELI, A., C. ATZORI, R. PIVA *et al.* 1999. Lack of apoptosis in mice with ALS. Nat. Med. **5:** 966–967.

In Vitro Systems as Simulations of *In Vivo* Conditions: The Study of Cognition and Synaptic Plasticity in Neurotoxicology[a]

M. E. GILBERT[b]

Neurotoxicology Division, National Health and Environmental Effects Research Laboratory, United States Environmental Protection Agency, Research Triangle Park, North Carolina, and Department of Psychology, University of North Carolina, Chapel Hill, North Carolina, USA

ABSTRACT: Neuroscientists have been engaged for decades in the search for brain regions and brain processes that underlie learning and memory. The effects of regional brain stimulation and ablation on behavior have been documented and inferences made on the impact of these manipulations on the psychological constructs of "learning" and "memory". Discovery of an electrophysiological property, long-term potentiation (LTP), greatly expanded the ability to probe cellular aspects of how memories are represented in the brain. The study of LTP serves as an excellent example of how *in vivo* phenomena can be taken to more simplified *in vitro* test systems to directly address cellular and biochemical mechanisms of information storage in brain.

Upon exposure to toxic substances, changes in behavior are often one of the first indications of impaired nervous system function. It has been well documented that agents such as lead, polychlorinated biphenyls, and solvents interfere with higher mental processing in humans (e.g., see references 1–5). Toxic substances that affect higher nervous system functions, such as learning, memory, and affect, most often are detected in the absence of knowledge of the underlying biological action of the toxicant. Learning, memory, and emotion are complex processes to study and remain areas of intensive research in the neurosciences. Thus, associating any toxicant-induced brain change to constructs as intangible as "cognition" or "affect", entities that can only be estimated by inference, adds an additional layer of complexity to any attempt to examine mechanisms of neurotoxicity.

---

[a]The information in this document has been funded by the U.S. Environmental Protection Agency. It has been subjected to review by the National Health and Environmental Effects Research Laboratory and approved for publication. Approval does not signify that the contents reflect the views of the Agency nor does mention of trade names or commercial products constitute endorsement or recommendation for use.

[b]Address for correspondence: M. E. Gilbert, Neurotoxicology Division (MD-74B), National Health and Environmental Effects Research Laboratory, U.S. Environmental Protection Agency, Research Triangle Park, NC 27711. Voice: 919-541-4394; fax: 919-541-4849.
gilbert.mary@epa.gov

Neuroscientists have been engaged for decades in the search for brain regions and brain processes that underlie learning and memory.[6–8] The effects of regional brain stimulation and ablation on behavior have been documented and inferences made on the impact of these manipulations on the psychological constructs of "learning" and "memory". These techniques have certainly been valuable in enhancing the ability to determine where in the brain certain types of learning processes may reside, but have told us little of how information is acquired and stored. Model systems have been developed to simplify this latter exploit. Long-term potentiation (LTP) is one such model system that has greatly expanded the ability to probe cellular aspects of how memories are represented in the brain.[9] The study of LTP serves as an excellent example of how *in vivo* phenomena can be taken to more simplified *in vitro* test systems to directly address cellular and biochemical mechanisms of information storage in brain.

WHAT IS LTP AND WHY IS IT IMPORTANT?

Synaptic transmission is the main mechanism by which neurons communicate. Environmental events are represented as spatiotemporal patterns of neural activity, and activity-dependent modification of synaptic strength is a means whereby representations of these events are stored. The notion that what is taking place in brain during learning is a change in the strength of synaptic connections has a long history,[10] but convincing evidence of a persistent enhancement in synaptic efficacy did not appear until the seminal report of LTP in the rabbit hippocampus by Bliss and Lomo.[9] These authors observed large, long-lasting augmentations in synaptic strength that followed application of high-frequency trains of electrical stimulation to incoming pathways of the hippocampus. The impact of their discovery was certainly not hindered by the fact that they had observed these changes in the hippocampus, a brain region known to be critical for certain forms of learning and memory.[6–8] Bliss and Lomo[9] postulated that this artificially induced augmentation in synaptic transmission reflected activation of processes that are actually used in the encoding of a memory. Intensive research since that time has revealed that LTP, or a similar process, appears to be a general property of many circuits in brain that are required for associative learning (see references 11–15).

PROPERTIES OF LTP

LTP has maintained its position as the most viable candidate for a memory storage mechanism in part because its properties are compliant with network theories of information storage (see references 16 and 17). These include the features of input specificity, cooperativity, saturability, and persistence. Input specificity indicates that only the pathways that are stimulated are potentiated. A change that is not localized to the synapses that were active would be too nonspecific to be useful as a memory model. Cooperativity among afferents is another feature of LTP based on observations that a certain threshold exists and a minimum period of stimulation must be achieved before LTP is induced. Thus, a minimal amount of presynaptic activity and postsynaptic activation is required to trigger LTP. Saturability indicates that LTP in the hippocampus is a memory storage mechanism with a finite capacity. This premise is based upon the observation that repetitive stimulation leads to an asymptotic level of LTP beyond which no further increase in synaptic strength can be induced. Finally, the durability of LTP in the hippocampus is certainly one of its most prominent features. LTP typically lasts as long as the preparation remains viable *in vitro*, and *in vivo* studies have demonstrated enhanced responses in hippocampus for several weeks.[15,18–20]

HOW MIGHT ENHANCED SYNAPTIC STRENGTH BE EXPRESSED?

A number of possible changes in synapse physiology and cell biophysical properties of activated neurons can lead to an enhancement in synaptic responsiveness. These include an increase in the amount of neurotransmitter released from the presynaptic terminal, more sensitive or a greater number of postsynaptic receptors, and an enlarged postsynaptic area. Changes in the physical structure of the postsynaptic spine or in the actual formation of new synapses resulting from LTP may also serve to enhance synaptic output. Evidence for each of these scenarios has been reported.[13,17,21–23]

BIOCHEMISTRY OF LTP

Many excellent reviews[17,24–30] of the biochemical substrates of LTP are available and the following provides a very simplified overview of the primary biochemical processes believed to contribute to this type of synaptic plasticity. Learning is based on increases in associative strength between previously unrelated events. In synaptic terms, strengthening of synaptic contacts requires the coincident activation of both pre- and postsynaptic elements. The lamellar structure of hippocampus with densely packed neurons, well-defined neurochemistry and neuroanatomy, and visual identification of distinct inputs has made this model system experimentally accessible for *in vitro* study. Glutamate is the primary excitatory neurotransmitter in the hippocampus. A boost to the field of LTP as a biological substrate of learning and memory occurred with the discovery of the properties of a subset of postsynaptic glutamate receptors, the *N*-methyl-D-aspartate (NMDA) receptors.[11,31–33] This voltage-gated ion channel is held closed during low-frequency activation by the presence of magnesium ions bound within the channel. Glutamate binds to the metabotropic receptor on the postsynaptic site to transduce normal synaptic communication. However, with sufficient postsynaptic depolarization, the magnesium block of the NMDA receptor channel is relieved and calcium and sodium are permitted to flow into the postsynaptic cell. Thus, the NMDA receptor has been characterized as a "coincidence detector", a means whereby a neuron can gauge the coincident pre- and postsynaptic activity across a synapse.

Calcium entry through voltage-sensitive NMDA channels is a critical step in the induction of LTP.[31,34] This rapid rise in intracellular calcium triggers a cascade of biochemical signaling events, the complexity of which is currently under intensive investigation in neuroscience.[27,28] Multiple kinase systems are activated by the receptor-mediated increase in intracellular calcium; the primary ones studied to date include protein kinase A (PKA), protein kinase C (PKC), and calcium-calmodulin kinase II (CAMKII). The cascade and sequence of kinase activation are critical for the encoding of synaptic information and the formation of a memory. Each kinase system appears to display a time-dependent profile of activation with respect to the learning event (see references 26 and 29). A variety of specific proteins are phosphorylated as a direct consequence of kinase activation and work in concert to produce both short-term and long-term modifications at the synapse.[24,25,30] Short-term modifications include the phosphorylation of additional receptors and ion channels to produce enhanced postsynaptic response amplitudes. Other proteins phosphorylated by kinase activation alter the cytoskeletal architecture to facilitate release of transmitter or postsynaptic activation. Phosphorylation of additional kinase systems induces more enduring modifications in synaptic transmission. Kinases of this class activate transcription factors of early and late effector genes that control synaptic growth and promote the persistence of LTP and presumably of memory.[17,26]

LTP AND LTD

A related form of synaptic plasticity, discovered in the cerebellum, but also demonstrated in hippocampal circuits, is long-term depression (LTD).[35–38] As the name implies, long-lasting suppression rather than enhancement of synaptic transmission characterizes LTD. Stimulation parameters required to produce LTP and LTD are distinct, but it appears that similar biochemical substrates are accessed by both processes.[17,38–40] In the case of LTP, strong depolarization and the large influx of calcium induced by high-frequency stimulation preferentially activate protein kinases and subsequent phosphorylation events that lead to strengthening of synaptic connections. In the case of LTD, small influxes of calcium over a more protracted period of time are induced by low-frequency stimulation. Selective activation of phosphatases that work on the same proteins and kinase systems as LTP serve to "dephosphorylate" these substrates and lead to a synaptic depression.

EVIDENCE FOR A ROLE OF THESE BIOCHEMICAL PROCESSES IN LEARNING AND MEMORY

When relying upon *in vitro* phenomena to study mechanisms of behavior, it is essential to take the observations back to the living organism. The issue of LTP as a memory model must deal with two levels of extrapolation: (1) Do the phenomena of LTP and LTD so well studied in the isolated *in vitro* preparation actually occur *in vivo*? (2) Do these phenomena truly represent a mechanism for memory formation *in vivo*? The first level of extrapolation is relatively easy to handle. Although the bulk of LTP studies have been conducted in brain slices maintained *in vitro*, the hippocampus is well suited for extrapolation from the *in vitro* to *in vivo* preparation. Its initial discovery was made in the dentate gyrus of the anesthetized rabbit and since that time LTP has been demonstrated in several brain regions in the fully con-

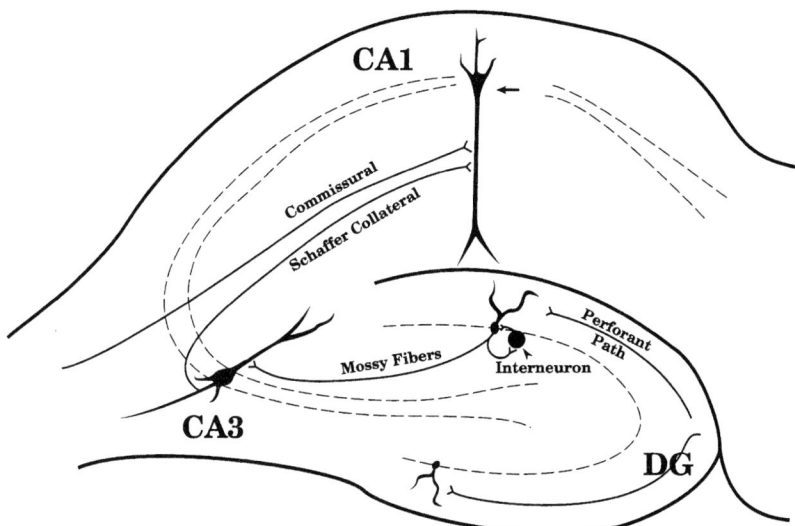

FIGURE 1. Schematic of the trisynaptic circuit in the dorsal rat hippocampus. Long-term potentiation (LTP) is typically induced in *in vitro* preparations by stimulating the axons of CA3 neurons, the Schaffer collaterals, which synapse directly onto the dendrites of CA1 pyramidal cells. The pyramidal cell layer is indicated by an arrow. LTP *in vivo* is typically induced by stimulating axons of neurons originating in the entorhinal cortex that course together to form the perforant path. These axons synapse directly onto the dendrites of dentate gyrus granule cells.

scious animal. The lamellar structure of the hippocampus, with well-defined inputs and outputs, permits recordings of large extracellular field potentials that very faithfully reflect the intracellular activity in the intact, unanesthetized animal.[41,42] Although hippocampal LTP appears to generally exhibit the same properties and constraints *in vivo* and *in vitro*, it has typically been investigated in two different subregions of the hippocampus by these two approaches. The dentate gyrus is the hippocampal subregion most accessible *in vivo*, whereas *in vitro* studies have largely focused on the pyramidal cells of hippocampal area CA1. Nonetheless, the underlying biochemical substrates of LTP in both of these hippocampal regions appear to be comparable. The ease of accessibility for experimental investigation *in vitro* (see FIG. 1) has promoted a detailed cellular and biochemical dissection of the underlying processes of use-dependent plasticity in hippocampus.

The second level of extrapolation concerns the degree to which LTP-like phenomena actually reflect the changes that occur during learning. The rodent hippocampus is critical for the processing of spatial information and contextual relationships between stimuli and events in the environment.[6,7] The bulk of evidence for LTP as a memory storage device derives from pharmacological manipulations that impair both LTP and spatial learning (e.g., see references 43–49). Similarly, detailed histochemical analysis of receptors and enzymes in hippocampus at various time points after training or after LTP (*in vitro* or *in vivo*) demonstrates comparable changes as a result of learning and LTP.[26,50] More recently, genetically altered mice with gene knockouts for specific receptors (e.g., NMDAR1), enzymes (e.g., CAMKII), or proteins (e.g., adhesion cell molecules) thought to be critical for hippocampal learning and hippocampal LTP show spatial learning deficits and LTP impairments *in vivo* and *in vitro* (see references 51 and 52). Despite these positive correlations, numerous reports have also appeared in which there is a lack of correspondence between electrophysiological and behavioral indices of learning; that is, treatments may impair hippocampal LTP, but fail to alter spatial learning, while others may disrupt spatial learning in the presence of robust hippocampal LTP (see reference 53). This lack of correlation has led to a certain amount of skepticism about the role of LTP in learning and memory.

WHY MIGHT LTP NOT MAP DIRECTLY ONTO SPATIAL LEARNING?

There are a number of reasons why such a correlational approach might fail (see reference 54 for review). One of the potential pitfalls may lie in the complexity of the behavioral tasks that have come to be the "hallmark" of hippocampal function.[6,7,49] Radial arm maze (RAM) and Morris water maze (MWM) learning are two standard tests of spatial learning that show dependence upon the hippocampus. In the RAM task, animals are placed in a center platform with arms emanating from it like the spokes on a wheel. The animal is to retrieve a food pellet from the end of each arm (typically 8 or 12 arms) without visiting each arm more than once.[7] In the MWM, animals are placed in a large tank of water and required to locate an escape platform hidden beneath the surface of the water. Rodents are very effective in utilizing the extramaze spatial cues to guide themselves to the untraversed arm or the correct position of the hidden platform.[45] These types of instrumental learning tasks, although well characterized pharmacologically and shown convincingly to require the hippocampus for their resolve, are limited as tools to relate specific brain activity to learning. The learning is protracted and the experimenter has little control over the temporal and configurational domain that guides the animal's response pattern to solve these spatial tasks. The quantity and quality of information available to the test subject are determined not by the experimenter, but by the behavior of the test subject itself (see references 55 and 56). Under such conditions, relating characteristics of an animal's behavior in space and time to the activation of a defined neural circuit and to neurochemical indices of synaptic plasticity becomes a daunting, if not untenable, task.

CLASSICAL CONDITIONING

Given the complications of instrumental learning tasks, many researchers have turned to the study of classical conditioning. Classical conditioning is the simplest form of associative learning, in which one "meaningful" stimulus (unconditioned stimulus, US) that elicits a reflexive response is presented close together in time with a neutral stimulus (conditioned stimulus, CS). With repetition, the previously neutral stimulus comes to elicit a manifestation of the reflexive response previously evoked only by the meaningful stimulus. One such classical conditioning procedure that has been extensively studied to understand brain mechanisms of learning and memory is cerebellar eye blink conditioning (see references 57 and 58). In eye blink conditioning, a puff of air is delivered to the eye (US) and elicits an eye blink (unconditioned response, UR). Repeated pairing of a neutral tone CS with the eye puff US eventually promotes activation of the eye blink response to presentation of the tone CS alone. Advantages over more complex forms of learning ascribed for the hippocampus are that the stimuli are well defined, their presentation and intensity can be precisely controlled, and the anatomical loci and circuitry activated by the tone, the air puff, and the reflexive arc driving the motor eye blink response have been identified (see FIG. 2). The neurological substrates underlying each component of this learning task have been deduced using a number of lesion, recording, and microstimulation techniques and have been found to involve the brain stem–cerebellar circuitry depicted in FIGURE 2.

HOW CLOSELY DO LTP AND LTD MIRROR "LEARNING" IN THE EYE BLINK CONDITIONING PARADIGM?

Armed with specific information on the requisite circuitry that drives the learning in cerebellar eye blink conditioning, at least two potential sites of synaptic plasticity exist whereby convergence between US and CS pathways can occur (see FIG. 2). One of these sites is a deep cerebellar nucleus, the nucleus interpositus; the second resides in the Purkinje cells of the cerebellar cortex. The nucleus interpositus receives sensory information about the air puff US via the inferior olivary nucleus in the brain stem. Sensory information about the tone CS also converges upon the nucleus interpositus via the brain stem pontine nucleus. The nucleus interpositus is directly connected to the output circuitry that drives the motor eye blink response. Thus, changes in synaptic strength at this site are pivotal to the control of the conditioned eye blink response.[58] Although not extensively studied, LTP has been observed in the nucleus interpositus in the intact animal.[59]

The other potential site of synaptic plasticity, the Purkinje cells of the cerebellar cortex, will also receive US information via the inferior olive. CS information is relayed from the pontine nucleus to the granule cells of the cerebellar cortex and then to the Purkinje cells. The Purkinje cells display synaptic LTD upon stimulation of the climbing fibers, axons emanating from the inferior olive, and the parallel fibers, the cerebellar granule cell axons. The Purkinje cells exert an inhibitory influence on the deep cerebellar nuclei, including the nucleus interpositus. Thus, a depression in synaptic strength in the Purkinje cells produces a "disinhibition" of interpositus output to the motor eye blink circuitry (see FIG. 2).

LTD was discovered and is best characterized in the cerebellum *in vitro*. However, demonstration of LTD in cerebellum has not been easy in the intact preparation (see references 37, 38, and 40). Although cerebellar LTP/LTD-like synaptic plasticity as a function of eye blink conditioning has not been directly demonstrated, Schreurs *et al.*[60] recently reported learning-specific changes in Purkinje cell membrane excitability in rabbit cerebellar slices *ex vivo* following conditioning. The strength of the cerebellar conditioning model system, one that contrasts sharply with hippocampal learning paradigms, is that the brain circuitry that drives the behavior has been well established. One of the limitations in bridging behavioral to electrophysiological indices of learning in this paradigm, however, is the relative inaccessibility of the circuitry under study for *in vivo* or *in vitro* analyses of use-dependent synaptic plasticity.

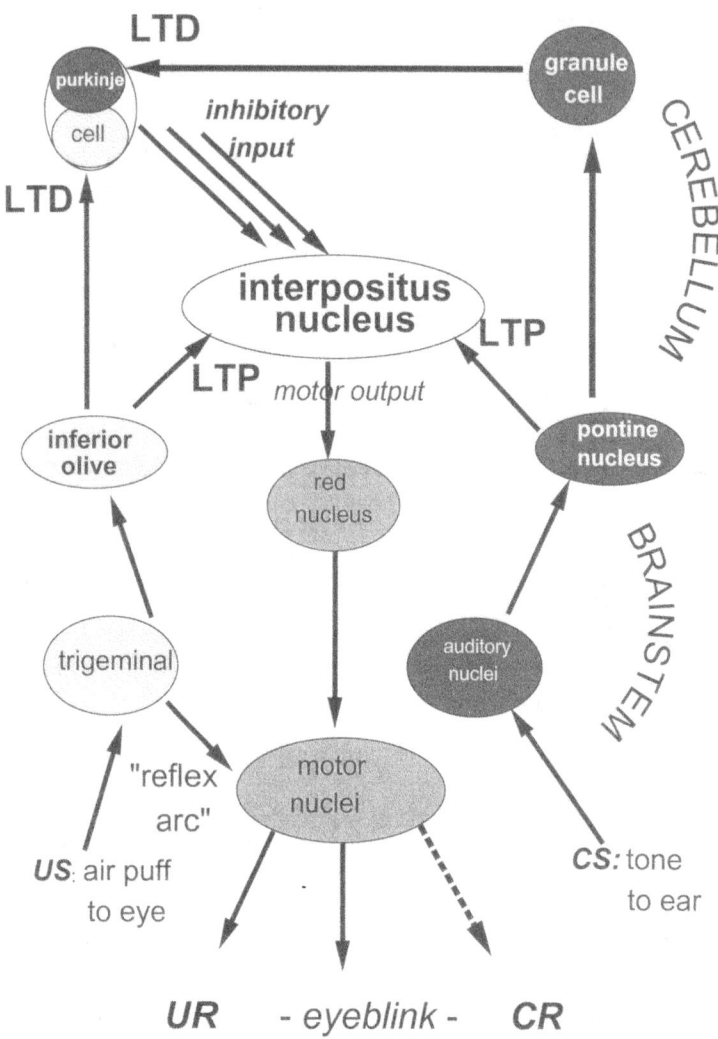

FIGURE 2. Circuitry involved in cerebellar eye blink conditioning. Information about the unconditioned stimulus (US) is transferred to the deep cerebellar nucleus, the nucleus interpositus, and the Purkinje cells of the cerebellar cortex via the inferior olive. Information about the conditioned stimulus (CS) also converges on the nucleus interpositus via the pontine nucleus. Purkinje cells receive CS information indirectly from the pontine nucleus via cerebellar granule cells. The nucleus interpositus is well positioned to modulate the motor output of the conditioned eye blink response (CR) by its connections to motor nuclei of the brain stem via the red nucleus. Long-term potentiation (LTP) and long-term depression (LTD) occur at points where the CS and US information converge, that is, the nucleus interpositus and the Purkinje cells of the cerebellar cortex. LTP has been observed in the interpositus nucleus *in vivo*.[57] Purkinje cells preferentially display LTD, which serves to dampen the inhibitory influence that these cells have on the interpositus nucleus, rendering them in a state of relative disinhibition. See text for additional details. Modified from Thompson and Krupa.[58]

FEAR CONDITIONING AND THE AMYGDALA

The limitations of the cerebellar model to link synaptic plasticity with learning may be overcome in another brain region for which a physiology of conditioning circuits has more recently emerged. In the amygdala fear conditioning model, the strength of the classical conditioning behavioral paradigm and the ease of accessibility of the amygdala circuitry for study of synaptic plasticity converge to directly address the role of LTP in learning. In this conditioning paradigm, a neutral tone CS is paired with a foot-shock US, and the learned behavioral "fear" response is indexed by the amount of "freezing" elicited in the animal by subsequent presentation of the tone alone. The amygdala has long been implicated in the control of affective behavior, and stimulation, lesioning, and recording studies have documented its role in fear behavior.[61,62] Afferents from the medial geniculate nucleus (MGN) of the thalamus, a relay station for sensory information from the periphery, synapse directly onto neurons in the lateral nucleus of the amygdala. High-frequency stimulation of these axons induces LTP in the amygdala and, as with hippocampal LTP, this synaptic plasticity is also NMDA-dependent.[61–63] In two recent reports, fear conditioning itself was shown to produce an enhancement in synaptic transmission in the amygdala akin to LTP induced by electrical stimulation.[64,65] This endogenous, behaviorally induced LTP was demonstrated in recordings from intact animals, as well as in tissue excised from animals following conditioning and studied *in vitro*. In the intact preparation, auditory evoked potentials were recorded in the amygdala when a tone CS was delivered to the animal. After a series of tone/foot-shock pairings, the synaptic potential evoked by the tone was potentiated in animals relative to preconditioning baseline amplitudes. No such augmentation in auditory evoked responses was observed in similarly treated animals who received the tone/shock combinations in an unpaired fashion.[65] Another group of investigators, following a similar behavioral paradigm, prepared slices containing the thalamic MGN and the lateral amygdala from animals the day after conditioning. In the *ex vivo* preparation, synaptic currents of amygdala neurons, a more direct measure of synaptic efficacy than field potentials, were increased in conditioned animals relative to unpaired controls.[64] Manipulation of the constituents of the external bathing medium revealed an increase in evoked transmitter release in amygdala slices from conditioned relative to unpaired control subjects. Thus, augmentations in presynaptic transmitter release may contribute to the enhanced postsynaptic currents that occur coincident with learning. These complementary *in vivo* and *in vitro* investigations of synaptic plasticity provide the most compelling evidence that a process like LTP may well serve as a learning mechanism.

WHAT IS THE RELEVANCE OF MECHANISMS OF SYNAPTIC PLASTICITY TO NEUROTOXICOLOGY?

One of the values of the LTP model system approach in general is to provide an interface between behavioral studies of cognition at the organismal level and studies of the neurochemical, cellular, and molecular substrates that drive the learned response. As discussed above, although direct linkages between the use-dependent synaptic plasticity and learning have been equivocal in the hippocampus, clear evidence that LTP-like plasticity accompanies learning has been recently provided in the classical fear conditioning paradigm and amygdala LTP. A process like LTP is also likely to serve a role in hippocampal learning and the challenge in neuroscience will be to design the appropriate behavioral and electrophysiological experimental conditions under which it can be observed.

In toxicology, we have moved from lethality (LD-50) studies to simple behavioral assessments of locomotor activity and neurological batteries to examine the potential for toxicants to impact upon nervous system function.[66] Standard operant conditioning paradigms have provided sensitive indicators and a wealth of information on chemically induced disruptions of behavior.[67] However, the underlying neurobiological substrates of these measures remain uncertain. Paralleling the track taken in the neurosciences, the hippocampus has been the primary focus of the limited number of neurotoxicology studies investigating synaptic plasticity as a surrogate for cognitive function. Reductions in the capacity to support LTP *in vivo* and *in vitro* have been demonstrated for neurotoxicants such as lead, PCBs, and ethanol (e.g., see references 19 and 68–79). As in neuroscience, a direct link between perturbance in synaptic plasticity and disruption of simple behavioral tasks dependent upon the hippocampus has been more difficult to demonstrate (e.g., see references 80 and 81).

The challenge to bridge this behavioral/electrophysiological gap in neurotoxicology is similar to the challenge faced in the neurosciences at large. Toxicological investigations are further complicated by the relative lack of toxicokinetic information and limited understanding of the cellular mechanisms through which most neurotoxicants act. In the next millennium, the means whereby xenobiotics interfere with induction, expression, and persistence of synaptic plasticity may serve us well in our understanding of how such chemicals perturb complex brain processes like cognition. Increased sophistication in our approach to study the neurobiological basis of toxicant-induced disruption of behavior and the physiological substrates that support that behavior will be required to accomplish this goal.

REFERENCES

1. BELLINGER, D., J. SLOMAN, A. LEVITON, M. RABINOWITZ, H.L. NEEDLEMEN & C. WATERNAUX. 1991. Low-level lead exposure and children's cognitive function in the preschool years. Pediatrics **87:** 219–227.
2. BUSHNELL, P.J. & K.M. CROFTON. 1999. Neurobehavioral toxicology of organic solvents. *In* Introduction to Neurobehavioral Toxicology: Food and Environment, pp. 395–428. CRC Press. Boca Raton, FL.
3. JACOBSON, J. & S.W. JACOBSON. 1996. Intellectual impairment in children exposed to polychlorinated biphenyls *in utero*. N. Engl. J. Med. **335:** 783–789.
4. PATANDIN, S., C.I. LANTING, P.G. MULDER, E.R. BOERSMA, P.J. SAUER & N. WEISGLAS-KUPERUS. 1999. Effects of environmental exposure to polychlorinated biphenyls and dioxins on cognitive abilities in Dutch children at 42 months of age. J. Pediatr. **134:** 33–41.
5. RIESS, J.A. & H.L. NEEDLEMAN. 1992. Cognitive, neural, behavioral effects of low-level lead exposure. *In* The Vulnerable Brain and Environmental Risks. Volume 2: Toxins in Food, pp. 111–126. Plenum. New York.
6. O'KEEFE, J. & L. NADEL. 1978. The Hippocampus as a Cognitive Map. Oxford University Press. London/New York.
7. OLTON, D.S., J.T. BECKER & G.E. HANDELMANN. 1979. Hippocampus, space, and memory. Behav. Brain Sci. **2:** 313–365.

8. SQUIRE, L.R. 1992. Memory and the hippocampus: a synthesis from findings with rats, monkeys, and humans. Psychol. Rev. **99:** 195–231.
9. BLISS, T.V.P. & T. LOMO. 1973. Long-lasting potentiation of synaptic transmission in the dentate area of the anaesthetized rabbit following stimulation of the perforant path. J. Physiol. (Lond.) **232:** 331–356.
10. HEBB, D.O. 1949. Organization of Behavior. Wiley. New York.
11. BLISS, T.V.P. & G.L. COLLINGRIDGE. 1993. A synaptic model of memory: long-term potentiation in the hippocampus. Nature **361:** 31–39.
12. MALENKA, R.C. & R.A. NICOLL. 1999. Long-term potentiation—a decade of progress? Science **285:** 1870–1874.
13. MARTINEZ, J.L. & B.E. DERRICK. 1996. Long-term potentiation and learning. Annu. Rev. Psychol. **47:** 173–203.
14. MCNAUGHTON, B.L. 1983. Activity dependent modulation of hippocampal synaptic efficacy: some implications for memory processes. *In* Neurobiology of the Hippocampus, pp. 233–251. Academic Press. New York.
15. RACINE, R.J., N.W. MILGRAM & S. HAFNER. 1983. Long-term potentiation phenomena in the rat limbic forebrain. Brain Res. **260:** 217–231.
16. MCNAUGHTON, B.L. 1993. The mechanism of expression of long-term enhancement of hippocampal synapses: current issues and theoretical implications. Annu. Rev. Physiol. **55:** 375–396.
17. WANG, J-H., G.Y.P. KO & P. KELLY. 1997. Cellular and molecular bases of memory: synaptic and neuronal plasticity. J. Clin. Neurophysiol. **14:** 264–293.
18. ABRAHAM, W.C., S.E. MASON-PARKER, J. WILLIAMS & M. DRAGUNOW. 1995. Analysis of the decremental nature of LTP in the dentate gyrus. Mol. Brain Res. **30:** 367–372.
19. GILBERT, M.E. & C.M. MACK. 1998. Chronic developmental lead exposure accelerates decay of long-term potentiation in rat dentate gyrus *in vivo*. Brain Res. **789:** 139–149.
20. JEFFERY, K.J., W.C. ABRAHAM, M. DRAGUNOW & S.E. MASON. 1990. Induction of fos-like immunoreactivity and the maintenance of long-term potentiation in the dentate gyrus of unanesthetized rats. Mol. Brain Res. **8:** 267–274.
21. EDWARDS, F.A. 1995. Anatomy and electrophysiology of fast central synapses lead to a structural model for long-term potentiation. Physiol. Rev. **75:** 759–787.
22. GEINISMAN, Y., L. DETOLEDO-MORRELL, F. MORRELL, I.S. PERSINA & M.A. BEATTY. 1996. Synapse restructuring associated with the maintenance phase of hippocampal long-term potentiation. J. Comp. Neurol. **368:** 413–423.
23. LYNCH, G., M. KESSLER, A. ARAI & J. LARSON. 1996. The nature and causes of hippocampal long-term potentiation. Prog. Brain Res. **183:** 233–250.
24. BENOWITZ, L.I. & A. ROUTTENBERG. 1997. GAP-43: an intrinsic determinant of neuronal development and plasticity. Trends Neurosci. **20:** 84–91.
25. GERENDASY, D.D. & J.G. SUTCLIFFE. 1997. RC3/neurogranin, a postsynaptic calpacitin for setting the response threshold to calcium influxes. Mol. Neurobiol. **15:** 131–163.
26. IZQUIERDO, I. & J.H. MEDINA. 1997. Memory formation: the sequence of biochemical events in the hippocampus and its connection to activity in other brain structures. Neurobiol. Learning Memory **68:** 285–316.
27. MICHEAU, J. & G. RIEDEL. 1999. Protein kinases: which one is the memory molecule? Cell. Mol. Life Sci. **55:** 534–548.
28. PASINELLI, P., G.M.J. RAMAKERS, I.J.A. URBAN, J.J.H. HENS, A.B. OESTREICHER, P.N.E. DEGRAAN & W.H. GISPEN. 1995. Long-term potentiation and synaptic protein phosphorylation. Behav. Brain Res. **66:** 53–59.
29. SILVA, A.J., K.P. GIESE, N.B. FEDOROV, P.W. FRANKLAND & J.H. KOGAN. 1998. Molecular, cellular, and neuroanatomical substrates of place learning. Neurobiol. Learning Memory **70:** 44–61.
30. SODERLING, T.R. 1997. Phosphorylation of non-NMDA glutamate receptor ion channels: implications for synaptic plasticity and their membrane topology. *In* The Ionotropic Glutamate Receptors, pp. 121–134. Humana Press. Totowa, NJ.
31. COLLINGRIDGE, G.L. 1992. The mechanism of induction of NMDA receptor–dependent long-term potentiation in the hippocampus. Exp. Physiol. **77:** 771–797.
32. COLLINGRIDGE, G.L. & T.V.P. BLISS. 1987. NMDA receptors—their role in long-term potentiation. Trends Neuropharmacol. **10:** 288–293.

33. MASSICOTTE, G. & M. BAUDRY. 1991. Triggers and substrates of hippocampal synaptic plasticity. Neurosci. Biobehav. Rev. **15:** 415–423.
34. MALENKA, R.C. 1992. The role of postsynaptic calcium in the induction of long-term potentiation. Mol. Neurobiol. **5:** 289–295.
35. CUMMINGS, J.A., R.M. MULKEY, R.A. NICOLL & R.C. MALENKA. 1996. Ca^{2+} signaling requirements for long-term depression in the hippocampus. Neuron **16:** 825–833.
36. DOYER, V., M.L. ERRINGTON, S. LAROCHE & T.V.P. BLISS. 1996. Low-frequency trains of paired stimuli induce long-term depression in area CA1, but not in dentate gyrus of the intact rat. Hippocampus **6:** 52–57.
37. ITO, M. 1989. Long-term depression. Annu. Rev. Neurosci. **12:** 85–102.
38. LEVENES, C., H. DANIEL & F. CREPEL. 1998. Long-term depression of synaptic transmission in the cerebellum: cellular and molecular mechanisms revisited. Prog. Neurobiol. **55:** 79–91.
39. DEBANNE, D. & S.M. THOMPSON. 1994. Calcium: a trigger for long-term depression and potentiation in the hippocampus. NIPS **9:** 256–260.
40. LINDEN, D.J. & J.A. CONNOR. 1995. Long-term synaptic depression. Annu. Rev. Neurosci. **18:** 319–357.
41. ANDERSEN, P. 1983. Operational principles of hippocampal neurons. *In* Neurobiology of the Hippocampus, pp. 81–86. Academic Press. New York.
42. LOMO, T. 1971. Patterns of activation in a monosynaptic cortical pathway: the perforant path to the dentate area of the hippocampal formation. Exp. Brain Res. **12:** 18–45.
43. BANNERMAN, D.M., M.A. GOOD, S.P. BUTCHER, M. RAMSEY & R.G.M. MORRIS. 1995. Distinct components of spatial learning revealed by prior training and NMDA receptor blockade. Nature **378:** 182–186.
44. DAVIS, S., S.P. BUTCHER & R.G.M. MORRIS. 1992. The NMDA receptor antagonist D-2-amino-5-phosphonopentanoate (D-AP5) impairs spatial learning and LTP *in vivo* at intracerebral concentrations comparable to those that block LTP *in vitro*. J. Neurosci. **12:** 21–34.
45. MORRIS, R.G.M., E. ANDERSON, G.S. LYNCH & M. BAUDRY. 1986. Selective impairment of learning and blockade of long-term potentiation by an N-methyl-D-aspartate receptor antagonist, AP5. Nature **319:** 774–776.
46. MORRIS, R.G.M. 1989. Synaptic plasticity and learning: selective impairment of learning in rats and blockade of long-term potentiation *in vivo* by the N-methyl-D-aspartate antagonist AP5. J. Neurosci. **9:** 3040–3057.
47. O'DELL, T.J., S.G.N. GRANT, K. KARL, P.M. SORIANO & E.R. KANDEL. 1992. Pharmacological and genetic approaches to the analysis of tyrosine kinase function in long-term potentiation. Cold Spring Harbor Symp. Quant. Biol. **52:** 517–526.
48. RIEDEL, G. & K.G. REYMANN. 1996. Metabotropic glutamate receptors in hippocampal long-term potentiation and learning and memory. Acta Physiol. Scand. **157:** 1–19.
49. STEELE, R.J. & R.G.M. MORRIS. 1999. Delay-dependent impairment of a matching-to-place task with chronic intrahippocampal infusion of the NMDA-antagonist, D-AP5. Hippocampus **9:** 118–136.
50. IZQUIERDO, I. & J.H. MEDINA. 1995. Correlation between pharmacology of long-term potentiation and the pharmacology of memory. Neurobiol. Learning Memory **63:** 19–32.
51. CHEN, J. & S. TONEGAWA. 1997. Molecular genetic analysis of synaptic plasticity, activity-dependent neural development, learning, and memory in the mammalian brain. Annu. Rev. Neurosci. **20:** 157–184.
52. MAYFORD, M., I.M. MANSUY, R.U. MULLER & E.R. KANDEL. 1997. Memory and behavior: a second generation of genetically modified mice. Curr. Biol. **7:** 580–589.
53. SHORS, T. & L.D. MATZEL. 1997. Long-term potentiation: what's learning got to do with it? Behav. Brain Sci. **20:** 597–655.
54. BARNES, C. 1995. Involvement of LTP in memory: are we "searching under the street light"? Neuron **15:** 751–754.
55. KEITH, J.R. & J.W. RUDY. 1990. Why NMDA-receptor-dependent long-term potentiation may not be a mechanism of learning and memory: reappraisal of the NMDA-receptor blockade strategy. Psychobiology **18:** 251–257.
56. RUDY, J.W. & J.R. KEITH. 1997. LTP and memory: déjà vu. Behav. Brain Sci. **20:** 629.

57. THOMPSON, R.F., S. BAO, L. CHEN, B.D. CIPRIANO, J.S. GRETHE, J.J. KIM, J.K. THOMPSON, J. TRACY, M.S. WENINGER & D.J. KRUPA. 1997. Associative learning. Int. Rev. Neurobiol. **41:** 151–189.
58. THOMPSON, R.F. & D.J. KRUPA. 1994. Organization of memory traces in the mammalian brain. Annu. Rev. Neurosci. **17:** 519–549.
59. RACINE, R.J., D.A. WILSON, R. GINGELL & D. SUNDERLAND. 1986. Long-term potentiation in the interpositus and vestibular nuclei in the rat. Exp. Brain Res. **63:** 158–162.
60. SCHREURS, B.G., P.A. GUSEV, D. TOMSIC, D.L. ALKON & T. SHI. 1998. Intracellular correlates of acquisition and long-term memory of classical conditioning in Purkinje cell dendrites in slices of rabbit cerebellar lobule HVI. J. Neurosci. **18:** 5498–5507.
61. DAVIS, M. 1992. The role of the amygdala in fear and anxiety. Annu. Rev. Neurosci. **15:** 353–375.
62. MARIN, S. 1996. Synaptic transmission and plasticity in the amygdala: an emerging physiology of fear conditioning circuits. Mol. Neurobiol. **13:** 1–22.
63. FANSELOW, M.S. & J.J. KIM. 1994. Acquisition of contextual Pavlovian fear condition is blocked by application of an NMDA receptor antagonist D,L-2-amino-5-phosphonovaleric acid to the basolateral amygdala. Behav. Neurosci. **108:** 210–212.
64. MCKERNAN, M.G. & P. SHINNICK-GALLAGHER. 1997. Fear conditioning induces a lasting potentiation of synaptic currents *in vitro*. Nature **390:** 607–611.
65. ROGAN, M.T., U.V. STAUBLI & J. LEDOUX. 1997. Fear conditioning induces associative long-term potentiation in the amygdala. Nature **390:** 604–607.
66. KULIG, B.M. & R.M.A. JASPERS. 1999. Assessment techniques for detecting neurobehavioral toxicity. *In* Introduction to Neurobehavioral Toxicology: Food and Environment, pp. 70–113. CRC Press. Boca Raton, FL.
67. CORY-SLECHTA, D.A. 1994. Neurotoxicant-induced changes in schedule-controlled behavior. *In* Principles of Neurotoxicology, pp. 313–344. Dekker. New York.
68. ALTMANN, L., M. GUTOWSKI & H. WIEGAND. 1994. Effects of maternal lead exposure on functional plasticity in the visual cortex and hippocampus of immature rats. Dev. Brain Res. **81:** 50–56.
69. ALTMANN, L., H. LILIENTHAL, J. HANY & H. WIEGAND. 1998. Inhibition of long-term potentiation in developing rat visual cortex, but not hippocampus by *in utero* exposure to polychlorinated biphenyls. Dev. Brain Res. **110:** 257–260.
70. ALTMANN, L., H. WEINAND-HAERER, H. LILIENTHAL & H. WIEGAND. 1995. Maternal exposure to polychlorinated biphenyls inhibits long-term potentiation in the visual cortex of adult rats. Neurosci. Lett. **202:** 53–56.
71. GILBERT, M.E. 1997. Towards the development of a biologically-based dose-response model for lead neurotoxicity. Am. Zool. **37:** 389–398.
72. GILBERT, M.E. & K.M. CROFTON. 1999. Developmental exposure to a complex PCB mixture (Aroclor 1254) produces a persistent impairment in long-term potentiation in the dentate gyrus *in vivo*. Brain Res. In press.
73. GILBERT, M.E. & D. LIANG. 1998. Alterations in synaptic transmission and plasticity in hippocampus by a complex PCB mixture, Aroclor 1254. Neurotoxicol. Teratol. **20:** 383–389.
74. GILBERT, M.E., C.M. MACK & S.M. LASLEY. 1999. The influence of developmental period of lead exposure on long-term potentiation in the rat dentate gyrus *in vivo*. Neurotoxicology **20:** 71–82.
75. GILBERT, M.E., C.M. MACK & S.M. LASLEY. 1999. Chronic developmental lead exposure impairs hippocampal long-term potentiation *in vivo*: a dose-response analysis. Neurotoxicology **20:** 57–70.
76. NIEMI, W.D., J. AUDI, B. BUSH & J.O. CARPENTER. 1998. PCBs reduce long-term potentiation in the CA1 region of rat hippocampus. Exp. Neurol. **151:** 26–34.
77. SUTHERLAND, R.J., R.J. MCDONALD & D.D. SAVAGE. 1997. Prenatal exposure to moderate levels of ethanol can have long-lasting effects on hippocampal synaptic plasticity in adult offspring. Hippocampus **7:** 232–238.
78. WONG, P.W., R.M. JOY, T.E. ALBERTSON, S.L. SCHANTZ & I.N. PESSAH. 1997. *Ortho*-substituted 2,2′,3,5′,6-pentachlorobiphenyl (PCB 95) alters rat hippocampal ryanodine receptors and neuroplasticity *in vitro*: evidence for altered hippocampal function. Neurotoxicology **18:** 443–456.

79. ZAISER, A.E. & V. MILETIC. 1997. Prenatal and postnatal chronic exposure to low levels of inorganic lead attenuates long-term potentiation in the adult rat hippocampus *in vivo*. Neurosci. Lett. **239:** 128–130.
80. ELLIOTT, A. & V. MILETIC. 1997. A disconnection between spatial learning and LTP in young rats chronically exposed to lead. Toxicologist **36:** 57.
81. SAMSAM, T. & M.E. GILBERT. 1999. Developmental lead (Pb) exposure fails to disrupt spatial learning in the Morris water maze. Toxicol. Sci. **48:** 360.

Transgenic Zebrafish as Sentinels for Aquatic Pollution

MICHAEL J. CARVAN III,[a] TIMOTHY P. DALTON,[a] GARY W. STUART,[b] AND DANIEL W. NEBERT[a,c]

[a]*Center for Environmental Genetics (CEG) and Department of Environmental Health, University of Cincinnati Medical Center, Cincinnati, Ohio 45267-0056, USA*

[b]*Department of Life Sciences, Indiana State University, Terre Haute, Indiana 47809, USA*

ABSTRACT: Using the *golden* mutant zebrafish having a decrease in interfering pigmentation, we are developing transgenic lines in which DNA motifs that respond to selected environmental pollutants are capable of activating a reporter gene that can be easily assayed. We have begun with three response elements that recognize three important classes of foreign chemicals. Aromatic hydrocarbon response elements (AHREs) respond to numerous polycyclic hydrocarbons and halogenated coplanar molecules such as 2,3,7,8-tetrachlorodibenzo-*p*-dioxin (TCDD; dioxin) and polychlorinated biphenyls. Electrophile response elements (EPREs) respond to quinones and numerous other potent electrophilic oxidants. Metal response elements (MREs) respond to heavy metal cations such as mercury, copper, nickel, cadmium, and zinc. Soon, we will include estrogen response elements (EREs) to detect the effects of environmental endocrine disruptors, and retinoic acid response elements (RARE, RXRE) to detect the effects of retinoids in the environment. Each of these substances is known to be bioconcentrated in fish to varying degrees; for example, 10^{-17} M TCDD in a body of water becomes concentrated to approximately 10^{-12} M TCDD in a fish, where it would act upon the AHRE motif and turn on the luciferase (*LUC*) reporter gene. The living fish as a sentinel will not only be assayed intact in the luminometer, but—upon several days or weeks of depuration—would be usable again. To date, we have established that zebrafish transcription factors are able to recognize both mammalian and trout AHRE, EPRE, and MRE sequences in a dose-dependent and chemical-class-specific manner, and that expression of both the *LUC* and jellyfish green fluorescent protein (*GFP*) reporter genes is easily detected in zebrafish cell cultures and in the intact live zebrafish. Variations in sensitivity of this model system can be achieved by increasing the copy number of response elements and perhaps by altering the sequence of each core consensus response element and flanking regions. This transgenic technology should allow for a simple, exquisitely sensitive, and inexpensive assay for monitoring aquatic pollution. We have already initiated studies using sentinel zebrafish to monitor a public drinking water source.

[c]Corresponding author: Daniel W. Nebert, Department of Environmental Health, University of Cincinnati Medical Center, P.O. Box 670056, Cincinnati, OH 45267-0056. Voice: 513-558-4347; fax: 513-558-3562.
dan.nebert@uc.edu

INTRODUCTION

Exposure to numerous man-made and natural environmental agents poses a significant threat to human health. For many of these dangerous toxic agents, aquatic environments serve as the major route of distribution, and their sediments represent the ultimate sink. Human exposure to many aquatic pollutants occurs primarily through the ingestion of contaminated fish and/or shellfish.[1] Fish accumulate environmental contaminants by absorption across the gill epithelium and primarily by bioconcentration in the food chain. It has been demonstrated that this bioconcentration can be in excess of 40,000 times for Hg^2 and 100,000 times for TCDD.[3] Humans, unfortunately, are at the end of the food chain.

In order to protect human health, regulatory agencies have set limits on the concentration levels and kinds of pollutants allowed to enter bodies of water. These water-quality criteria are established on the basis of correlations between the concentration of a pollutant in a body of water and the accumulation of that pollutant in fish; ultimately, these data are extrapolated to risk assessment methodologies in humans. There is no mathematical formula in which the concentration of a particular contaminant, measured at its source, can be correlated to a concentration of that contaminant in fish.[1,4]

In this article, we first discuss the traditional methods for environmental monitoring of aquatic systems, including biological-impact analyses of complex mixtures. Next, we describe the principle of "bioconcentration" and the genetic/genomic reasons behind our choice of using zebrafish. We then describe our transgenic zebrafish model system and its successes in zebrafish cell culture, as well as the intact fish. Last, we describe our ongoing field tests, using these sentinel zebrafish to monitor drinking water in Clermont County, Ohio.

ENVIRONMENTAL MONITORING OF WATER SOURCES

In monitoring the quality of the aquatic environment, a major approach involves the quantitation of water, sediment, or tissue residue levels by analytical chemical methods; these are generally expensive, labor-intensive, and slow. This process usually includes the acquisition of a sample in the field, transport back to the analytical facility, sample processing, data collection, and finally data analysis. This is the more straightforward of the methods used, but also the more expensive, requiring extensive technical expertise in the analysis of pesticide, inorganic, nonpesticide organic, physical, and radiological parameters.[5]

Wild-caught fish are often used as a biomonitor to indicate the potential for human exposure to polycyclic hydrocarbon, oxidant, and metal contaminants. This method is proposed to circumvent problems related to correlating effluent concentrations at the source to concentrations in fish tissues. The evaluation of fish tissues for the presence of dangerous foreign chemical(s) is also quite expensive and labor-intensive and of limited utility because the bioavailability of a particular chemical(s) in the body of water is often unknown.

HOW TO ESTIMATE THE BIOLOGICAL IMPACT OF COMPLEX MIXTURES

Three types of biological-impact analyses are performed and each requires varying levels of technical expertise, specialized facilities and equipment, and time: (a) the exposure of test organisms in the laboratory to effluents and receiving waters can be carried out in order to estimate the toxicity of the sample;[6] (b) an estimate of the quality of the biological community at a given site is often performed; this involves evaluation of species richness and composition, trophic composition, and individual abundance and condition;[7] and (c) the alteration of biomolecules and/or changes in simple biochemical physiological responses can be measured and can serve as early warning systems as the most sensitive biological response for delineating potential areas of pollution impact.[8]

In fish, the most common assays require the collection of specimens and preparation of the appropriate tissue and/or biochemical samples (i.e., liver homogenate, DNA, etc.). Specific assays have traditionally involved the analysis of DNA damage, factors that regulate redox potential in the cell (glutathione, ascorbic acid, and α-tocopherol), or quantitation of the activity of enzymic defenses such as superoxide dismutase, catalase, and glutathione peroxidase.[9] Changes in the expression of pollutant-inducible genes have also been used to indicate the exposure to a wide variety of contaminants.[10–13] Such analyses require specialized equipment found in most laboratories that use the latest molecular biological tools, specialized training in the use of such tools, and great care in sample handling to limit denaturing relevant mRNA and proteins.

Although environmental pollutants are known to act upon several fish enzyme systems, there are inherent limitations in the interpretation of such data because a number of physiological, genetic, and metabolic factors have an impact on these multifunctional enzyme complexes.[8,10,14–18] Individual variability is likely to be striking when measurements from several fish are taken. Moreover, the fish tissues require great care in handling so as to try to limit denaturation and/or proteolysis.

BIOCONCENTRATION

It has long been established that environmental contaminants are bioconcentrated in fish and other aquatic organisms. The degree of bioconcentration will vary, depending upon the species, type of contaminant (due to solubility in water), the organism's capacity for metabolism and excretion, and chemical properties of the water (e.g., concentration of ionic and organic material affecting solubility). However, related chemical contaminants under standard conditions will be bioconcentrated to a similar degree for most species of fish. Contaminant levels in wild fish are often 1000 to 100,000 times higher than levels in their environment. For example, mercury levels can be more than 40,000 times higher in fish muscle tissue as compared with that in the surrounding water.[2] TCDD has been reported[3] to become bioconcentrated 100,000-fold in fish. This means that 10^{-17} M TCDD in the water or sediments would be bioconcentrated in fish to about 10^{-12} M (0.32 parts per trillion) and might activate the transcription of at least some of the dioxin-inducible genes, of which there are several dozen genes.[19] It is this process of gene induction, combined in an organism that bioconcentrates polluting chemicals, that we have exploited in our transgenic zebrafish model system.

WHY USE ZEBRAFISH?

The zebrafish is an efficient vertebrate model system because of its relatively short reproductive cycle, the large number of progeny that can be produced, and the relatively small space needed to maintain large numbers of offspring at low cost. Zebrafish embryos are also transparent and accessible throughout development, which allows for easy microinjection and other manipulations. Moreover, the zebrafish is becoming a powerful system for genetic analysis, with the development of a high-density genome map[20] and intentions of the Zebrafish Genome Project to completely sequence this (comparatively small) genome within the next several years.

Relatively simple and reliable methods for the production of transgenic zebrafish have also been developed.[21,22] Gene transfer into embryos has improved with the use of retroviral vectors[23] and transposons,[24,25] and the use of border elements has stabilized the expression of transgenes in subsequent generations.[26]

OVERVIEW OF OUR TRANSGENIC ZEBRAFISH MODEL SYSTEM

We are developing a model system that uses transgenic zebrafish with an easily assayable reporter gene under the control of pollutant-inducible DNA response elements (FIG. 1). Transgenic zebrafish, carrying pollution-inducible response elements, are placed in the water to be tested, and the contaminants become bioconcentrated (generally 1000- to 40,000-fold, relative to the water) in the tissues of the fish, thereby activating specific response elements, which upregulate the *LUC* reporter gene. Fish are then removed from the test water and placed immediately in a luminometer cuvette and incubated with luciferin. Luciferin is rapidly taken up into the tissues of the fish and oxidized by luciferase, and light is produced. The luminescence is proportional to the environmental concentration of the pollutant (to which the fish had been exposed), which drives the expression of the *LUC* gene by means of the various DNA motifs. The luminescence is quantitated in the luminometer. In each response element–containing construct, the expression of the *LUC* gene is activated by a specific class of polluting chemicals, allowing for differential identification of pollutants in a complex mixture. This assay does not require killing the fish and allows for repeated analysis of the same site with the same fish. The sensitivity of the system can be manipulated by varying the sequence of the response element.

This zebrafish model system will provide sensitive, economical, and practical biological monitors for specific common aquatic pollutants and should be able to differentiate between chemical classes within a complex mixture. The only equipment required to detect luciferase activity is a luminometer. In this living system, the only reagent needed is luciferin.

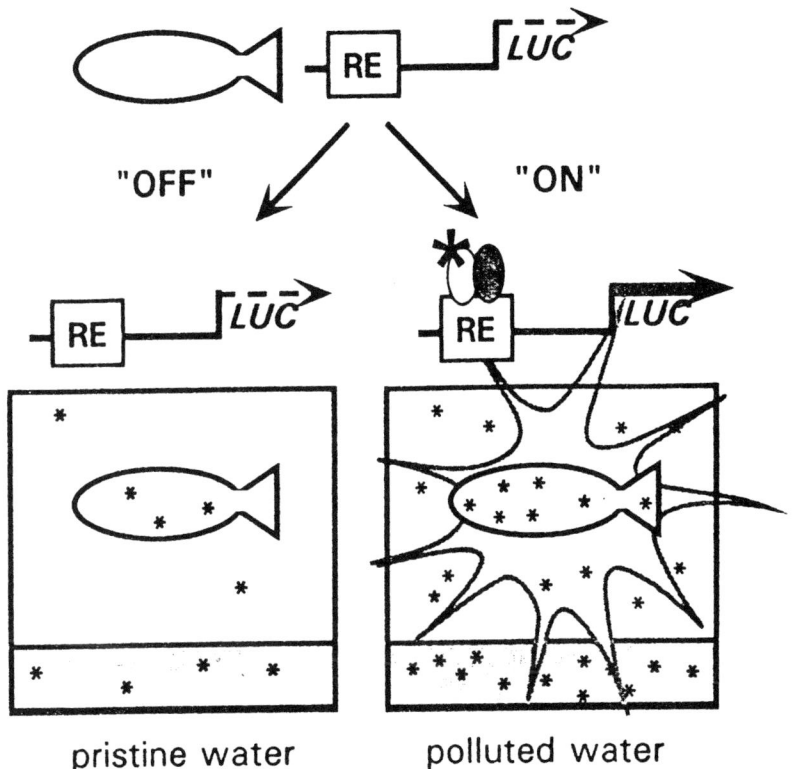

FIGURE 1. Schematic diagram of the transgenic zebrafish model system as a sentinel for monitoring of aquatic pollution. Transgenic zebrafish, carrying pollution-inducible response elements, are placed in the water to be tested, and the contaminants (*) are bioconcentrated in the tissues of the fish, thereby activating any specific response element (RE), which then upregulates the *LUC* gene. The higher the concentration of pollutant, the greater the luminescence in this assay. In each response element–containing construct, the expression of the *LUC* gene is activated by a specific class of polluting chemicals, allowing for the differential identification of pollutants in a complex mixture. The sensitivity of the system can be manipulated by varying the copy number, and the nucleotide sequence, of the response element.

BENEFITS OF THIS TRANSGENIC ZEBRAFISH MONITORING SYSTEM

There are several advantages of this model system in the detection of aquatic pollutants. First, data analysis is much faster. Environmental agents generally become bioconcentrated in fish in a matter of minutes.[3] Luciferase readings from 20 zebrafish, which might indicate (for example) a specific increase in Hg concentrations, can be achieved in less than 30 min, including the time required for luciferin uptake. Traditional analytical chemical methods take days from the time of sampling to the determination of pollutant values. Second, data acquisition is significantly cheaper and thus allows for the sampling of more sites. Traditional analytical chemical equipment is expensive. Shipping samples to a central analytical facility might reduce the cost per sample, but greatly increases the time required for data acquisition and analysis. Luciferase readings from these zebrafish can be analyzed in the back of a truck, or in a boat, with a $5000 luminometer and a laptop computer, connected to a regular automobile (or boat) battery. Third, *in vivo* bioaccumulation in fish is a much better indicator of potential exposure via consumption of contaminated fish than is the analysis of water and/or sediment samples. Fish are the direct source of most pollutant exposure and, as described above, fish are able to bioconcentrate pollutants in their environment. If water-borne pollution, rather than fish consumption, is the concern for estimating human exposure, then analyzing fish for biological effects will also give us a better understanding of the bioavailability of aquatic pollutants.

MODULAR ENHANCER UNITS, OR "RESPONSE ELEMENTS"

In the past 15 years, there has been a growing number of identified and characterized sequence-specific DNA motifs, located in the regulatory regions of all genes, that respond to an intracellular or extracellular stimulus by means of a signal transduction cascade—resulting in activated transcription factors that bind to the motif and that either up- or downregulate gene expression.[27,28] These stimuli not only can be endogenous compounds or changes in homeostasis, but also can be exogenous substances (e.g., environmental pollutants). Inducible response elements consist of a core consensus sequence, which usually is influenced by its flanking sequences and/or nearby multiple response elements (i.e., cooperativity) in causing maximal induction. The six DNA motifs—plus their core consensus sequences and basic properties—that we are using, or plan to use soon, in our transgenic zebrafish model system are summarized in TABLE 1 and described briefly below.

Aromatic Hydrocarbon Response Element (AHRE)

Ligands for the Ah receptor (AHR) activate the AHRE and cause many adverse biological effects, including immunosuppression, teratogenesis, tumor promotion, endocrine disruption, and cardiovascular disease.[29,30] Upon binding ligand, the AHR translocates to the nucleus and binds to AHRE motifs located in the promoter region of the mammalian *CYP1A1* and probably more than a dozen other genes (reviewed in references 19, 31, and 32). Halogenated and nonhalogenated polycyclic hydrocarbons (e.g., polychlorinated biphenyls, TCDD, benzo[a]pyrene) are ligands for the AHR and thus activate genes via AHREs. In fact, the observation that the level of inducible *CYP1A1* activity—in the nonmigrant cunner (*Tautogolabrus adspersus*) fish—varies as an inverse function of the distance from petroleum-contaminated waters near Newfoundland, Canada,[10] led to our original conception of designing this transgenic zebrafish model system.

Electrophile Response Element (EPRE)

Also called "antioxidant response element" (ARE), the EPRE is activated following treatment with potent oxidants and electrophiles, leading to the induction of numerous stress-inducible genes (reviewed in references 32 and 33). Electrophilic

TABLE 1. Six DNA motifs that respond to environmental pollutants

Response element	Consensus sequence 5′–3′	Activating agents	Transcription factors	Normal genes upregulated
AHRE	TWGCGTG	Dibenzo-*p*-dioxins, dibenzofurans, planar polychlorinated biphenyls, and polycyclic aromatic hydrocarbons	AH receptor + ARNT heterodimer	Cytochromes P450 1 (CYP1A, 1B), quinone oxidoreductase, glutathione transferase, UDP glucuronosyl-transferases
EPRE	RTGACNNNGC	Planar aromatic hydrocarbons, potent electrophiles (heavy metals, arsenicals, diphenols, quinones, azo dyes)	NF-E2-related factor 1 (?), NF-E2-related factor 2 (?), small Maf (?), ARE-BP (?)	Heme oxygenase, γ-glutamate-cysteine ligase, quinone oxidoreductase, glutathione transferase, UDP glucuronosyl-transferase
MRE	TGCRCNCGG	Heavy metals	MTF-1	Metallothioneins, γ-glutamate-cysteine ligase
ERE	GGTCANNNTGACC	Estrogen, pharmaceuticals, pesticides, chlorinated aromatic hydrocarbons, phytoestrogens	Estrogen receptor homodimer	Estrogen-responsive finger protein, vitellogenin, glucose-6-phosphatase, lactoferrin
RARE	RGGTCA(N$_{0-8}$)RGGTCA	Retinoic acid and other retinoids—natural and pharmaceutical	Retinoic acid receptor homodimers, heterodimers with retinoid X receptor	*Hoxa1*, retinoic acid receptor-β, cellular retinoic acid binding protein II, α-fetoprotein
RXRE	GGGGTCAAAGGTCA GGGGTCATGGGGTCA	Retinoic acid and other retinoids—natural and pharmaceutical	Retinoid X receptor homodimers	Apolipoprotein A1

NOTE: Several properties of the pollution-inducible response elements are listed. Extended flanking sequences, which may be necessary for maximal response, are highly variable and not shown. As indicated, some genes can be induced by several response elements due to the complexity of their 5′ flanking sequences or the oxidative properties of the inducing pollutant. Within each consensus sequence: N = A, T, G, or C; R = A or G; W = A or T.

compounds and metabolites that activate EPREs also react with nucleophilic centers on macromolecules and are involved in mutagenesis, carcinogenesis, and aging.[34] Inducing agents include not only reactive hydrogen peroxide, phenols, and quinones, but also metabolites of phase I metabolism such as oxygenated benzo[a]pyrene or β-naphthoflavone.[35] EPRE sequences have been found upstream of phase II drug-metabolizing genes[34,35] and other genes that respond to oxidative stress.[36,37]

Metal Response Element (MRE)

MREs were first identified upstream of the mouse metallothionein (*Mt1*, *Mt2*) genes.[38] Heavy metal cations that induce via the MRE include cadmium, zinc, mercury, cobalt, and nickel. Several heavy metals are potent electrophiles, thus activating the EPRE as well as the MRE, leading to mutagenesis and carcinogenesis.[39] Induction of genes via MREs occurs upon exposure to heavy metals such as cadmium, silver, copper, cobalt, mercury, and nickel; zinc and heavy metal toxicity has been demonstrated in virtually every organ system.[40]

Estrogen Response Element (ERE)

The estrogen receptor (ER-α, -β) binds a number of estrogenic compounds and forms a transcription complex with the ERE as a homodimer. Environmental and dietary "endocrine disruptors" bind (to varying degrees) to the ER-α, -β and are purported to disrupt normal cellular signaling and lead to reproductive tissue abnormalities and/or cancer.[41] Several environmental and pharmaceutical chemicals exhibit varying degrees of estrogenicity, including diethylstilbestrol, tamoxifen, dietary phytoestrogens, phthalate plasticizers, insecticides (e.g., *p,p'*-DDT, *p,p'*-DDE, dieldrin, methoxychlor, toxaphene, and endosulfan), 4-nonylphenol, *bis*-phenol-A, and kepone.[42]

Retinoic Acid and Retinoid X Response Elements (RAREs, RXREs)

Both retinoic acid receptors (RARs) and retinoid X receptors (RXRs) bind with high affinity to 9-*cis*-retinoic acid, but show striking differences in their affinity for other retinoids.[43] Many retinoic acid analogues have been developed as therapeutic and chemopreventive agents and bind preferentially to specific RAR and/or RXR isoforms, activating RAREs and RXREs.[43,44] The popular insecticide methoprene has been found to be a potent RXR agonist.[45] An imbalance in the normal levels of retinoic acid (vitamin A) and/or its derivatives can cause striking deformities in limbs and other organs during embryonic development or regeneration. Environmental retinoids have been implicated in frog deformities in the Great Lakes area, where a powerful teratogen appears to exist in groundwater and well water.[46]

RESPONSE ELEMENTS ARE FUNCTIONAL IN ZEBRAFISH CELL CULTURE

Following initial characterization of two zebrafish cell lines, we determined that the ZEM2S line—derived from an embryonic stem cell culture[47]—grew better and responded to inducers better than the ZFL line.[48] We then examined whole-cell and nuclear extracts of ZEM2S cells, using electrophoretic mobility shift analysis, for their capacity to bind AHRE, EPRE, or MRE motifs; we concluded that ZEM2S cells indeed appear to contain all the factors necessary to specifically bind to these response elements, within well-defined limits of ligand concentrations, salt requirements, and temperature.

For transient transfection of the pGL3-control plasmid (SV40 promoter and enhancer, driving the *LUC* gene) into ZEM2S cells, we compared the calcium phosphate method with Lipofectin (Life Technologies, Grand Island, NY), Lipofectamine (Life Technologies), Lipofectamine Plus (Life Technologies), GenePORTER (Gene Therapy Systems, San Diego, CA), and the Perfect Lipids Transfection Kit (Invitrogen, Carlsbad, CA). Lipofectamine Plus was most suitable in our hands and used for all subsequent transfections. Although stable transfectants are preferable to transiently transfected cells, we have been unsuccessful in generating stably transfected ZEM2S cells.

Comparing the potency of various mammalian and trout promoters for their capacity to confer dose-dependent *LUC* induction, we examined four AHRE, three EPRE, and two MRE constructs (FIG. 2). All nine promoters that we tested demonstrated dose-dependent *LUC* induction upon treatment with the appropriate environmental agent (not shown). For the prototypic inducers of the three classes of environmental inducers, we decided to use dioxin, tBHQ, and cadmium, respectively (FIG. 2). From the magnitude of successful responses in the ZEM2S cell line, we chose the *AHRDtk*, *EPREmt1*, and *MREd5mt1* constructs[49] as the best three candidates for developing transgenic zebrafish. Interestingly, the trout-derived constructs failed to respond as well as those with mammalian enhancers.

TRANSGENE ACTIVITIES ARE DETECTABLE IN LIVE ZEBRAFISH

Zebrafish embryos are essentially transparent and hence make excellent model systems for the introduction of luminous and/or fluorescent markers.[50] It was reported that *LUC* activity can be detected within the deep tissues of adult mice.[51,52] Therefore, we felt there should be no problem detecting *LUC* activity within the tissues of an adult zebrafish. The advancement of successfully expressing the jellyfish green fluorescent protein (*GFP*) reporter gene[53,54] has also allowed for the rapid development of this probe in the zebrafish. Thus, we also plan to incorporate into our studies the "gene-swapping" methods described elsewhere in this volume,[55] that is, swapping a heterotypic *lox*-flanked gene for *gfpzeo* in zebrafish embryos.

Because we wished to assay luminescence or fluorescence in the living intact fish, we searched for zebrafish lines lacking pigmentation. Initial studies with a mutant albino line revealed that this line would be difficult due to chronic poor breeding. Since then, we have been successful in establishing a robust breeding colony, using the *golden, long-fin* zebrafish *(gol/lof)* zebrafish line. The very long fins are an excellent source of tissue for genotyping, whereas the *golden* mutant is useful because it has reduced amounts of body pigmentation.

For the insertion of plasmids into the zebrafish embryo, we compared electroporation with microinjection and found the latter to be much more efficient. We have also been most successful by using constructs containing the locus control region

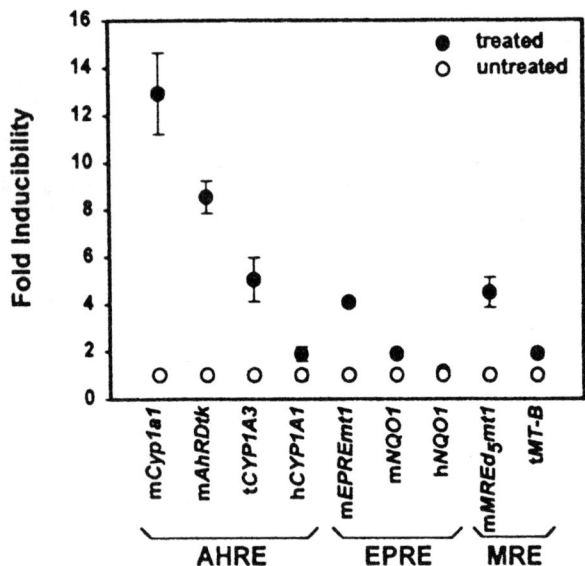

FIGURE 2. Comparison of inducible promoters in zebrafish ZEM2S cells. Reporter constructs included DNA sequences from the 5' regulatory regions of mammalian and trout genes, cloned into the pGL3-basic firefly luciferase (*LUC*) reporter construct. Promoter/enhancer sequences (left to right) were derived from the following: mouse *CYP1A1* (−1646 to +57); mouse *AhRDtk* [−1100 to −896 of mouse *CYP1A1* containing four AHREs, fused to the herpes simplex virus type I thymidine kinase (*tk*) minimal promoter (−79 to +53) from which the SP1-binding site was removed]; rainbow trout *CYP1A3* (−1987 to +78); human *CYP1A1* (−1604 to +88); mouse *EPREmt1* [single EPRE from the mouse *Gsta1* enhancer region (−722 to −682) fused to the minimal mouse *Mt1* promoter]; mouse *Nqo1* (from the *Mlu* I restriction site at approximately −3000 to +109); human *NQO1* (−1539 to +115); mouse *MREd$_5$mt1* [concatamer of five MREd' sequences from the mouse *Mt1* enhancer fused to the minimal mouse *Mt1* promoter (−42 to +60)]; and the trout *MT-B* promoter/enhancer sequences (−137 to +8). Further details and sources of these constructs are given in reference 49. Following transient transfection, we determined that maximal *LUC* activity was achieved in AHRE reporter constructs by 10 nM TCDD, in EPRE constructs by 10 μM tBHQ, and in MRE constructs by 30 μM CdCl$_2$. The data represent the means of duplicate determinations from at least six independent transfections, and brackets denote standard errors of the mean (modified from reference 49).

(LCR) of the mouse *Mt1* gene in order to create an artificial locus. If the zebrafish species contains a more rigorous "genome surveillance system" than the mouse, it may be difficult to maintain transgenes through many subsequent generations. Insulating border elements, such as the *Mt1*-LCR, have been used to stabilize the expression of transgenes in zebrafish for several generations.[26]

Even though *LUC* has been the reporter gene of choice for these studies, development of the jellyfish green fluorescent protein (*GFP*) reporter gene as a tool in molecular/cellular biology has assisted in the rapid development and analysis of our methods for making transgenic zebrafish. *GFP* expression allows for direct visualization of the gene product; this allows us to determine the relative level of gene ex-

TABLE 2. Generation of transgenic zebrafish with a variety of constructs

Construct	Fish injected	Survival (%)	Transgene positive (%)
CMV-*gfpzeo*-MTLCR	356	26	58
EF1α-*gfpzeo*-MTLCR	534	69	58
EF1α-βGal	118	58	35
pGL3-control	56	34	68
AHRDtk*luc3*	144	63	81

NOTE: The constructs were microinjected into 1- or 2-cell embryos, and transgene expression was determined visually 24 h later. CMV = human cytomegalovirus promoter; EF1α = *Xenopus* elongation factor α promoter; *gfpzeo* = fusion between the *GFP* gene and the Zeocin-resistance gene; βGal = β-galactosidase; MTLCR = locus control region of the mouse *Mt1* gene; pGL3 = basal construct containing the *LUC* gene.

pression in various tissues, as well as the proportion of cells in which the gene is being expressed—both of which vary widely between embryos.

F_0 Transgenic Zebrafish Express Transgenes into Adulthood

Embryos were microinjected with supercoiled plasmid at the 1- or 2-cell stage and visualized or assayed 24 h later. The rate at which embryos survived microinjection and expressed the transgene is shown in TABLE 2. The EF1α-GFPZ-MTLCR construct gave the best embryo survival rate and also produced a very high number of embryonic cells expressing GFPzeo. High levels of expression in these zebrafish have been maintained for more than 180 days, and the transgene has been successfully transmitted into the F_1 and sometimes the F_2 generation, following which it is lost. Other laboratories have had the same difficulties in sustaining transgene expression beyond the F_2 generation in zebrafish for reasons not known, but possibly due to an efficient genome surveillance system in this species. Another possible explanation might be related to gene silencing in mammals, plants, and *Drosophila*, which has been observed when multiple transgene copies are incorporated into a single site.[55]

USE OF SENTINEL ZEBRAFISH TO MONITOR DRINKING WATER

Using sentinel zebrafish, we have begun field tests in Clermont County, east of Cincinnati. After we are satisfied that the fish can live under these field conditions, we will then switch to our transgenic zebrafish of the F_0, F_1, and F_2 generations. The east fork of the Little Miami River is a major source of drinking water for Clermont County and is proposed to be the sole source in the future for drinking water supplied to the new residential areas. Directly upstream of the reservoir from which drinking water will be pumped is a hazardous toxic waste dump site that is known to be leaching toxic waste, PCBs in particular, into the watershed. This has given us a unique opportunity to examine the utility of the transgenic zebrafish model system as a living biomonitor and early warning system for the presence of environmental pollutants. Furthermore, we are comparing our model system with the more traditional technologies currently operating on-site.

We are evaluating three different modes of contaminant exposure—cages, flow-through tanks, and sediment exposure. The fish will be held in aluminum cages anchored to cement blocks submersed within specific bodies of water. Flow-through tanks are being constructed within the Village of Williamsburg Water Works facility and within the Harshaw Lake water intake tower, which is the water source for the Bob McEwan Water Treatment Plant with a capacity of 10 million gallons/day that serves about 30,000 customers. Sediments are being collected from areas near the aluminum cages and transported to the laboratory for embryo exposures.

Clermont County maintains 32 chemical monitoring stations on the east fork of the Little Miami River for biweekly to monthly analysis of water-quality parameters. At present, biological data are being collected at 6 to 9 of the 32 sites. There are currently 3 sites where the cages are tentatively scheduled to be deployed, where recent deterioration of the biological community structure has been significant.

SUMMARY

First, in cell culture, we have determined that the zebrafish possesses those transcription factors necessary to recognize both mammalian and trout pollution-inducible DNA response elements.

Second, in ZEM2S cell culture, we have shown that AHRE, EPRE, and MRE sequences drive the *LUC* reporter gene in a dose-dependent, chemical-class-specific manner in response to the more than 20 environmental pollutants so far tested. As expected, some AHR ligands activate the AHRE and, following metabolism, activate the EPRE; some heavy metals not only activate the MRE, but also (as potent electrophiles) activate the EPRE.

Third, the *LUC*, *GFP*, and β*GAL* reporter genes have been inserted into the zebrafish genome via microinjection of embryos, and expression of GFP is easily detected into adulthood and in the F_1 and F_2 generations.

Fourth, sentinel zebrafish are already being used to monitor drinking water sources in Clermont County, east of Cincinnati. Ultimately, our transgenic model system should be useful in identifying distinct individual classes of environmental pollutants within complex mixtures, providing an inexpensive biomonitor for the protection of drinking water sources, and detecting chemical pollutants introduced into sensitive aquatic environments.

Fifth, and last, for quantitating pollutants in water sources, traditional analytical techniques are expensive and time-consuming and do not address bioavailability; biological-impact analyses are time-consuming and require the examination of several biological parameters in a variety of organisms. This transgenic zebrafish model system, on the contrary, will be a rapid, sensitive, and simple assay, which might be the best system yet for assessing complex mixtures. We predict that this transgenic model system, and others based on similar principles, will likely become commonplace during the first decade of the new millennium.

ACKNOWLEDGMENTS

We thank our colleagues for valuable discussions and critical reading of this manuscript. This work was supported in part by NIH Grant Nos. R01 ES07058, R01 ES08147, R01 ES06321, and P30 ES06096.

REFERENCES

1. RIFKIN, E. & J. LAKIND. 1991. Dioxin bioaccumulation: key to a sound risk assessment methodology. J. Toxicol. Environ. Health **33:** 103.
2. KANNAN, K., R.G. SMITH, JR., R.F. LEE, H.L. WINDOM, P.T. HEITMULLER, J.M. MACAULEY & J.K. SUMMERS. 1998. Distribution of total mercury and methyl mercury in water, sediment, and fish from south Florida estuaries. Arch. Environ. Contam. Toxicol. **34:** 109.
3. FRAKES, R.A., C.Q. ZEEMAN & B. MOWER. 1993. Bioaccumulation of 2,3,7,8-tetrachlorodibenzo-*p*-dioxin (TCDD) by fish downstream of pulp and paper mills in Maine. Ecotoxicol. Environ. Saf. **25:** 244.
4. SHERMAN, W.R., R.E. KEENAN & D.G. GUNSTER. 1992. Reevaluation of dioxin bioconcentration and bioaccumulation factors for regulatory purposes. J. Toxicol. Environ. Health **37:** 211.
5. U.S. EPA. 1995. Whole effluent toxicity: guidelines establishing test procedures. Fed. Regist. **60:** 53529.
6. U.S. EPA. 1994. Short-Term Methods for Estimating the Chronic Toxicity of Effluents and Receiving Waters to Freshwater Organisms. Third edition.
7. BARBOUR, M.T., J. GERRITSEN, B.D. SNYDER & J.B. STRIBLING. 1997. Revision to rapid bioassessment protocols for use in streams and rivers: periphyton, benthic, macroinvertebrates, and fish. EPA 841-D-97-002.
8. PAYNE, J.F., L.L. FANCEY, A.D. RAHIMTULA & E.L. PORTER. 1987. Review and perspective on the use of mixed-function oxygenase enzymes in biological monitoring. Comp. Biochem. Physiol. **86C:** 233.
9. KELLY, S.A., C.M. HAVRILLA, T.C. BRADY, K.H. ABRAMO & E.D. LEVIN. 1998. Oxidative stress in toxicology: established mammalian and emerging piscine model systems. Environ. Health Perspect. **106:** 375.
10. PAYNE, J.F. 1976. Field evaluation of benzopyrene hydroxylase induction as a monitor for marine petroleum pollution. Science **191:** 945.
11. JANZ, D.M., M.E. MCMASTER, K.R. MUNKITTRICK & G. VAN DER KRAAK. 1997. Elevated ovarian follicular apoptosis and heat shock protein-70 expression in white sucker exposed to bleached kraft pulp mill effluent. Toxicol. Appl. Pharmacol. **147:** 391.
12. SCHLENK, D., Y.S. ZHANG & J. NIX. 1995. Expression of hepatic metallothionein messenger RNA in feral and caged fish species correlates with muscle mercury levels. Ecotoxicol. Environ. Saf. **31:** 282.
13. SOIMASUO, M.R., A.E. KARELS, H. LEPPPANEN, R. SANTTI & A.O. OIKARI. 1998. Biomarker responses in whitefish (*Coregonus lavaretus* L. s.l.) experimentally exposed in a large lake receiving effluents from pulp and paper industry. Arch. Environ. Contam. Toxicol. **34:** 69.
14. GILL, T.S., H. TEWART & J. PANDEE. 1990. Use of the fish enzyme system in monitoring water quality: effects of mercury in tissue enzymes. Comp. Biochem. Physiol. **97C:** 287.
15. GOKSØYR, A., T. ANDERSSON, D.R. BUHLER, J.J. STEGEMAN, D.E. WILLIAMS & L. FÖRLIN. 1991. Immunochemical cross-reactivity of α-naphthoflavone-inducible cytochrome P450, P450IA, in liver microsomes from different fish species and rat. Fish Physiol. Biochem. **9:** 1.
16. GOKSØYR, A., H.E. LARSEN & A.M. HUSOY. 1991. Application of a cytochrome P-450 IA1-ELISA in environmental monitoring and toxicological testing of fish. Comp. Biochem. Physiol. **100C:** 157.

17. HAASCH, M.L., P.J. WEJKSNORA, J.J. STEGEMAN & J.J. LECH. 1989. Cloned rainbow trout liver $P_1 450$ complementary DNA as a potential environmental monitor. Toxicol. Appl. Pharmacol. **98:** 362.
18. RODRÍGUEZ-ARIZA, A., G. DORADO, J.I. NAVAS, C. PUEYO & J. LÓPEZ-BAREA. 1994. Promutagen activation by fish liver as a biomarker of littoral pollution. Environ. Mol. Mutagen. **24:** 116.
19. NEBERT, D.W., A.L. ROE, M.Z. DIETER, W.A. SOLIS, Y. YANG & T.P. DALTON. 2000. Role of the aromatic hydrocarbon receptor and [Ah] gene battery in the oxidative stress response, cell cycle control, and apoptosis. Biochem. Pharmacol. **59:** 65.
20. GEISLER, R., G.J. RAUCH, H. BAIER, F. VAN BEBBER, L. BROBETA, M.P. DEKENS, K. FINGER, C. FRICKE, M.A. GATES, H. GEIGER, S. GEIGER-RUDOLPH, D. GILMOUR et al. 1999. A radiation hybrid map of the zebrafish genome. Nat. Genet. **23:** 86.
21. ALESTROM, P., G. KISEN, H. KLUNGLAND & O. ANDERSON. 1992. Fish gonadotropin-releasing hormone gene and molecular approaches for control of sexual maturation: development of a transgenic fish model. Mol. Mar. Biol. Biotechnol. **1:** 376.
22. MOAV, B., Z. LIU, L.D. CALDOVIC, M.L. GROSS, A.J. FARAS & P.B. HACKETT. 1993. Regulation of expression of transgenes in developing fish. Transgen. Res. **2:** 153.
23. GAIANO, N., M. ALLENDE, A. AMSTERDAM, K. KAWAKAMI & N. HOPKINS. 1996. Highly efficient germ-line transmission of proviral insertions in zebrafish. Proc. Natl. Acad. Sci. U.S.A. **93:** 7777.
24. LAM, W.L., T.S. LEE & W. GILBERT. 1996. Active transposition in zebrafish. Proc. Natl. Acad. Sci. U.S.A. **93:** 10870.
25. FADOOL, J.M., D.L. HARTL & J.E. DOWLING. 1998. Transposition of the mariner element from *Drosophila mauritiana* in zebrafish. Proc. Natl. Acad. Sci. U.S.A. **95:** 5182.
26. CALDOVIC, L. & P.B. HACKETT, JR. 1995. Development of position-independent expression vectors and their transfer into transgenic fish. Mol. Mar. Biol. Biotechnol. **4:** 51.
27. DYNAN, W.S. & R. TJIAN. 1985. Control of eukaryotic messenger RNA synthesis by sequence-specific DNA-binding proteins. Nature **316:** 774.
28. PTASHNE, M. & A. GANN. 1997. Transcriptional activation by recruitment. Nature **386:** 569.
29. SAFE, S. 1991. Polychlorinated dibenzo-*p*-dioxins and related compounds: sources, environmental distribution, and risk assessment. Environ. Carcinog. Ecotoxicol. Rev. **C9:** 261.
30. BIRNBAUM, L.S. 1994. Endocrine effects of prenatal exposure to PCBs, dioxins, and other xenobiotics: implications for policy and future research. Environ. Health Perspect. **102:** 676.
31. HANKINSON, O. 1995. The aryl hydrocarbon receptor complex. Annu. Rev. Pharmacol. Toxicol. **35:** 307.
32. WHITLOCK, J.P., JR., C.H. CHICHESTER, R.M. BEDGOOD, S.Y. OKINO, H.P. KO, Q. MA, L. DONG, H. LI & R. CLARKE-KATZENBERG. 1997. Induction of drug-metabolizing enzymes by dioxin. Drug Metab. Rev. **29:** 1107.
33. DALTON, T.P., H.G. SHERTZER & A. PUGA. 1999. Regulation of gene expression by reactive oxygen. Annu. Rev. Pharmacol. Toxicol. **39:** 67.
34. JAISWAL, A.K. 1994. Antioxidant response element. Biochem. Pharmacol. **48:** 439.
35. RUSHMORE, T.H., R.G. KING, K.E. PAULSON & C.B. PICKETT. 1990. Regulation of glutathione S-transferase Ya subunit gene expression: identification of a unique xenobiotic-responsive element controlling inducible expression by planar aromatic compounds. Proc. Natl. Acad. Sci. U.S.A. **87:** 3826.
36. TALALAY, P., J.W. FAHEY, W.D. HOLTZCLAW, T. PRESTERA & Y. ZHANG. 1995. Chemoprotection against cancer by phase 2 enzyme induction. Toxicol. Lett. **82/83:** 173.
37. MOINOVA, H.R. & R.T. MULCAHY. 1998. An electrophile response element (EpRE) regulates β-naphthoflavone induction of the human γ-glutamylcysteine synthetase regulatory subunit gene: constitutive expression is mediated by an adjacent AP-1 site. J. Biol. Chem. **273:** 14683.
38. STUART, G.W., P.F. SEARLE & R.D. PALMITER. 1985. Identification of multiple metal regulatory elements in mouse metallothionein-I promoter by assaying synthetic sequences. Nature **317:** 828.

39. THIELE, D.J. 1992. Metal-regulated transcription in eukaryotes. Nucleic Acids Res. **20:** 1183.
40. TEMPLETON, D.M. & M.G. CHERIAN. 1991. Toxicological significance of metallothionein. Methods Enzymol. **205:** 11.
41. CHEEK, A.O., P.M. VONIER, E. OBERDORSTER, B.C. BUROW & J.A. MCLACHLAN. 1998. Environmental signaling: a biological context for endocrine disruption. Environ. Health Perspect. **106**(suppl. 1): 5.
42. SONNENSCHEIN, C. & A.M. SOTO. 1998. An updated review of environmental estrogen and androgen mimics and antagonists. J. Steroid Biochem. Mol. Biol. **65:** 143.
43. MINUCCI, S., J.P. SAINT-JEANNET, R. TOYAMA, G. SCITA, L.M. DELUCA, M. TIARA, A.A. LEVIN, K. OZATO & I.B. DAWID. 1996. Retinoid X receptor–selective ligands produce malformations in *Xenopus* embryos. Proc. Natl. Acad. Sci. U.S.A. **93:** 1803.
44. CASTALEIN, H., A. JANSSEN, P.E. DECLERCQ & M. BAES. 1996. Sequence requirements for high-affinity retinoid X receptor-α homodimer binding. Mol. Cell. Endocrinol. **119:** 11.
45. HARMON, M.A., M.F. BOEHM, R.A. HEYMAN & D.J. MANGELSDORF. 1995. Activation of mammalian retinoid X receptors by the insect growth regulator methoprene. Proc. Natl. Acad. Sci. U.S.A. **92:** 6157.
46. MANUEL, J. 1997. Frog deformities research not leaping to conclusions. Environ. Health Perspect. **105:** 1046.
47. GHOSH, C. & P. COLLODI. 1994. Culture of cells from zebrafish (*Brachydanio rerio*) blastula-stage embryos. Cytotechnology **14:** 21.
48. COLLODI, P., C.L. MIRANDA, X. ZHAO, D.R. BUHLER & D.W. BARNES. 1994. Induction of zebrafish (*Brachydanio rerio*) P450 *in vivo* and in cell culture. Xenobiotica **24:** 487.
49. CARVAN, M.J., III, W.A. SOLIS, L. GEDAMU & D.W. NEBERT. 2000. Activation of transcription factors in zebrafish cell cultures by environmental pollutants. Arch. Biochem. Biophys. **376:** 320.
50. CHALFIE, M., Y. TU, G. EUSKIRCHEN, W.W. WARD & D.C. PRASHER. 1994. Green fluorescent protein as a marker for gene expression. Science **263:** 802.
51. CONTAG, C.H., S.D. SPILMAN, P.R. CONTAG, M. OSHIRO, B. EAMES, P. DENNERY, D.K. STEVENSON & D.A. BENARON. 1997. Visualizing gene expression in living mammals using a bioluminescent reporter. Photochem. Photobiol. **66:** 523.
52. CONTAG, P.R., I.N. OLOMU, D.K. STEVENSON & C.H. CONTAG. 1998. Bioluminescent indicators in living mammals. Nat. Med. **4:** 245.
53. AMSTERDAM, A., S. LIN & N. HOPKINS. 1995. The *Aequorea victoria* green fluorescent protein can be used as a reporter in live zebrafish embryos. Dev. Biol. **171:** 123.
54. PETERS, K.G., P.S. RAO, B.S. BELL & L.A. KINDMAN. 1995. Green fluorescent fusion proteins: powerful tools for monitoring protein expression in live zebrafish embryos. Dev. Biol. **171:** 252.
55. NEBERT, D.W., T.P. DALTON, G.W. STUART & M.J. CARVAN III. 2000. "Gene-swap knock-in" cassette in mice to study allelic differences in human genes. This volume.
56. GARRICK, D., S. FIERING, D.I. MARTIN & E. WHITELAW. 1998. Repeat-induced gene silencing in mammals. Nat. Genet. **18:** 56.

"Gene-Swap Knock-in" Cassette in Mice to Study Allelic Differences in Human Genes

DANIEL W. NEBERT,[a,b] TIMOTHY P. DALTON,[a] GARY W. STUART,[c] AND MICHAEL J. CARVAN III[a]

[a]*Center for Environmental Genetics (CEG) and Department of Environmental Health, University of Cincinnati Medical Center, Cincinnati, Ohio 45267-0056, USA*

[c]*Department of Life Sciences, Indiana State University, Terre Haute, Indiana 47809, USA*

ABSTRACT: Genetic differences in environmental toxicity and cancer susceptibility among individuals in a human population often reflect polymorphisms in the genes encoding drug-metabolizing enzymes (DMEs), drug transporters, and receptors that control DME levels. This field of study is called "ecogenetics", and a subset of this field—concerning genetic variability in response to drugs—is termed "pharmacogenetics". Although human-mouse differences might be 3- to perhaps 10-fold, human interindividual differences can be as great as 20-fold or more than 40-fold. It would be helpful, therefore, to study toxicokinetics/pharmacokinetics of particular environmental agents and drugs in mice containing these "high-" and "low-extreme" human alleles. We hope to use transgenic "knock-in" technology in order to insert human alleles in place of the orthologous mouse gene. However, the knock-in of each gene has normally been a separate event requiring the following: (a) construction of the targeting vector, (b) transfection into embryonic stem (ES) cells, (c) generation of a targeted mouse having germline transmission of the construct, and (d) backcross breeding of the knock-in mouse (at least 6–8 times) to produce a suitable genetically homogeneous background (i.e., to decrease "experimental noise"). These experiments require 1½ to 2 years to complete, making this very powerful technology inefficient for routine applications. If, on the other hand, the initial knock-in targeting vector might include sequences that would allow the knocked-in gene to be exchanged (quickly and repeatedly) for one new allele after another, then testing distinctly different human polymorphic alleles in transgenic mice could be accomplished in a few months instead of several years. This "gene-swapping" technique will soon be done by zygotic injection of a "human allele cassette" into the sperm or fertilized ovum of the parental knock-in mouse inbred strain or by the cloning of whole mice from cumulus ovaricus cells or tail-snip fibroblasts containing the nucleus wherein each new human allele has already been "swapped." In mouse cells in culture using heterotypic lox sites, we and others have already succeeded in gene swapping, by exchanging one gene, including its regulatory regions, with a second gene (including its regulatory regions). It is anticipated that mouse lines carrying numerous human alleles will become commonplace early in the next millennium.

[b]Address for correspondence: Department of Environmental Health, University of Cincinnati Medical Center, P.O. Box 670056, Cincinnati, OH 45267-0056. Voice: 513-558-4347; fax: 513-558-3562.

dan.nebert@uc.edu

INTRODUCTION

The past several years have seen an increasing appreciation for the marked genetic variability among humans. Between 6 million and 30 million single-nucleotide polymorphisms (SNPs) are believed to exist among the 3 billion bases in the human genome; the precise number of SNPs will soon be known because the entire human genome will have been sequenced during the next several years. Each gene is expected to exhibit between 4 and perhaps greater than a dozen coding SNPs (cSNPs) that change an amino acid and alter the function of the gene product; each gene is also anticipated to have a similar number of perigenic SNPs (pSNPs)—found in noncoding regions, introns, and 5′ and 3′ flanking regions—which may or may not affect function of the gene product.[1]

Interindividual differences in susceptibility to environmental toxicity and cancer among human populations have been demonstrated to be associated with polymorphisms in genes encoding drug-metabolizing enzymes (DMEs), drug transporters, and receptors that control DME levels. This field of study is termed "ecogenetics," and a subset of this field—which concerns genetic variability in response to pharmaceuticals—is called "pharmacogenetics."

Regulatory agencies are constantly required to extrapolate from toxicity and cancer data in laboratory animals to human populations in order to provide guidelines for risk assessment. However, interindividual human differences (which can be from 20- to greater than 40-fold) are often greater than differences between humans and laboratory animals (3- to perhaps 10-fold). It is important to understand the mechanism(s) of toxicity and carcinogenesis and to study the toxicokinetics of specific environmental agents and the pharmacokinetics of particular drugs. In the study of these mechanisms, it would be advantageous if "high-" and "low-extreme" human alleles of DME, drug transporter, or DME receptor genes could be inserted efficiently into mouse lines. We could then determine, for example, what the target organ(s) is when the agent is given by a particular route of administration. We could also measure any changes in these effects on the target organ as a function of dose or exposure.

To this end, we have begun to develop methods for "gene swapping," with an ultimate goal of introducing specific human alleles in place of the orthologous mouse gene. Eventually, more than one mouse gene will have been replaced by uniquely interesting human genes. As mouse lines become more and more "humanized," therefore, the kinetics of uptake, binding and distribution, biotransformation, and excretion can be studied for any environmental or pharmaceutical agent as a function of dose and the route of administration.

In this article, we first review briefly the field of ecogenetics and pharmacogenetics. Next, the Cre recombinase/*loxP* transgenesis methodology is described. Then, our successes and failures in gene swapping to date are detailed. Finally, we present our predictions as to where this field is expected to go during the first decade of the new millennium.

ECOGENETICS AND PHARMACOGENETICS DEFINED

"Ecogenetics," or "environmental genetics," is the study of heritable variability in response to environmental agents. The entire field of gene-environment inter-

TABLE 1. Classification of some human pharmacogenetic differences

A. Less enzyme/defective protein
  1. N-Acetylation polymorphisms (*NAT2*, *NAT1*)
  2. Increased susceptibility to chemical-induced hemolysis (G6PD deficiency) (*G6PD*)
  3. P450 monooxygenase polymorphisms (oxidation deficiencies):
      Debrisoquine (*CYP2D6*), *S*-mephenytoin (*CYP2C19* & *2C9*), phenytoin (*CYP2C9* & *2C19*), nifedipine (*CYP3A4*), coumarin and nicotine (*CYP2A6*), theophylline (*CYP1A2*), acetaminophen (*CYP2E1*)
  4. Null mutants of glutathione transferase, mu class (*GSTM1*); theta class (*GSTT1*)
  5. Thiopurine methyltransferase (*TPMT*)
  6. Paraoxonase deficiency, sarinase (*PON1*)
  7. UDP glucuronosyltransferase [Gilbert's disease, *UGT1A1*; (*S*)-oxazepam, *UGT2B7*]
  8. NAD(P)H:quinone oxidoreductase (*NQO1*)
  9. Epoxide hydrolase (*HYL1*)
  10. Atypical or absent aldehyde dehydrogenase (*ALDH2*)
  11. Alpha-one (α_1)–antitrypsin (*PI*)
  12. Dihydropyrimidine dehydrogenase (*DPD*)
  13. Succinyl sensitivity, atypical or absent serum cholinesterase (*CHE1*)
  14. Butyrylcholinesterase (*BCE1*)
  15. Dubin-Johnson syndrome; multispecific organic anion transporter (*MOAT*, *MRP*)
  16. Altered serotonin transporter (*5HHT*)
  17. Altered dopamine transporter (*DAT*)
  18. Defective drug transporters (e.g., *MDR1*), resistance to chemotherapeutic agents

B. Increased resistance to chemicals
  1. Inability to taste phenylthiourea
  2. Vasopressin resistance (*AVPR2*)
  3. Increased metabolism—atypical liver alcohol dehydrogenase (*ADH*)
  4. Defective receptor—malignant hyperthermia/general anesthesia (Ca^{++}-release channel ryanodine receptor) (*RYR1*, *MHS1*)

C. Change in response due to enzyme induction
  1. Porphyrias (esp. cutanea tarda)
  2. Aryl hydrocarbon receptor (*AHR*) polymorphism (*CYP1A1*, *CYP1A2* inducibility polymorphism):
      Cancer, immunosuppression, birth defects, chloracne, porphyria, (?) eye toxicity, (?) ovarian toxicity

D. Abnormal metal distribution
  1. Iron (hemochromatosis, *HFE*), copper (Wilson's disease, Menkes' disease), (?) lead, (?) cadmium, (?) others

E. Disorders of unknown etiology (known to run in families)
  1. Corticosteroid (eye drops)–induced glaucoma
  2. Halothane-induced hepatitis
  3. Chloramphenicol-induced aplastic anemia
  4. Beryllium-induced lung disease
  5. Beeturia; red urine after eating beets
  6. Malodorous urine after eating asparagus

NOTE: A list of more than six dozen ecogenetic differences is provided in reference 1.

actions includes differences in response to agents as diverse as ionizing radiation, heavy metals, chemicals in the workplace, pesticides and herbicides, foods, food additives, drugs, and alcohol. "Pharmacogenetics" is the study of genetic variability in response to pharmaceuticals and is regarded as a subset of ecogenetics. In the past several years, "pharmacogenomics," emphasizing the development of novel drugs, based on newly discovered genes as the entire human genome becomes sequenced, has been described. "Pharmacoanthropology" and "ethnopharmacology" are terms used to describe the study of ethnic differences in variable drug response (reviewed in references 2–12).

DEFINITION OF A "POLYMORPHISM"

Generally agreed upon by epidemiologists, a genetic polymorphism exists in a human population when allelic variants occur with a frequency of 1% or greater. When chemicals, foodstuff, heavy metals, or drugs enter the body, their fate depends upon (a) the rate of uptake, (b) transport, binding, and distribution, (c) biotransformation (metabolism), and (d) the rate of excretion. Of the more than six dozen ecogenetic differences that have so far been described (TABLE 1), the majority represent variability in DME metabolism; most of the remaining appear to represent alterations in receptor affinity, transporters, or protein binding (see references 1–9). Pharmacogenetic differences in metabolism can be striking—for example, the metabolic ratio (metabolite/parent drug) of the CYP2D6-poor metabolizer and the ultrametabolizer phenotypes can differ by more than 10,000-fold.[4] On the other hand, differences in binding and transport are generally less than 20-fold.[1,13] Ecogenetic differences in uptake or excretion of environmental chemicals are relatively uncommon. Vitamin B_{12} malabsorption or hemochromatosis, and certain aminoacidurias (e.g., cystinuria), might be regarded as ecogenetic differences in uptake and excretion, respectively.[1,2,9]

PHASE I AND PHASE II METABOLISM

The vast majority of environmental agents are metabolized by "phase I" (functionalization, often cytochromes P450) followed by "phase II" (conjugation) DMEs. The human genome is expected to contain probably several thousand DME genes; for example, 49 human cytochrome P450 (*CYP*) genes are known to exist.[14] Most incoming environmental agents might be regarded as "exogenous signals" that are "detected" by the cell, either by means of well-characterized endogenous receptors or by "reception mechanisms" not yet understood (FIG. 1); these chemicals/signals can displace the naturally occurring endogenous ligands and act as either agonists or antagonists to up- or downregulate phase I and phase II DME genes.[15] For example, benzo[a]pyrene and phenytoin are both known to upregulate their own phase I metabolism; dioxin or phenobarbital each induces particular subsets of genes of both the phase I and phase II categories.

The oxygenated reactive intermediates following phase I metabolism, as well as many incoming nonmetabolized chemicals (and even conjugated products whose conjugation group has been cleaved), are capable of causing oxidative stress, toxic-

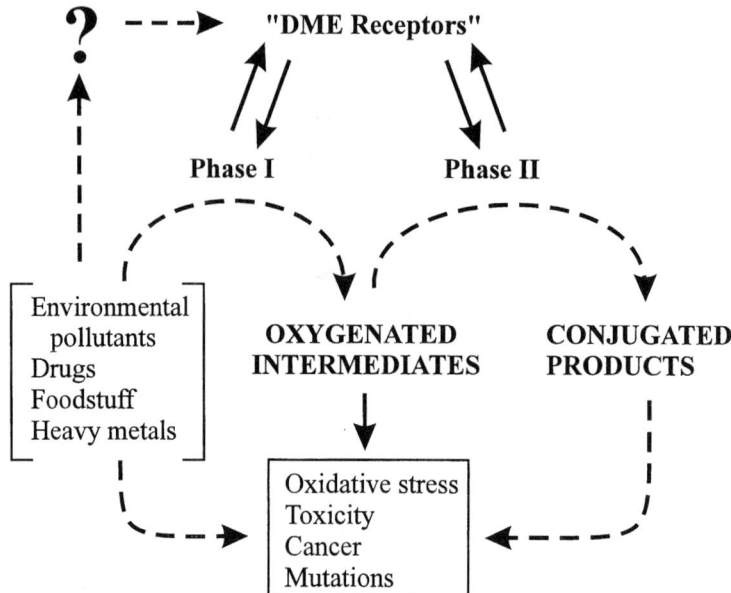

FIGURE 1. Diagram of the fate of environmental agents. Heavy metals or chemicals can enter the cell by either passive diffusion or active transporters. The parent (nonmetabolized chemical), metabolite, or conjugated product is capable of causing oxidative stress, toxicity, cancer, and/or mutations. Reception mechanisms (denoted by question mark) are able to detect the incoming chemical as a "signal" and sometimes can up- or downregulate phase I and phase II DMEs.[15] Transporter proteins can also assist in moving the parent chemical, metabolite, or conjugated product out of the cell (modified from reference 13).

ity, mutation, and cancer (FIG. 1). Toxicity occurs fundamentally via two mechanisms: (a) covalent binding to cellular proteins and nucleic acids, and (b) oxidative stress, leading to perturbation of the cell cycle.[1] Oxidative stress, disturbance of the cell cycle, and covalent binding can lead to mutations or cancer. Heavy metals and chemicals can be passively and actively transported into the cell; nonmetabolized environmental agents, reactive intermediates, and conjugated products can all be transported out of the cell. Genes encoding phase I and phase II DMEs, drug transporters, and the DME receptors are known to be highly polymorphic and, thus, allelic differences can be responsible for genetic variation in response to environmental chemicals and drugs (reviewed in references 2–13). Although genes involved in the oxidative stress response and cell cycle regulation are also expected to exhibit polymorphisms, these variant alleles are less well understood or appreciated at the present time.[1]

CLINICAL PHARMACOLOGY

In a recent meta-analysis of 39 prospective studies in U.S. hospitals, the overall incidence of adverse drug reactions (ADRs) was about 6.7% and that of fatal ADRs was about 0.32%.[16] The year 1994 alone, for example, saw 2,216,000 hospitalized patients with "serious ADRs" and 106,000 patients with fatal ADRs; these data therefore rank "adverse drug reactions" between the fourth and sixth leading causes of death in the United States. It is well known that, when several patients receive the same "recommended" prescribed dosage of a particular drug, the effect can be efficacious in most, of little or no consequence in others, and toxic—even fatal—to a third subset. Genetic differences in DMEs, drug transporters, and DME receptors are likely to be a major reason for these clinical differences in drug response. Understanding the interaction between each drug (or other environmental agent) and the underlying genetic predisposition of the individual is therefore extremely important in clinical medicine.

ALL CELLS IN THE BODY EXPRESS AT LEAST SOME DMEs

DMEs, drug transporters, and DME receptors are commonly believed to exist largely, if not completely, in the liver; this probably stems from classical pharmacology courses, but could not be further from the truth.[15] For example, CYP3A4, the most abundant hepatic cytochrome P450, is expressed at high levels in the gastrointestinal tract.[17] Many DMEs exist in the vascular endothelial cells and contribute to the arachidonic acid cascade, cell division, cell migration, inflammatory response, vasoconstriction, and numerous other homeostatic mechanisms.[15] DMEs exist in the brain and play roles in neuroendocrine functions.[18] Particular P450 activities have been found to be as much as 50-fold greater in the human oral mucosa than in liver.[19] A number of DMEs exist at high concentrations in the nasal mucosa.[20] We must therefore keep in mind that variability in risk of environmental toxicity or cancer can occur in any tissue and need not be determined by DME, drug transporter, or DME receptor expression only in liver. This concept is of central importance if we wish to study the toxicokinetics/pharmacokinetics of environmental agents or drugs given to mouse lines having high- and low-extreme human alleles; for example, should the inserted human alleles be controlled by mouse or human regulatory sequences that might include the regulation of tissue-specific expression that differs between mouse and human?

THE NEED TO STUDY HUMAN ALLELIC VARIANTS IN MICE

As described above, recent advances in clinical medicine and molecular biology during the past two decades have led to the identification and characterization of more than six dozen polymorphisms in human ecogenetics. Due to the lack of appropriate animal model systems, however, the functional and toxicokinetic significance of many of these polymorphisms remains elusive.

There are important differences in DME activities between the mouse and human: for example, using the baculovirus expression vector driving mouse and human CYP1A2, we have determined that uroporphyrinogen oxidation by mouse CYP1A2 is 5 times higher (per unit of CYP1A2) than that by human CYP1A2 (in collaboration with Peter Sinclair, White River Junction, VT), N-hydroxylation of 4-aminobiphenyl by human CYP1A2 is more than 3 times greater than that by mouse CYP1A2 (in collaboration with Glenn Talaska, Cincinnati, OH), and N-hydroxylation of 2-amino-1-methyl-6-phenylimidazo[4,5-*b*]pyridine (PhIP, derived from charcoal-broiled meat) by human CYP1A2 is 6–10 times higher than that by mouse CYP1A2 (in collaboration with James S. Felton, Livermore, CA). Compared with these 3- to 10-fold interspecies differences, however, human interindividual variability in DME activities has often been shown to vary 20- to more than 40-fold, as detailed above. Hence, for a particular DME gene, it would seem most efficient to develop mouse lines having individual human alleles—expressing the "highest" and "lowest" activities—in place of the mouse orthologous gene. This same strategy has been used for dissecting the genes involved in blood pressure homeostasis—for example, studying the genetic profile of individuals having the 2.5th-percentile highest and 2.5th-percentile lowest blood pressure and not studying the 95% of patients in between.[21,22] Toxicokinetic and pharmacokinetic studies of environmental agents or drugs in such mouse lines would help regulatory agencies in establishing risk assessment policy.

Transgenic "knock-in" technology, which employs gene targeting to replace mouse genes with their human counterparts, appears to be an extremely promising approach for understanding the contribution of human alleles in causing environmental toxicity and cancer susceptibility.[23] The knock-in of each gene is a separate targeting event, however, requiring (a) construction of the targeting vector, (b) transfection into embryonic stem (ES) cells, (c) generation of a targeted mouse having germline transmission of the construct, and (d) backcross breeding of the knock-in mouse (at least 6–8 times) to produce a suitable genetically homogeneous background (i.e., to decrease "experimental noise"). These experiments require years to complete, making this very powerful technology inefficient for routine applications. If, on the other hand, the initial knock-in targeting vector were to include sequences that would allow the knocked-in gene to be exchanged (quickly and repeatedly) for yet another new allele, and if this could be done by zygotic injection into a particular cell derived from the parental knock-in mouse inbred strain of your choice, then testing a battery of human polymorphic alleles in transgenic mice could be accomplished in several months and would be relatively simple.

STANDARD PROCEDURES FOR MAKING A KNOCKOUT MOUSE LINE

The protocol for the generation of chimeric mice, in which the coat color phenotype is used for selection, is well established.[24] Briefly described, targeted ES cells (almost always derived from 129/SV mice, agouti) are injected into the blastocoele cavity of 3.5-day (usually C57BL/6J) embryos bearing the nonagouti phenotype (FIG. 2). The resulting chimeric blastocysts are then transferred to a pseudopregnant female's uterus. Identification of chimeric pups can be determined by presence of the agouti coat color as early as 7–10 days of age. For trying to achieve germline transmission, males are generally used instead of females because of the enormous number of offspring that the males can generate, compared with females; also, the XY chromosome–containing ES cells produce more than 50% males, making it more likely that the ES cells have contributed to the male reproductive tract. After subsequent crosses, a completely agouti coat color usually—but not always (discussed in reference 25)—denotes there has been germline transmission of the ES cell construct by the father into the offspring.

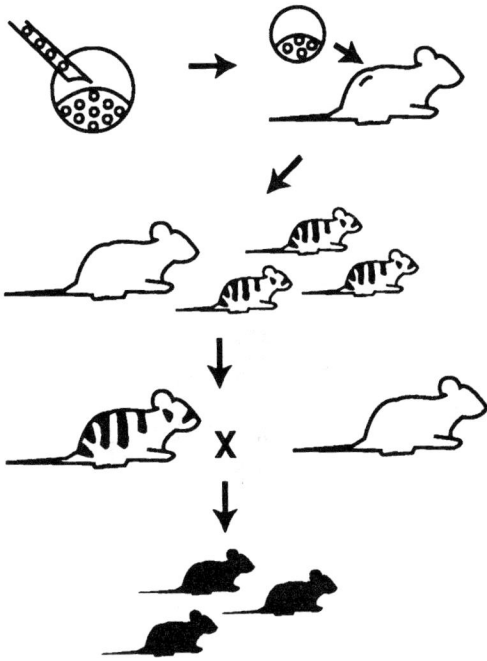

FIGURE 2. Illustration of the generation of a knockout mouse line. ES cells, derived from the 129/J mouse (agouti) that have been genetically engineered, are injected into the blastocoele cavity of the C57BL/6J mouse (nonagouti) and then placed into the uterus of a pseudopregnant foster mother. The chimeric offspring will represent a mixture of the two inbred mouse strains, as manifested by the agouti (shown here as black) and nonagouti (white) coat color. Germline transmission of the agouti coat color is usually associated with germline transmission of the genetically engineered gene construct.

The mouse line at first contains approximately half its genome from the agouti and half its genome from the nonagouti inbred mouse strains. TABLE 2 lists the mathematical estimations of percent inbred mouse background, comparing the original knockout mouse with one to eight backcrosses into the parent line. It can be seen that the mouse line theoretically becomes >99% genetically homogenous after six crosses. Because each cross takes a minimum of 10 weeks of generation time, eight backcrosses would take at least 1½ years under ideal conditions.

FIGURES 3A and 3B illustrate two examples in which the phenotype of a knockout mouse line can vary dramatically, based on genetic background. The percent of $Tgfb1(-/-)$ mice surviving beyond birth ranges from >80% in the NIH background to 0% in the C57BL/6J background (FIG. 3A). We found that the degree of variability in hepatic uroporphyrin in treated $Cyp1a2(+/+)$ littermates having 75% to 87.5% C57BL/6J background is striking, compared with that in treated $Cyp1a2(+/+)$ littermates having >99% C57BL/6J background (FIG. 3B). Dozens of other such phenotypes influenced by the "neighborhood effect" have now been described (reviewed in reference 28).

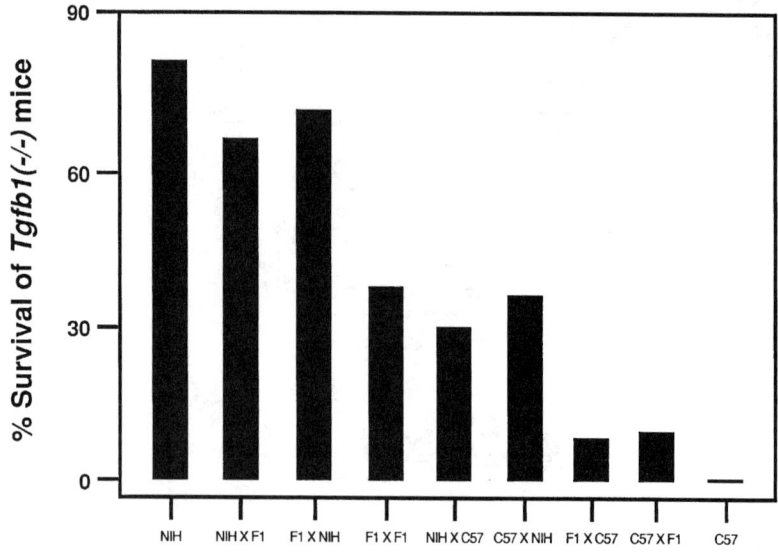

FIGURE 3A. An example of striking differences in phenotype as a function of the genetic background: Percent survival to birth of *Tgfb1(−/−)* knockout mice, comparing the NIH with the C57BL/6J background (modified from reference 26).

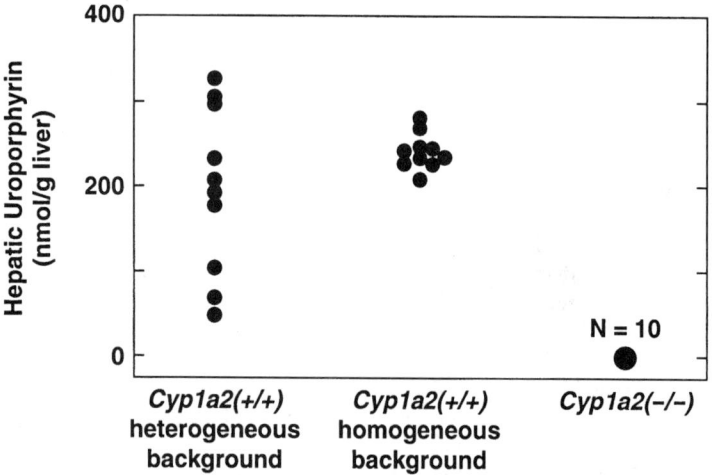

FIGURE 3B. An example of striking differences in phenotype as a function of the genetic background: Liver uroporphyrin concentrations in *Cyp1a2(+/+)* mice having a heterogeneous background (75% to 87.5% C57BL/6J), compared with that in *Cyp1a2(+/+)* mice having a homogeneous background (>99% C57BL/6J). The CYP1A2 enzyme is absolutely required for porphyria, as shown in the *Cyp1a2(−/−)* mice.[27]

TABLE 2. Number of breedings needed to obtain a (theoretical) percentage of genetically homogeneous background

Beginning knockout mouse	50%
First cross	75%
Second cross	87.5%
Third cross	93.75%
Fourth cross	96.875%
Fifth cross	98.4375%
Sixth cross	99.21875%
Seventh cross	99.609385%
Eighth cross	99.8046875%[a]

NOTE: These percentages are simple mathematical calculations; the actual amount of genetically homogeneous background may become asymptotic as these mouse lines approach 98% and above.

[a] If the mouse genome contains 80,000 genes, this value would represent ~79,844 genes from the homogeneous background and ~156 genes from the other mouse line.

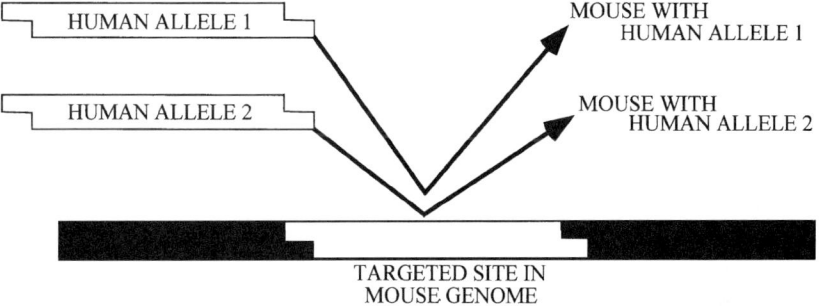

FIGURE 4. Illustration of the gene-swapping technique for placing one human allele after another into the same targeted site in the mouse genome.

These data underscore the importance of having a genetically homogeneous background if one wishes to carry out the most informative and precise experiments in laboratory animals. It would thus be to the investigator's advantage if one human allele after another could be inserted into an appropriate targeted site in the genome of an inbred mouse line (FIG. 4). In our lab, we have always chosen C57BL/6J for breeding into the genetically homogeneous background because this inbred mouse line has been selected for sequencing by the Mouse Genome Project (Cambridge, MA).

HETEROTYPIC LOX SITES

Cre recombinase is an enzyme from the bacteriophage P1 that catalyzes the site-specific recombination of DNA through the recognition of 34-bp motifs called *lox*

```
ATAACTTCGTATA ATGTATGC TATACGAAGTTAT
TATTGAAGCATAT TACATACG ATATGCTTCAATA      loxP
| inverted repeat | directional spacer | inverted repeat |
ATAACTTCGTATA GAAAGGTA TATACGAAGTTAT
TATTGAAGCATAT CTTTCCAT ATATGCTTCAATA      loxY
```

FIGURE 5A. The 34-bp sequences of the *loxP* and *loxY* sites. The inverted 13-bp repeats are the same, whereas the 8-bp spacer region differs.

sites. The naturally occurring site in the bacteriophage P1 is called the *loxP* site. The *loxP* site represents an inverted repeat of 13 bp, plus the 8-bp spacer sequence (FIG. 5A) that imposes directionality (same orientation = excision; opposite orientation = inversion) to the recombination event. It was discovered that two *loxP* sites, as far apart as 200 kb,[29] can be recognized by the Cre recombinase, which then excises all the DNA between these two *loxP* sites (FIG. 5B). Intriguingly, Cre recombinase has even been shown to mediate recombination and excision between nonhomologous chromosomes.[30,31]

Cre-mediated excision is reversible such that circular DNA containing a *loxP* site can be site-specifically integrated via a *loxP* site into linear DNA. This process has been used to catalyze the integration of reporter genes into target *loxP* sites in chromosomes.[32] This strategy has some problems, however, because Cre recombinase is so efficient that the integrated DNA is quickly excised; also, the circular DNA product of excision has no selection advantage and thus becomes lost quickly. This shortcoming limits the usefulness of genomic targeting with Cre recombinase.

Using heterospecific *lox* sites, though, we have developed a method of segmental replacement of *lox*-flanked DNA that will allow not only targeting of a specific site in the genome, but (at the same time) the site-specific replacement of one sequence of DNA with another. We have chosen to call this technique "gene swapping."

GENE SWAPPING

Heterotypic *lox* sites differ in the sequence of their 8-bp spacer regions (FIG. 5A). It has been shown that the sequence of the spacer is important—both in imparting directionality to a *lox* site, as mentioned above, and in exhibiting compatibility of two *lox* sites in recombination. Thus, two *loxP* sites will recombine as shown in FIGURE 5B. If the sequence of the spacer is changed so that we create a *loxY* site, however, then *loxY* sites can be catalyzed to recombine. It should be emphasized that a *loxY* site usually will not recombine with a *loxP* site. With this rule in mind, consider the sequence of events presented in FIGURE 6. Heterotypic *lox* sites (i.e., *loxP* and *loxY*) flank a gene and its regulatory sequences integrated into a chromosome. In the presence of Cre recombinase activity, either the *loxP* site can recombine with the *loxP* site, or the *loxY* site can recombine with the *loxY* site. In either case, both genes are integrated at the target locus. As mentioned above, the efficient action of Cre recombinase will resolve this locus—either through recombination of *loxP* sites or

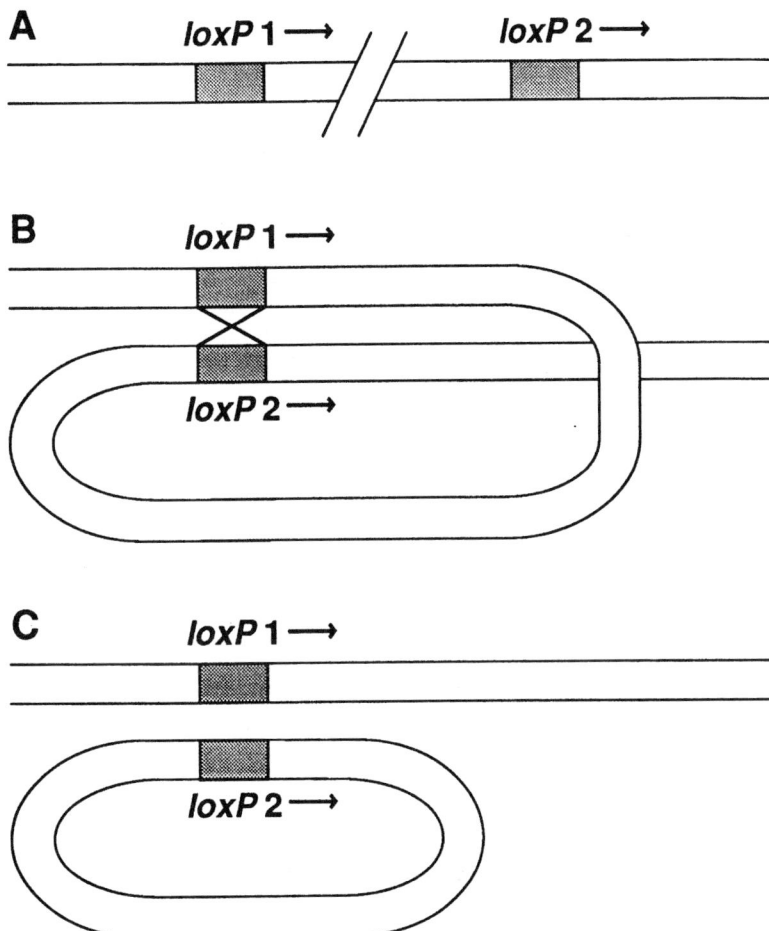

FIGURE 5B. Mechanism of action of Cre recombinase. Two *loxP* sites in the same orientation lead to excision of all DNA between the two sites by Cre recombinase (modified from reference 30).

through recombination of *loxY* sites. In one scenario, the locus of integration ("Gene A") is left unchanged; in the other scenario, our gene of interest ("Gene B") replaces the original gene. Thus, "gene swapping" has occurred. As an example of further versatility, the *loxP* and *loxY* sites can also flank a gene of interest in a large vector (e.g., cosmid, bacteriophage P1, bacterial artificial chromosome, etc.; FIG. 7).

CONFIRMATION THAT GENE SWAPPING WORKS

Experimentally, we have recently confirmed the ability to gene-swap in cultured mouse hepatoma Hepa-1c1c7 cells. In these experiments (TABLE 3), we tested the

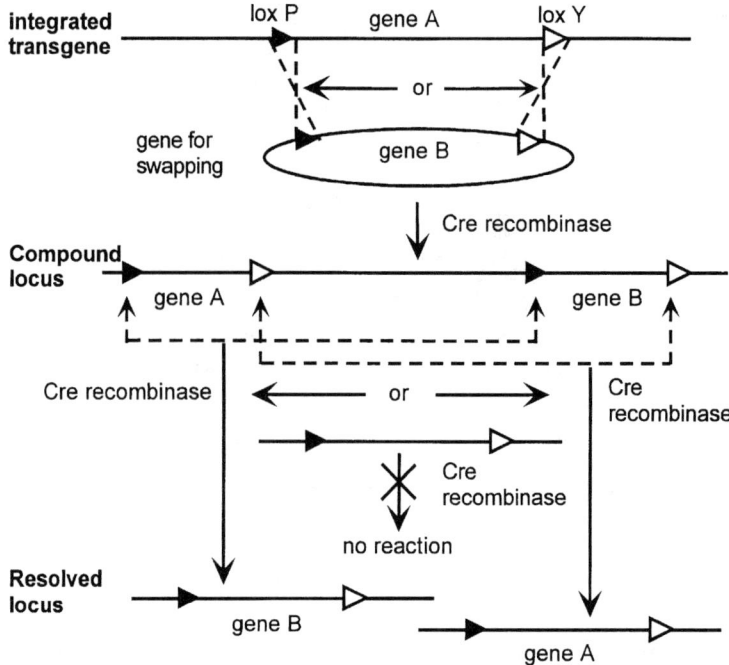

FIGURE 6. Illustration of the gene-swapping technique. Use of heterotypic *lox* sites, followed by Cre recombinase action, will result in either retention of "Gene A" or replacement of "Gene A" with "Gene B" that had been introduced into the cell on a circular construct.

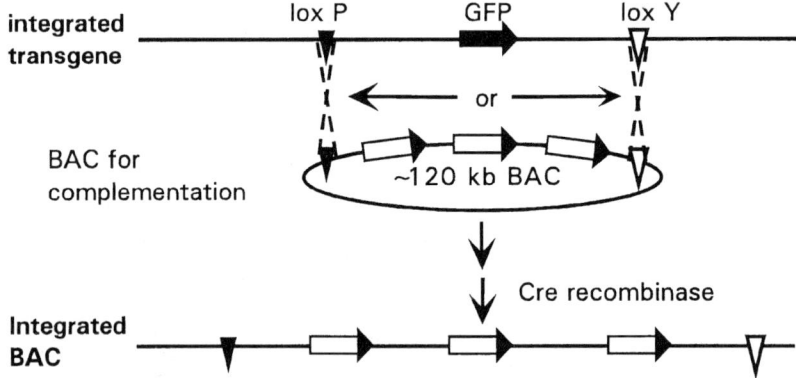

FIGURE 7. Scheme to demonstrate the use of heterotypic *lox* sites for replacing the jellyfish green fluorescent protein (*GFP*) gene with a genetically engineered human gene located on a bacterial artificial chromosome (BAC), which is generally 40 to 400 kb in size. Ultimately, a newborn mouse that does not fluoresce green would be a mouse having had a successful gene swap.

TABLE 3. Demonstration of one gene replaced by another

Cell line	Transfection	Fluorescence	zeo^R	βGAL activity	neo^R	Rel. # neo^R colonies
gfpzeo	—	green	yes	nil	no	
gfpzeo	β*geo* swap	green	yes	0.79 ± 0.78	yes	1
gfpzeo	β*geo* swap + CRE	none	no	1.71 ± 0.17	yes	10

ability of a *loxP/loxY*-flanked β-galactosidase–neomycin phosphotransferase fusion gene *(βgeo)* to swap with a *loxP/loxY*-flanked green fluorescent protein–zeocin resistance fusion gene (*gfpzeo*). In other words, *gfpzeo* is "Gene A" and β*geo* is "Gene B" (FIG. 6). To accomplish this, the cells were first stably transfected with a *loxP/loxY*-flanked *gfpzeo* gene. These cells were resistant to zeocin and displayed green fluorescence (TABLE 3). Next, we transfected with the β*geo* gene, with and without Cre recombinase activity present, and selected for G418 resistance (neo^R). In the absence of Cre recombinase, all G418-resistant colonies remained fluorescent green and resistant to zeocin. In the presence of Cre recombinase, the number of G418-resistant colonies increased 10-fold, despite 2-fold lower transfection efficiency. In addition, more than 70% of the G418-resistant colonies no longer displayed green fluorescence. Furthermore, these colonies were no longer resistant to zeocin.

β-Galactosidase activity in individual clones from the transfection without Cre recombinase was variable, with the standard deviation larger than the mean. This result is to be expected since the β*geo* gene presumably integrates randomly and its expression is in large part dependent on its site of integration and copy number. In distinct contrast, β-galactosidase activity in colonies from the transfection with Cre recombinase present was consistent between colonies, with the standard deviation less than 10% of the mean. This result is only possible if β*geo* became integrated as a single-copy gene into a single locus, in short, was "gene-swapped" for *gfpzeo*. After we had begun our studies, the Sauer laboratory[32] reported similar results, using an approach quite similar to that described above.

GENE SWAPPING IN THE INTACT MOUSE

To test the plausibility of gene swapping directly in a zygote of an inbred mouse strain, it seems most logical, in the interest of saving time and effort, to first generate a transgenic mouse using conventional zygotic microinjection and to then use transgenic zygotes from these animals for gene swapping. For this purpose, we have generated a *loxP/loxY*-flanked *CMV-gfpzeo* gene, which is cloned into the mouse metallothionein locus control regions (FIG. 8). The locus-control regions have previously been demonstrated to impart copy number–dependent and integration site–independent expression of transgenes.[34] Therefore, almost all transgenic animals will express the transgene. Furthermore, as previously demonstrated, the transgenic animals should be easy to identify because they will glow green under fluorescent light.[35] The *gfpzeo* gene in this metallothionein LCR construct has been shown to function in mammalian cells.[34] To date, we have been successful in mouse transfect-

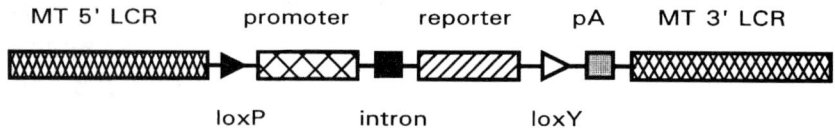

FIGURE 8. Illustration of the floxed *CMV-gfpzeo* gene that has been cloned into the mouse metallothionein (*Mt1*) locus control regions (LCR). The *hCMV* promoter is the promoter, and *gfpzeo* is the reporter gene. "Intron" denotes the two introns from SV40, which normally are used to splice out the viral 16S and 19S late mRNAs.[33] The polyadenylation (polyA) signal is 3'-ward of the *loxY* site.

ed Hepa-1c1c7 cells and in zebrafish embryos, but so far we have been unsuccessful in detecting this construct in the newborn mouse.

Using the *loxP/loxY-gfpzeo* mice, we are attempting gene swapping with four quite different strategies. The *loxP/loxY*-β*geo* incoming gene is being injected with four delivery systems for Cre recombinase: (a) with the pCAGGS–Cre recombinase expression plasmid[36] and similar expression construct,[37] successful and efficient removal of *loxP*-flanked sequences in the mouse fertilized egg has been achieved; (b) with an mRNA encoding Cre recombinase, this strategy has also been reported to remove *loxP*-flanked sequences in mouse zygotes;[38] (c) with the Cre recombinase protein itself, although this approach has not been attempted in the zygote, a maltose-binding protein–Cre recombinase (MBP/CR) fusion protein is known to function successfully in recombination, following electroporation into cultured cells;[39] and (d) finally, *loxP/loxY-gfpzeo* mice will be bred with mice that express Cre recombinase during early development. We are using the "deleter-Cre" and the "balancer-Cre" mouse lines;[40,41] these mice express Cre recombinase under the control of the human *CMV* and the rat *nestin* gene promoters, respectively. Mice that express Cre recombinase under the control of a *CMV* promoter have been shown to successfully recombine *loxP* sequences at the zygote stage.[42]

Integration site effects have been a major roadblock in expression studies using transgenic animals and have been even more deleterious when comparing transgenic animals having different genetic backgrounds.[28] Further, Cre recombinase–mediated processes are very efficient, including Cre recombinase–mediated recombination in zygotes. Hence, generation of transgenic mice using this approach might be much more efficient than standard techniques for generating transgenic mice. Finally, identification and selection of a gene-swapped mouse, derived from the inbred strain of your choice, should be as simple as shining a fluorescent light on mouse newborns; those mice that do not fluoresce green are those in which gene swapping has occurred.

CONVENTIONAL PLUS CONDITIONAL KNOCKOUT MOUSE LINES

The use of the Cre/*loxP* system to generate conventional plus conditional knockout mouse lines has provided a quantum leap in our understanding of the function of many genes and, undoubtedly, there will be expanded use of this system as we enter the next millennium. Thus, to study a gene essential for embryonic development (such that conventional knockout animals die during embryogenesis), one can create an animal that manifests the knockout genotype only conditionally at some time after birth or in adulthood (see reference 30). This same technology allows for the tissue-specific ablation of genes. The basis of this powerful approach is the combination of conventional gene targeting procedures and Cre-mediated recombination.

The usual strategy in making a conditional knockout mouse line, starting with ES cells, has two essential components: (1) A targeting construct of your gene of choice is made such that sequences essential for gene function are flanked by *lox* sites existing as direct repeats, and a selectable marker (e.g., *hprt*, *tk*) gene minicassette flanked by *lox* sites is also included (FIG. 9). Such a gene is called a "floxed gene." The *lox* sites are engineered into portions of the gene believed to be without function, meaning that the floxed gene will behave normally in the animal. (2) Following injection of the ES cells into the blastocoele cavity and germline transmission as described above, mice heterozygous for the type I and II deletions (i.e., carrying both alleles) are called "floxed mice." These mice can then be bred with a mouse that expresses Cre recombinase under the control of a promoter, which will, in turn, generate the gene ablation pattern desired. For example, to generate a conditional knockout of a gene in the liver, one could breed floxed mice with mice that express Cre recombinase under control of the albumin (liver-specific) promoter. Likewise, using tissue-specific or cell type–specific promoters driving the Cre recombinase gene, the conditional gene disruption could be designed to occur only in endothelial cells of the vascular system or in the substantia nigra of the brain. Alternatively, one

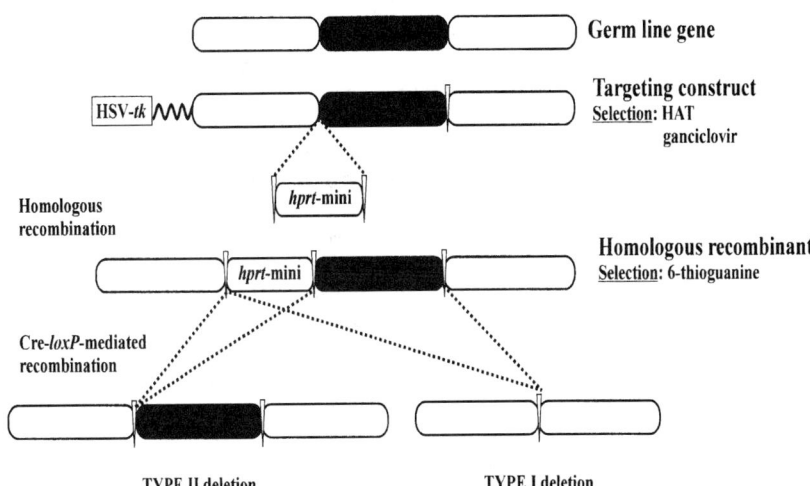

FIGURE 9. Strategy for generating a gene segment (closed bar) flanked by *loxP* sites in ES cells. Shown are the germline gene, a corresponding targeting construct generated *in vitro*, the resulting homologous recombinant in ES cells, and the two types of Cre/*loxP*-mediated deletions that will be isolated. The *loxP* sequences are represented by thin triangles. The position of the selection marker cassette containing the *hprt* minigene is indicated. ES cells containing the floxed *hprt* minigene are selected against due to 6-thioguanine in the medium (modified from reference 30).

could infect mice with a Cre recombinase–expressing virus and generate conditional ablation of a gene only in virally infected cells. Most of these approaches have been successful.

BYPASS THE ES CELLS AND GO DIRECTLY TO THE ANIMAL

An alternative to constructing the type I and type II alleles in ES cells is to generate them directly in the animal. Using this strategy, targeted ES cell clones would be used to develop mouse lines. As described above, Cre recombinase would then be introduced, or expressed, in the animal in such a way that the type I and II alleles would be present in the animal's germline. Type I and II alleles would then be detected by Southern or PCR analysis of the offspring. Our lab is attempting two approaches, hoping to succeed in the germline transmission of Cre recombinase–recombined alleles: (a) injection of zygotes carrying the floxed conditional knockout allele together with Cre recombinase, its mRNA, or an expression plasmid; and (b) breeding a Cre recombinase–expressing mouse line with a mouse line that carries the floxed conditional knockout allele.

We have used the pCAGGS–Cre recombinase expression plasmid, which has previously been shown to be successful for effecting Cre-mediated recombination in mouse zygotes.[36,37] We have also synthesized Cre recombinase mRNA using *in vitro* transcription with T7 RNA polymerase (IRES-Cre nRNA). Microinjection of Cre recombinase mRNA has been demonstrated to result in the successful recombination of *loxP* sites in mouse zygotes.[38] Finally, we have obtained a plasmid that expresses the MBP/CR fusion protein.[39] This protein can be easily purified over an amylose affinity column and contains a nuclear localization signal. Furthermore, the catalytic activity of MBP/CR is indistinguishable from Cre recombinase, and the MBP/CR fusion protein is even more stable than Cre recombinase. Because it has clearly been shown that Cre recombinase can function in the mouse fertilized egg, injection of the MBP/CR may be the most controlled approach for generating Cre recombinase–mediated deletions in the mouse zygote.

As discussed above, Cre recombinase–mediated deletion of *lox*-flanked sequences can also be accomplished by breeding a floxed mouse with a mouse that expresses Cre recombinase. There exist two transgenic mouse lines that are suitable for this purpose. As described earlier, the "deleter" Cre mouse expresses Cre recombinase under the control of the strong viral CMV promoter;[40] this promoter is expressed in most cell types and Cre expression is high and/or persistent enough to produce recombination in most or all cells in a given tissue, including testis. The "balancer" Cre mouse, on the other hand, in which Cre recombinase is expressed under the control of the *nestin* gene's promoter generates mosaic recombination in all tissues tested, including testis.[41] These data suggest the presence of no more than one Cre recombinase–mediated event per cell. Since the terminal event of Cre-mediated recombination (in a scenario such as that illustrated in FIG. 9) is a type I deletion (i.e., one remaining *lox* site), an animal that expresses a low level of Cre recombinase would theoretically be most suitable for production of the type II deletion. However, to err on the side of caution, we hope to use both types of the Cre recombinase-expressing animals.

Although generation of the type I plus type II alleles by expression of Cre recombinase in the intact animal has not yet been reported, the reports described above demonstrate that Cre recombinase does function in the zygote, early embryo, and newborn—as well as the adult animal—indicating that Cre-mediated recombination events can be successful in the germline of adult animals. Also, as discussed above, among the most common rate-limiting steps in generating a targeted mouse line is the effective germline transmission of constructs in our targeted ES cells that had been injected into the blastocoele cavity of mice. Furthermore, there is an inverse correlation between the amount of manipulation of ES cells in culture and the degree of successful germline transmission. The traditional procedure for the generation of a conditional knockout mouse line requires that ES cells spend twice the time in culture, compared with that of a conventional knockout mouse line. Therefore, conditional knockout procedures can be particularly problematic in providing ES cell clones that are capable of going germline. Use of ES clones immediately following the initial targeting event, in order to generate transgenic animals, should therefore optimize our chances that a given targeted ES cell line will go germline.

THE *CYP1A1(–/–)* KNOCKOUT LINE AS AN EXAMPLE

The construct shown in FIGURE 10 is a schematic of the mouse *Cyp1a1* gene that has recently been targeted in our laboratory. After targeting, and then screening 242

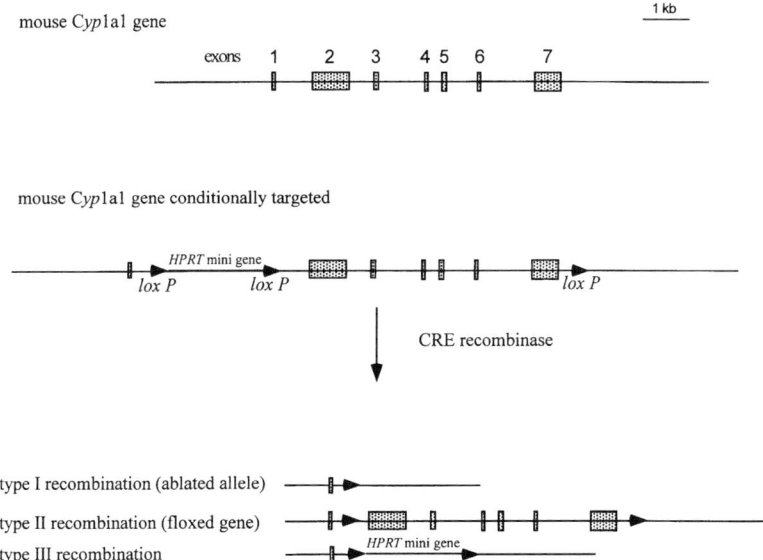

FIGURE 10. Diagram of the floxed *Cyp1a1* gene, having seven exons, from which the *Cyp1a1(–/–)* knockout mouse line has now been generated.[43] Differing Cre recombinase actions should result in the conventional knockout (type I), conditional knockout (type II), and the type III recombination event in which the *hprt* minigene cassette is retained. To date, we have succeeded in obtaining only the type I knockout.

colonies, we identified 9 ES cell clones that contained the complete targeting construct—including the distal nonselectable *loxP* site. To test the above-described methods of Cre expression, we injected zygotes heterozygous for the floxed *Cyp1a1* gene with either the pCAGGS-Cre plasmid or the IRES-Cre mRNA. We have not yet microinjected the MBP/CR fusion protein.

Of 12 heterozygous pups born that had been injected as zygotes with the pCAGGS–Cre recombinase plasmid, 3 (25%) were knockouts (type I deletion). By Southern blot analysis, these animals were not chimeric for the other form (e.g., type II deletion). The low rate of recombination (25%), coupled with the fact that we had injected plasmid DNA, suggests that the animals that were positive for recombination might have integrated successfully and are expressing Cre. If the only variable were plasmid expression (and not the low-efficiency integration event), then why do we have all-or-none (type I only) recombination at such low frequency? We have not yet tested the possibility that Cre is being expressed in these animals.

Of 3 heterozygous animals injected with the IRES-Cre mRNA, 2 (67%) were type I (conventional) knockouts. Again, these animals exhibited recombinational events until only one *lox* site remained (i.e., no type II recombination); however, since the RNA was used as a source of Cre expression, we do know that these animals are not Cre-expressing transgenics. To avoid Cre transgenesis and because of the high recombinational frequency, we conclude that the injection of Cre mRNA seems more promising than use of the pCAGGS–Cre recombinase expression plasmid. By titrating the amount of mRNA injected, we should now be able to generate the type II (floxed) deletion. These experiments are under way. We believe that use of the IRES–Cre recombinase mRNA can be successful in the fertilized ovum because both type I and type II deletions have been produced in ES cells in culture.

TROUBLESHOOTING AND FUTURE APPROACHES

Both the work of our laboratory and that of Sauer[44,45] suggest that gene swapping using heterotypic *lox* sites should become successful in the intact animal and highly popular during the first few years of the next millennium. However, one of us (G. W. Stuart, unpublished) has recently found rare, but significant, recombination between heterotypic *lox* sites present in bacteria that chronically express Cre recombinase. Conceptually, this would limit the utility of our currently designed gene-swapping approach. At the very least, this finding would suggest that we will need to select carefully the *lox* sites—such that recombination between heterotypic *lox* sites is kept to a minimum.

Another approach might be to use both Cre recombinase and FLP recombinase[46] together to swap genes. With this approach, the *loxY* site would be replaced with an FLP recombinase target (FRT). By using the coexpression of both Cre and FLP, one might succeed in the integration by one recombinase, and excision by the other. In this version of gene swapping, crossovers between *lox* and FLP sites would not be an issue because they are dissimilar. Also, one could titrate the ratio of Cre/FLP to determine what worked best in swapping. Although it was once believed that FLP recombination did not work well in mice, there are currently modified versions that have been optimized for higher temperature.[47]

USEFUL CONSTRUCTS AND MOUSE LINES

In collaboration with Fred Kadlubar (Jefferson, AR) and Henry Lin (UCLA, Los Angeles, CA), we have begun experiments to generate mouse lines containing the "high-" and "low-extreme" human *CYP1A2* alleles in place of the mouse orthologous *CYP1A2* gene. In the alleles we have chosen, the difference between the "high" and "low" constitutive *CYP1A2* activity is between 35- and 40-fold. We are inserting ample amounts of human *CYP1A2* upstream regulatory sequences, plus all introns and some 3' sequence, in an attempt to make the mouse lines exhibit tissue-specific *CYP1A2* expression like the human rather than the mouse. For example, although *CYP1A2* is found in both the human and mouse liver and gastrointestinal tract, human *CYP1A2* is found in brain, but not lung, and mouse *CYP1A2* is found in lung, but not brain (reviewed in reference 48). Hence, when these mouse lines are ultimately examined for the toxicokinetics/pharmacokinetics of *CYP1A2* substrates, it is hoped that the patterns of distribution and tissue-specific expression of the enzyme throughout the intact mouse will be more "human-like" than "mouse-like". As with β-galactosidase activity (discussed in TABLE 3), integration of the human *CYP1A2* gene, as a single copy and at a single locus, should provide an experimental system with exceedingly low error ascribed to differences in expression level of the human *CYP1A2* allele that had been inserted. During the first decade of the next millennium, we predict that the highest and lowest human *CYP2C9*, *CYP2C19*, *CYP2D6*, *CYP2E1*, and *CYP3A4* alleles[11,49] will also be incorporated into mouse lines.

After these transgenic mouse lines are generated and characterized, they should provide a stable resource for conducting innumerable possible experiments. Should this approach succeed, we would of course make our protocols and reagents available to colleagues worldwide. As discussed above, these lines could allow the expression of any transgene at the gene-swapping locus. Technically, this means that the integration site will be the same for all genes swapped.

SUMMARY

First, a growing number of human genetic polymorphisms in DME genes are being characterized; some of these have been demonstrated to be correlated with risk of toxicity or cancer, whereas others presently remain equivocal and require further study. Genetic differences in the regulation, expression, and activity of environmental susceptibility genes can be decisive in defining cancer susceptibility and the toxic or carcinogenic power of environmental chemicals.

Second, differences in DME genes between humans and mice (3- to perhaps 10-fold) are often far less than interindividual human differences (20- to sometimes more than 40-fold). It would be advantageous to study the toxicokinetics of chemicals and the pharmacokinetics of drugs by inserting the "high-" and "low-extreme" human alleles in place of the orthologous mouse gene. We have begun to generate mouse lines lacking the *CYP1A2* gene, but containing either the "highest" or the "lowest" human *CYP1A2* allele. One obvious goal is to generate mouse lines having additional human alleles of numerous DME genes in place of the mouse orthologous genes.

Third, in mouse hepatoma Hepa-1c1c7 cells in culture, using heterotypic *lox* sites we have succeeded in swapping one reporter gene (and its control regions) with a second gene (and its control regions), and vice versa. Our successes and shortcomings in doing the same in the intact mouse have been discussed.

Fourth, use of *lox* sites in the intact zygote for the generation of type I (conventional knockout) and type II (conditional knockout) mouse lines is summarized. We have described in detail our current success to date, using as an example the development of our *Cyp1a1(−/−)* knockout mouse line.

Fifth, and last, we anticipate that "humanized" mouse lines will become valuable during the first decade of the next millennium—not only to the toxicologist and pharmacologist researcher, but to regulatory agencies as well, as they define policy issues concerning risk assessment to environmental and pharmaceutical agents.

ACKNOWLEDGMENTS

These data have been presented, in part, at the following: the First Annual Workshop on "Transgenic Model Systems and Molecular Toxicology", National Institute of Environmental Health Sciences, Research Triangle Park, North Carolina (March 1997); the Session on "Transgenic Animals to Predict Drug Metabolism", Twelfth International Symposium on Microsomes and Drug Oxidations, Montpellier, France (July 1998); and the National Institutes of Health/U.S. Food and Drug Administration Conference on "Biomarkers and Surrogate Endpoints: Clinical Research and Applications", Toxicology Biomarkers Breakout Session, Bethesda, Maryland (April 1999). We thank our colleagues for valuable discussions and critical reading of this manuscript. This work was supported in part by NIH Grant Nos. R01 ES07058, R01 ES08147, R01 ES06321, and P30 ES06096.

REFERENCES

1. NEBERT, D.W. 1999. Pharmacogenetics and pharmacogenomics: why is this relevant to the clinical geneticist? Clin. Genet. **56:** 247.
2. NEBERT, D.W. & W.W. WEBER. 1990. Pharmacogenetics. *In* Principles of Drug Action: The Basis of Pharmacology. Third edition, pp. 469–531. Churchill Livingstone. New York.
3. DALY, A.K., S. CHOLERTON, M. ARMSTRONG & J.R. IDLE. 1994. Genotyping for polymorphisms in xenobiotic metabolism as a predictor of disease susceptibility. Environ. Health Perspect. **102**(suppl. 9)**:** 55.
4. MEYER, U.A. 1994. Pharmacogenetics: the slow, the rapid, and the ultrarapid. Proc. Natl. Acad. Sci. U.S.A. **91:** 1983.
5. KALOW, W. & L. BERTILSSON. 1994. Interethnic factors affecting drug response. Adv. Drug Res. **23:** 1.
6. GONZALEZ, F.J. 1997. The role of carcinogen-metabolizing enzyme polymorphisms in cancer susceptibility. Reprod. Toxicol. **11:** 397.
7. NEBERT, D.W. 1997. Polymorphisms in drug-metabolizing enzymes: what is their clinical relevance and why do they exist? Am. J. Hum. Genet. **60:** 265.
8. NEBERT, D.W. 1997. Pharmacogenetics: 65 candles on the cake. Pharmacogenetics **7:** 435.
9. WEBER, W.W. 1997. Pharmacogenetics. Oxford University Press. London/New York.
10. KLEYN, P.W. & E.S. VESELL. 1998. Genetic variation as a guide to drug development. Science **281:** 1820.

11. NEBERT, D.W., M. INGELMAN-SUNDBERG & A.K. DALY. 1999. Genetic epidemiology of environmental toxicity and cancer susceptibility: human allelic polymorphisms in drug-metabolizing enzyme genes, their functional importance, and nomenclature issues. Drug Metab. Rev. **31:** 467.
12. WEINSHILBOUM, R.M., D.M. OTTERNESS & C.L. SZUMLANSKI. 1999. Methylation pharmacogenetics: catechol O-methyltransferase, thiopurine methyltransferase, and histamine N-methyltransferase. Annu. Rev. Pharmacol. Toxicol. **39:** 19.
13. NEBERT, D.W., R.A. MCKINNON & A. PUGA. 1996. Human drug-metabolizing enzyme polymorphisms: effects on risk of toxicity and cancer. DNA Cell Biol. **15:** 273.
14. NELSON, D.R. 2000. Cytochrome P450 home page [web site]. http://drnelson.utmem.edu/cytochromeP450.html//.
15. NEBERT, D.W. 1991. Proposed role of drug-metabolizing enzymes: regulation of steady state levels of the ligands that affect growth, homeostasis, differentiation, and neuroendocrine functions. Mol. Endocrinol. **5:** 1203.
16. LAZAROU, J., B.H. POMERANZ & P.N. COREY. 1998. Incidence of adverse drug reactions in hospitalized patients: a meta-analysis of prospective studies. J. Am. Med. Assoc. **279:** 1200.
17. GUENGERICH, F.P. 1999. Cytochrome P-450 3A4: regulation and role in drug metabolism. Annu. Rev. Pharmacol. Toxicol. **39:** 1.
18. MARTINEZ, C., J.A. AGUNDEZ, G. GERVASINI, R. MARTIN & J. BENITEZ. 1997. Tryptamine: a possible endogenous substrate for CYP2D6. Pharmacogenetics **7:** 85.
19. ZHOU, L.X., B. PIHLSTROM, J.P. HARDWICK, S.S. PARK, S.A. WRIGHTON & J.L. HOLTZMAN. 1996. Metabolism of phenytoin by the gingiva of normal humans: the possible role of reactive metabolites of phenytoin in the initiation of gingival hyperplasia. Clin. Pharmacol. Ther. **60:** 191.
20. GU, J., Q.Y. ZHANG, M.B. GENTER, T.W. LIPINSKAS, M. NEGISHI, D.W. NEBERT & X. DING. 1998. Purification and characterization of heterologously expressed mouse CYP2A5 and CYP2G1: role in metabolic activation of acetaminophen and 2,6-dichlorobenzonitrile in mouse olfactory mucosal microsomes. J. Pharmacol. Exp. Ther. **285:** 1287.
21. SCHORK, N.J., J.E. KRIEGER, M.R. TROLLIET, K.G. FRANCHINI, G. KOIKE, E.M. KRIEGER, E.S. LANDER, V.J. DZAU & H.J. JACOB. 1995. A biometrical genome search in rats reveals the multigenic basis of blood pressure variation. Genome Res. **5:** 164.
22. HALUSHKA, M.K., J.B. FAN, K. BENTLEY, L. HSIE, N. SHEN, A. WEDER, R. COOPER, R. LIPSHUTZ & A. CHAKRAVARTI. 1999. Patterns of single-nucleotide polymorphisms in candidate genes for blood-pressure homeostasis. Nat. Genet. **22:** 239.
23. JAISSER, F. & A.T. BEGGAH. 1998. Transgenic models in renal tubular physiology. Exp. Nephrol. **6:** 438.
24. BRADLEY, A., M. EVANS, M.H. KAUFMAN & E. ROBERTSON. 1984. Formation of germ-line chimeras from embryo-derived teratocarcinoma cell lines. Nature **309:** 255.
25. LIANG, H.C., H. LI, R.A. MCKINNON, J.J. DUFFY, S.S. POTTER, A. PUGA & D.W. NEBERT. 1996. $Cyp1a2(-/-)$ null mutant mice develop normally, but show deficient drug metabolism. Proc. Natl. Acad. Sci. U.S.A. **93:** 1671.
26. BONYADI, M., S.A. RUSHOLME, F.M. COUSINS, H.C. SU, C.A. BIRON, M. FARRALL & R.J. AKHURST. 1997. Mapping of a major genetic modifier of embryonic lethality in TGFβ1 knockout mice. Nat. Genet. **15:** 207.
27. SINCLAIR, P.R., N. GORMAN, T.P. DALTON, H.S. WALTON, W.J. BEMENT, J.F. SINCLAIR, A.G. SMITH & D.W. NEBERT. 1998. Uroporphyria produced in mice by iron and 5-aminolevulinic acid does not occur in $Cyp1a2(-/-)$ null mutant mice. Biochem. J. **330:** 149.
28. OLSON, E.N., H.H. ARNOLD, P.W. RIGBY & B.J. WOLD. 1996. Know your neighbors: three phenotypes in null mutants of the myogenic bHLH gene *MRF4*. Cell **85:** 1.
29. LI, Z.W., G. STARK, J. GÖTZ, T. RÜLICKE & U. MÜLLER. 1996. Generation of mice with a 200-kb amyloid precursor protein gene deletion by Cre recombinase–mediated site-specific recombination in embryonic stem cells. Proc. Natl. Acad. Sci. U.S.A. **93:** 6158.
30. NEBERT, D.W. & J.J. DUFFY. 1997. How knockout mouse lines will be used to study the role of drug-metabolizing enzymes and their receptors during reproduction, develop-

ment, and environmental toxicity, cancer, and oxidative stress. Biochem. Pharmacol. **53**: 249.
31. VAN DEURSEN, J., M. FORNEROD, B. VAN REES & G. GROSVELD. 1995. Cre-mediated site-specific translocation between nonhomologous mouse chromosomes. Proc. Natl. Acad. Sci. U.S.A. **92**: 7376.
32. BETHKE, B. & B. SAUER. 1997. Segmental genomic replacement by Cre-mediated recombination: genotoxic stress activation of the p53 promoter in single-copy transformants. Nucleic Acids Res. **25**: 2828.
33. OKAYAMA, H. & P. BERG. 1983. A cDNA cloning vector that permits expression of cDNA inserts in mammalian cells. Mol. Cell. Biol. **3**: 280.
34. PALMITER, R.D., E.P. SANDGREN, D.M. KOELLER & R.L. BRINSTER. 1993. Distal regulatory elements from the mouse metallothionein locus stimulate gene expression in transgenic mice. Mol. Cell. Biol. **13**: 5266.
35. OKABE, M., M. IKAWA, T. KOMINAMI & Y. NISHIMUNE. 1997. "Green mice" as a source of ubiquitous green cells. FEBS Lett. **407**: 313.
36. SUNAGA, S., K. MAKI, Y. KOMAGATA, K. IKUTA & J.I. MIYAZAKI. 1997. Efficient removal of *loxP*-flanked DNA sequences in a gene-targeted locus by transient expression of Cre recombinase in fertilized eggs. Mol. Reprod. Dev. **46**: 109.
37. LAKSO, M., J.G. PICHEL, J.R. GORMAL, B. SAUER, Y. OKAMOTO, E. LEE, F.W. ALT & H. WESTPHAL. 1996. Efficient *in vivo* manipulation of mouse genomic sequences at the zygote stage. Proc. Natl. Acad. Sci. U.S.A. **93**: 5860.
38. DE WIT, T., D. DRABEK & F. GROSVLED. 1998. Microinjection of Cre recombinase RNA induces site-specific recombination of a transgene in mouse oocytes. Nucleic Acids Res. **26**: 676.
39. KOLB, A.F. & S.G. SIDDELL. 1996. Genomic targeting with an MBP-Cre fusion protein. Gene **183**: 53.
40. SCHWENK, F., U. BARON & K. RAJEWSKY. 1995. A Cre-transgenic mouse strain for the ubiquitous deletion of *loxP*-flanked gene segments including deletion in germ cells. Nucleic Acids Res. **23**: 5080.
41. BETS, U.A.K., C.A.J. VONHENRICH, K. RAJEWSKY & W. MYELLER. 1996. Bypass of lethality with mosaic mice generated by Cre-*loxP*-mediated recombination. Curr. Biol. **6**: 1307.
42. SAKAI, K. & J. MIYAZAKI. 1997. A transgenic mouse line that retains Cre recombinase activity in mature oocytes irrespective of Cre transgene transmission. Biochem. Biophys. Res. Commun. **237**: 318.
43. DALTON, T.P., M.S. DIETER, R.S. MATLIB, N. CHILDS, H.G. SHERTZER, M.B. GENTER & D.W. NEBERT. 2000. Targeted knockout in the *Cyp1a1* gene does not alter hepatic constitutive expression of other genes in the mouse [*Ah*] battery. Biochem. Biophys. Res. Commun. **267**: 184.
44. SAUER, B. 1998. Inducible gene targeting in mice using the Cre/*lox* system. Methods **14**: 381.
45. SOUKHAREV, S., J.L. MILLER & B. SAUER. 1999. Segmental genomic replacement in embryonic stem cells by double *lox* targeting. Nucleic Acids Res. **27**: e21.
46. THEODOSIOU, N.A. & T. XU. 1998. Use of the FLP/FRT system to study *Drosophila* development. Methods **14**: 355.
47. BUCHHOLZ, F., P.O. ANGRAND & A.F. STEWART. 1998. Improved properties of FLP recombinase evolved by cycling mutagenesis. Nat. Biotechnol. **16**: 657.
48. DEY, A., J.E. JONES & D.W. NEBERT. 1999. Tissue- and cell type–specific expression of cytochrome P450 1A1 and cytochrome P450 1A2 mRNA in the mouse localized by *in situ* hybridization. Biochem. Pharmacol. **58**: 525.
49. INGELMAN-SUNDBERG, M., A.K. DALY, M. OSCARSON & D.W. NEBERT. 2000. Human cytochrome P450 (*CYP*) allele nomenclature home page [web site]. http://www.imm.ki.se/CYPalleles//.

The Use of Explant Lens Culture to Assess Cataractogenic Potential

MICHAEL D. ALEO,[a,b] MICHAEL J. AVERY,[c] WILLIAM P. BEIERSCHMITT,[a] CYNTHIA A. DRUPA,[a] JAY H. FORTNER,[d] ADAM H. KAPLAN,[a] KIMBERLY A. NAVETTA,[a] RICHARD M. SHEPARD,[c] AND COLLEEN M. WALSH[a]

[a]*Drug Safety Evaluation,* [c]*Drug Metabolism, and* [d]*Comparative Medicine and Biology Support, Pfizer Central Research, Groton, Connecticut 06340, USA*

ABSTRACT: Explanted cultures of crystalline lenses have been used to investigate mechanisms of xenobiotic-induced cataract formation. However, very few studies have utilized mechanistic information to predict the cataractogenic potential of structurally diverse xenobiotics. The present investigation outlines how visual assessment of lens clarity, biochemical endpoints of toxicity, and mechanisms of lenticular opacity formation can be used to select compounds with a lower probability of causing cataract formation *in vivo*. The rat lens explant culture system has been used to screen thiazolidinediones against ciglitazone for their direct cataractogenic potential *in vitro*. The two compounds that were selected as development candidates (englitazone and darglitazone) did not produce cataracts in rats exposed daily for 3 months. The culture system has also been used to illustrate that the lens is capable of metabolizing compounds to reactive intermediates. In this example, the toxicity of *S*-(1,2-dichlorovinyl)-L-cysteine (DCVC), a model cataractogen, was attenuated by inhibiting lenticular cysteine conjugate β-lyase metabolism using aminooxyacetic acid. Finally, this model was used retrospectively to investigate the cataractogenic potential of CJ-12,918 and CJ-13,454 in rats. These compounds showed differences in the incidence of cataract formation *in vivo* based on differences in hepatic metabolism and penetration of parent drug and metabolites into the lens. The rank order of cataractogenic potential *in vitro* correlated better with *in vivo* results when an induced S9 microsomal fraction was added to the culture media. However, the model did not correctly predict the cataractogenic potential of ZD2138, a structurally similar compound. These studies illustrate the use of explant culture to assess mechanisms of cataract formation and outline its use and limitations for predicting cataractogenic potential *in vivo*.

INTRODUCTION

When a new therapeutic drug candidate causes lenticular opacities (i.e., cataracts) during the conduct of preclinical toxicology studies in animals, it is typically suspended from development in favor of expediting the development of backup candidates. This is a prudent course of action in the face of limited human safety information since some drugs have been associated with an increased risk of cataract formation in humans.[1–3] However, the decision to suspend development may be overturned with further investigation. For example, several well-known pharmaceu-

[b]Voice: 860-441-3588; fax: 860-441-5499.
Michael_D_Aleo@groton.pfizer.com

ticals like verapamil, FK506, and lovastatin increased the incidence of cataract formation in animals, but have not been reported to increase the risk of cataract formation in humans. In these cases, further investigative studies have demonstrated a favorable risk-benefit analysis that supported continued development of the therapeutic candidate. For example, Greiner and Glonek[4] reported that the cataractogenic potential of verapamil in dogs was species-specific. Ishida *et al.*[5] showed that cataract formation by FK506 in the rat was due to a dose-dependent diabetogenic effect caused by pancreatic injury that would not occur at clinically relevant doses. Therefore, additional animal studies alone may aid in discerning the relative risk associated with prolonged human exposure.

Traditional animal toxicology studies can also be supplemented with *in vitro* models. Lenses obtained from rodent and nonrodent species have been used as a short-term mechanistically based *in vitro* model to aid in predictions of cataractogenic potential and to determine mechanisms of opacity formation. This approach was used to help develop hydroxymethylglutaryl-coenzyme A (HMG-CoA) reductase inhibitors after lovastatin was found to be cataractogenic in dogs.[6,7] In addition to its pharmacologic inhibition of hepatic HMG-CoA reductase, further mechanistic studies showed that lovastatin also reduced cholesterol synthesis within the lens. The cataractogenic potential of this class of compounds in dogs was eliminated by developing more selective inhibitors of the hepatic isoform. Therefore, investigating mechanisms of cataract formation by drug candidates either can lessen concern for the potential to produce cataracts in humans or can result in the selection of a backup candidate with a superior preclinical safety profile.

Cataracts are primarily caused by xenobiotics that either penetrate the lens and directly disrupt normal cellular processes or indirectly interact with the lens surface through the generation of reactive oxygen species.[8,9] Cataractogenic compounds that penetrate the lens have an intrinsic ability to adversely perturb the lenticular environment, resulting in opacification. This can be caused by at least two major mechanisms: (1) changes in the refractive properties of the lens due to osmotic stress (increased water content) or (2) denaturation of lens proteins that are critical for maintaining lens clarity.[9–11] With some xenobiotics, such as acetaminophen, the compound that penetrates the lens and causes the damage is a metabolite that appears to be formed distally in the liver.[12] In contrast, other compounds such as *S*-(1,2-dichlorovinyl)-L-cysteine (DCVC) and naphthalene appear to be converted to a toxic metabolite within the lens.[13,14]

The lens explant culture model is an interesting *in vitro* model to utilize in mechanistic research. Although harvesting the lens from the eye without inducing mechanical trauma to the lens is technically challenging, the lens explant culture is an extremely simple and flexible system to utilize. Assessing cataractogenic potential of test compounds can be as simple as periodic visual assessments of lens clarity in culture after exposure to utilizing a vast array of biochemical, electrophysiological, or molecular endpoints that are known to be involved in mechanisms of cataract formation.

This chapter will highlight the use of lens explant culture to investigate the cataractogenic potential of three thiazolidinediones (ciglitazone, darglitazone, and englitazone), DCVC, and three tetrahydropyrans (CJ-12,918, CJ-13,454, and ZD2138). Thiazolidinediones are orally efficacious hypoglycemic agents in several rodent models of non-insulin-dependent diabetes mellitus.[15,16] Thiazolidinediones potentiate the action of insulin in skeletal muscle and adipose tissue[15,17–20] without stimulating insulin secretion directly from functioning pancreatic β-islet cells.[21,22] In the late 1980s, the lead drug candidate in this chemical class, ciglitazone, was anecdotally reported to cause cataracts in animals.[23] The lens explant culture model was used to rank and select alternative development candidates for the potential to cause opacity formation *in vitro* and, more recently, was used to investigate mechanisms of toxicity.[24]

In the next example, mechanisms of cataract formation were investigated with DCVC. Although DCVC is widely recognized for its acute nephrotoxic properties, prolonged low-dose exposure is associated with cataract formation in rodents.[25] The nephrotoxic properties of DCVC require biotransformation by cysteine conjugate β-lyase, an enzyme localized within the proximal tubule, to a reactive thioketene and cause toxicity through covalent binding to cellular macromolecules.[26] However, it was unknown whether DCVC was metabolized by a similar pathway in the lens. Using the lens explant culture model, we investigated the role of lenticular β-lyase activity in the cataractogenic potential of DCVC. A more in-depth analysis of DCVC-induced cataract formation has been reported.[13]

Finally, a retrospective analysis of cataract formation caused by two different tetrahydropyrans that was observed in 1-month safety evaluation studies was conducted using lens explant cultures. CJ-12,918 was under preclinical development when its administration to rats at a dose of 250 mg/kg/day was associated with an increased incidence of cataract formation during a 1-month safety evaluation study. The pharmacokinetics of CJ-12,918 were such that, well before the appearance of cataracts, systemic exposure to the parent compound was essentially negligible due to broad and extensive induction of hepatic cytochrome P-450 mixed-function oxygenases. This effect provided indirect evidence that opacity formation may be related to sustained exposure to metabolites rather than the parent compound. Analysis of plasma and lenses by HPLC/MS/MS after drug exposure *in vivo* showed extensive metabolism of CJ-12,918 to at least 12 metabolites, of which 6 were detected in the lens along with the parent compound. Knowing that the lens was exposed to numerous metabolites of CJ-12,918 as well as the parent compound *in vivo*, we retrospectively investigated the limitations of the lens explant model in predicting the cataractogenic potential of CJ-12,918 and the structural analogs CJ-13,454 and ZD2138. An aroclor-induced S9 microsomal fraction was incorporated into the culture media to assess the possible role of metabolite formation in cataract formation.

This manuscript illustrates the use of the lens explant model to investigate mechanisms of cataract formation and, with some limitations, how the system has been used to predict the cataractogenic potential of a small subset of pharmaceutical candidates *in vivo*.

MATERIALS AND METHODS

Materials

CJ-12,918 (hydrochloride salt), CJ-13,454, and ZD2138 were synthesized at Pfizer Central Research, Taketoyo, Japan (FIG. 1). Ciglitazone, darglitazone, and en-

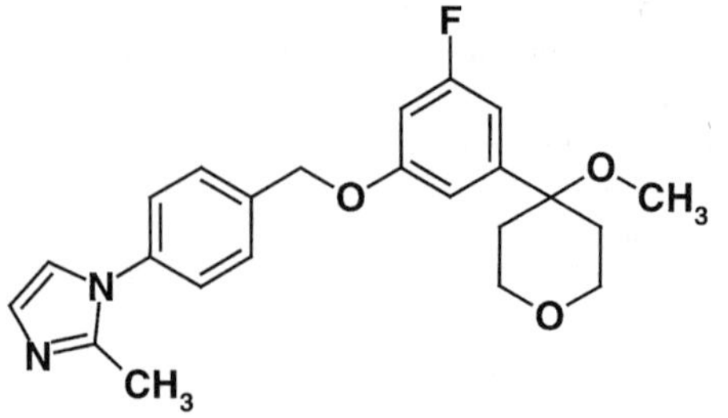

CJ-12,918: 4-[3-Fluoro-5-[4-(2-methylimidazol-1-yl)]benzyloxy]-phenyl-4-methoxy-3,4,5,6-tetrahydro-2H-pyran

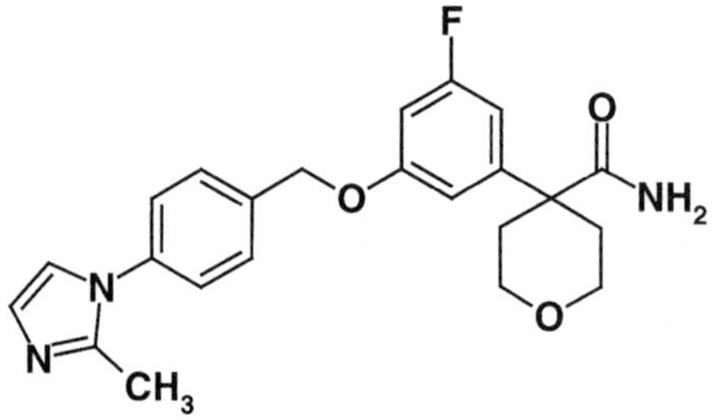

CJ-13,454: 4-[5-Fluoro-3-[4-(2-methylimidazol-1-yl)benzyloxy]phenyl]- 3,4,5,6-tetrahydro-2H-pyran-4-carboxamide

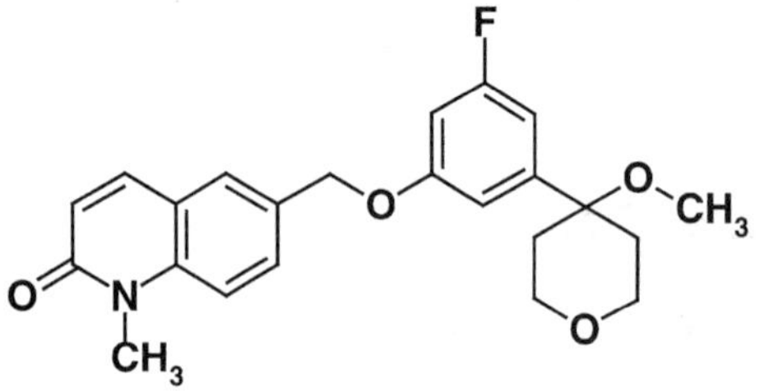

ZD2138: 4-methoxy-4-[3-(1-methyl-2-oxo-1,2-dihydroquinolin-6-ylmethoxy)phenyl] tetrahydropyran

FIGURE 1. Structures of three tetrahydropyrans—CJ-12,918, CJ-13,454, and ZD2138.

glitazone were synthesized at Pfizer Central Research, Groton, Connecticut (FIG. 2). DCVC was a kind gift from A. Jay Gandolfi and was synthesized in the laboratory of James L. Stevens. Dithiothreitol, 3-(4,5-dimethylthiazol-2-yl)-2,5-diphenyl tetrazolium bromide (MTT), methimazole, and aminooxyacetic acid were purchased from Sigma Chemical (St. Louis, MO). Ruthenium red was acquired from ICN (Cleveland, OH). Medium 199, glutamine, penicillin, and streptomycin were obtained from Gibco (Grand Island, NY). E64d and calpain inhibitor-II were purchased from Calbiochem (La Jolla, CA). All other reagents were the highest analytical grade commercially available.

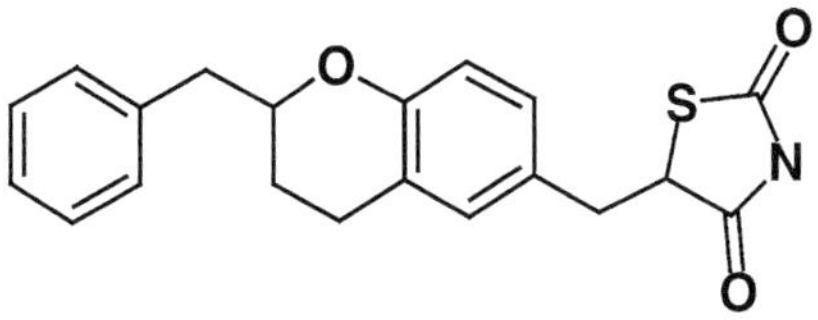

ENGLITAZONE: (±)-5-[3,4-dihydro-2-phenylmethyl-2H-1-benzopyran-6-yl)methyl] thiazolidine-2,4-dione

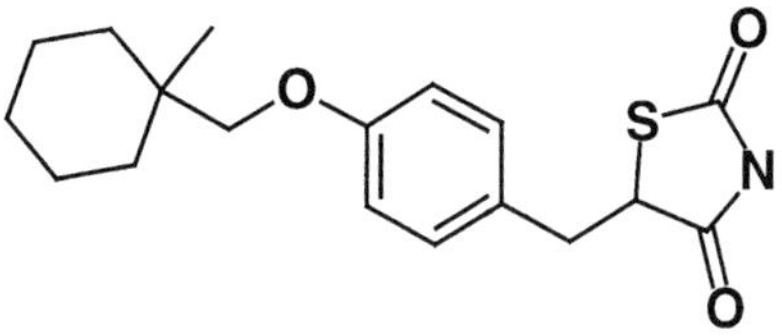

CIGLITAZONE: 5-(4-(1-methylcyclohexylmethoxy)benzyl)-thiazolidine-2,4-dione

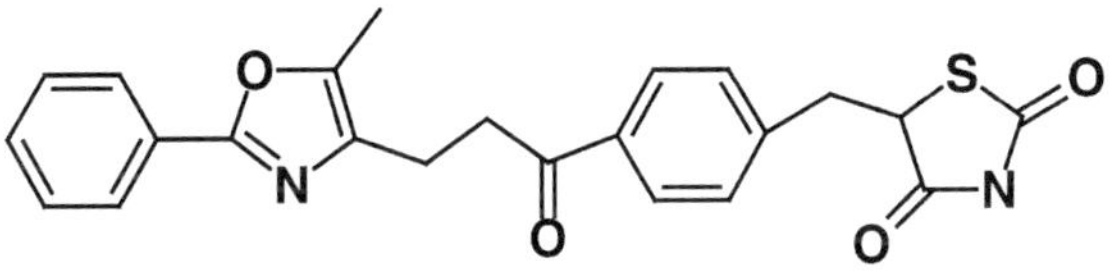

DARGLITAZONE: (±)-5-(4-(3-(5-methyl-2-phenyl-4-oxazolyl)-propionyl)phenyl methyl)-thiazolidine-2,4-dione

FIGURE 2. Structures of three thiazolidinediones—englitazone, ciglitazone, and darglitazone.

Animals

Sprague-Dawley rats (Charles River Inc., Kingston, NY) were housed individually in wire rack cages in an environmentally controlled room ($70 \pm 2°F$ and $50 \pm 5\%$ relative humidity) on a 12-h light/dark cycle with free access to food (Agway PRO-LAB RMH 3200) and reverse-osmosis purified water. Animal care and use were conducted in accordance with all applicable state and federal regulations and guidelines. These guidelines complied with or exceeded the Animal Welfare Act Regulation, 9 CFR parts 1–3, and the Association for Assessment and Accreditation of Laboratory Animal Care International Standards as set forth by the Guide for the Care and Use of Laboratory Animals (1996, National Academy Press, Washington, D.C.). Our facilities are registered as a research facility with the USDA-APHIS-REAC. All procedures conducted on animals were approved by an Institutional Animal Care and Use Committee.

In Vivo *Studies*

Compounds were administered by oral gavage (10 mL/kg) as a suspension in 0.5% (CJ-12,918, CJ-13,454, ZD2138) or 0.1% methylcellulose (englitazone), or dissolved in water (darglitazone), to rats (190–200 g) randomly assigned to groups and treated daily over a course of 1 (CJ-12,918, CJ-13,454, ZD2138) or 3 months (englitazone and darglitazone).

Lens Explant Culture

Male rats (100–250 g) were euthanized by CO_2 asphyxiation. After enucleation, lenses were extracted from the globes using a posterior approach and then placed in a 20-mL glass scintillation vial with a 2-mm hole in the cap. The vial contained 4 mL of warmed bicarbonate-based Medium 199 (Gibco) supplemented with L-glutamine (2 mM), penicillin (50,000 U/L), and streptomycin (50,000 mg/L). Final osmolality of the medium was adjusted to 295–300 mOsmol/kg. The medium was bubbled for 10 min with 95:5% air/CO_2, filter-sterilized, and stored at 4°C. The lenses were incubated on an orbital shaker in a humidified 37°C incubator in a 95:5% air/CO_2 environment.

After 24 h, only lenses without procedure-induced damage based on visual inspection (i.e., opacification of the lens or rupture of the capsule) were retained for further experimentation. Treatment began replacing with fresh supplemented media with or without test compounds. Lenses were incubated and appearance assessed daily in treated media containing vehicle (0.2% ethanol for all compounds, except DCVC) or test compound for 24 or 48 h. To assess the role of metabolites in producing cataracts, some lenses were incubated with test compounds in the presence of an S9 liver microsomal fraction obtained from arochlor 1254–induced Sprague-Dawley rats (Microbiological Associates, Rockville, MD). The S9 fractions were diluted 1:10 with a regenerating system containing 80 µM $MgCl_2$, 0.33 mM KCl, 10 mM NaH_2PO_4, 0.5 mM glucose-6-phosphate, and 0.41 mM NADP.[27] This mixture was diluted 1:5 with supplemented Medium 199. Control and compound-treated lenses were incubated in either the presence or absence of the S9 mixture. At the end of the incubation period, lenses were weighed and rinsed with saline prior to biochemical analysis [lenticular adenosine 5′-triphosphate (ATP), reduced glutathione (GSH), and MTT reduction].[13]

Parent Drug and Metabolite Analysis

Representative lenses, culture medium, and plasma were analyzed for parent compound concentrations and metabolite identification. Samples were prepared for analysis as follows: Lens samples were extracted by sonication in acetonitrile. Both lens homogenates and plasma were spiked with an internal standard before extraction with methyl *t*-butyl ether. The organic layer was dried and reconstituted in mobile phase. The aqueous layer was retained for parent drug analysis under isocratic conditions with ultraviolet light detection. Metabolite analysis was conducted in samples by gradient elution high pressure liquid chromatography using the electrospray interface of a Finnigan TSQ 7000 triple quadrupole mass spectrometer operated in the positive ion mode with optimized voltage parameters.

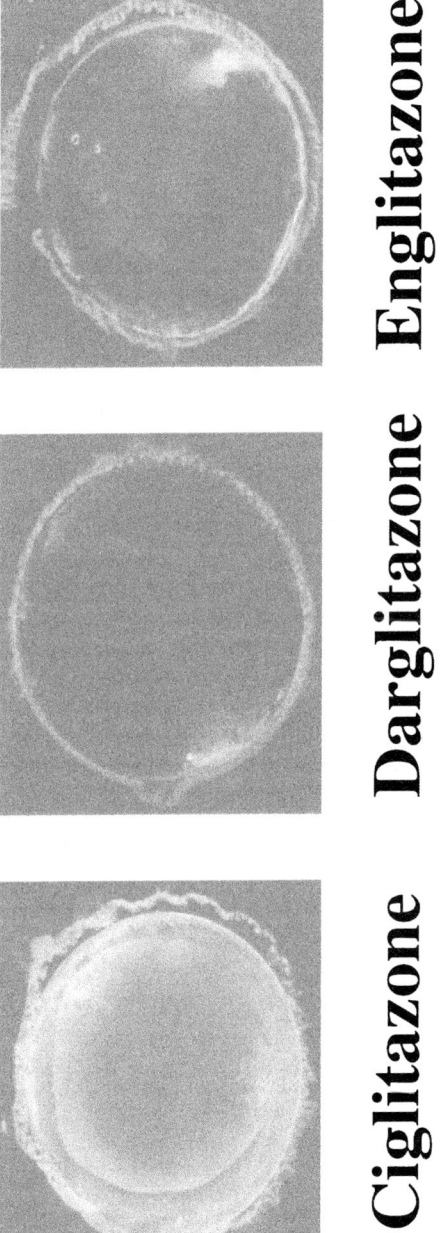

FIGURE 3. Appearance of rat lenses treated with thiazolidinediones, ciglitazone, darglitazone, and englitazone (15 μM), for 48 h.

Statistical Analysis

All results are expressed as the mean ± SEM. Student's t test or one-way analysis of variance followed by Fisher's Protected Least Significant Difference Test were used where appropriate. Levels of significance were based on a $p < 0.05$.

RESULTS

Rank Ordering of the Thiazolidinediones—Ciglitazone, Darglitazone, and Englitazone—in Vitro

Explanted lenses exposed to equivalent concentrations (15 µM) of the thiazolidinediones, ciglitazone, darglitazone, and englitazone, for 48 h showed marked differences in their clarity (FIG. 3). Ciglitazone-treated lenses were cloudy with the appearance of a distinct nucleus, while darglitazone- and englitazone-treated lenses were clear or only very slightly cloudy, respectively. Based on this single concentration comparison, the rank order of cataractogenic potential based on visual assessment was ciglitazone >> englitazone > darglitazone. Since both englitazone and darglitazone were less toxic to the lens compared to ciglitazone, both compounds were selected for further development. Unlike ciglitazone, neither darglitazone nor englitazone caused lenticular opacities during the 3-month rat safety studies at consecutive daily oral doses of up to 50 mg/kg (darglitazone) and 100 mg/kg (englitazone). These doses were associated with serum concentrations at C_{max} that ranged from 24 to 60 µM (darglitazone) and from 170 to 340 µM (englitazone) in male and female rats. This simple experiment illustrates that visual assessment alone can be useful in ranking the cataractogenic potential of structurally related compounds *in vitro*.

Mechanistic Studies of Ciglitazone-Induced Cataract Formation

Biochemical markers can also be helpful in showing toxicity earlier rather than relying on visual assessment alone. Significant reductions in lenticular ATP content (−57 ± 5%), GSH content (−42 ± 8%), and MTT reduction (−30 ± 28%) relative to controls ($N = 9$–32 lenses/treatment) can be observed within 24 h in lenses exposed to 7.5 µM ciglitazone. Lens weight increased 17 ± 4% relative to controls, while changes in the transparent quality of the lens were nearly imperceptible.

Major mechanisms of cataract formation can also be explored using prototypic inhibitors. For example, coincubation with the mitochondrial Ca^{2+} uniport inhibitor ruthenium red (100 µM) and the flavin monooxygenase inhibitor/antioxidant methimazole (1 mM) only partially protected ciglitazone-treated lenses from declines in lenticular ATP and GSH content and in MTT reduction, as well as the associated increase in lens weight (data not shown). These results suggest that ciglitazone may cause lenticular opacities by perturbing mitochondrial Ca^{2+} regulation. Changes in mitochondrial Ca^{2+} regulation may reflect metabolism of ciglitazone to a toxic metabolite by methimazole-sensitive enzymes (monooxygenases).

Although calpain activation plays a role in several rodent models of chemical-induced cataract formation, pretreatment with the selective and cell-permeant calpain inhibitors, calpain inhibitor-II (1 mM) and E64d (100 µM), were ineffective in preventing opacification of explanted lenses exposed to ciglitazone (data not shown). Although increased lens weight typically indicates stress caused by either oxidative damage or osmotic imbalance (i.e., abnormal polyol accumulation), inhibitors of these two pathways (2 mM dithiothreitol and 50 μM sorbinil, respectively) were also ineffective in protecting lenses from biochemical and morphological changes caused by ciglitazone (data not shown). Therefore, cataract formation by ciglitazone did not appear to be due to osmotic stress caused by either oxidative damage or polyol accumulation.

Role of Lenticular Biotransformation in DCVC-Induced Cataract Formation

Within 24 h of treatment, DCVC adversely affected the clarity of rat lenses in culture. Exposure to concentrations of DCVC ≤ 25 μM had no discernible adverse effect on lens clarity, while concentrations of ≥50 μM caused various grades of cloudiness. The incidence and severity of these changes were dependent on concentration (FIG. 4). Most lenses showed at the very least a slight cloudiness within 24 h at concentrations from 50 to 250 μM DCVC. Marked changes in lens clarity occurred after exposures of DCVC ≥ 500 μM for 24 h. These changes consisted of equatorial opacities and an overall cloudiness of the entire lens. The incidence of ad-

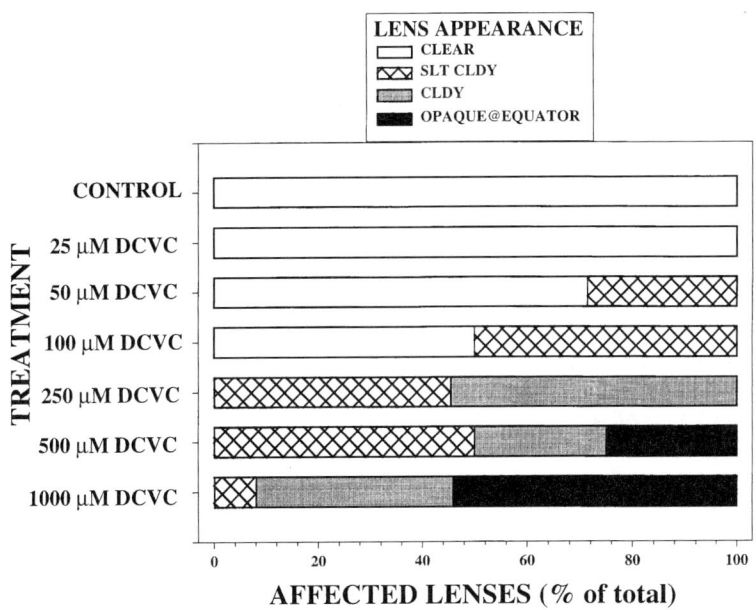

FIGURE 4. Concentration-dependent alterations in the clarity of cultured rat lenses treated with 2.5 to 1000 μM DCVC for 24 h. Gradation of shading represents percentage of lenses within each treatment group at the various stages of lens clarity indicated. SLT CLDY, slightly cloudy. Figure is based on the collective results of several independent experiments (11–58 lenses per treatment). Reproduced with permission from Academic Press.[13]

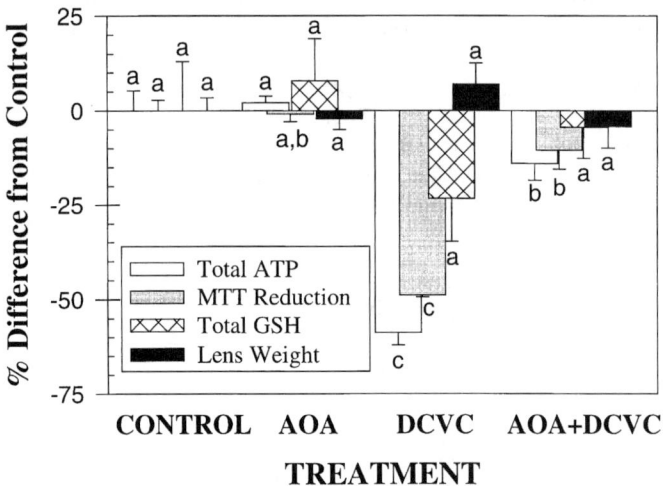

FIGURE 5. Effects of 1 mM aminooxyacetic acid (AOA) on ATP and GSH levels, mitochondrial MTT reduction, and lens weight in cultured rat lenses treated with 1 mM DCVC for 24 h. Lens clarity of AOA + DCVC–treated lenses was improved over DCVC treatment alone (clear to very slightly cloudy vs. slightly cloudy to opaque at the equator, respectively). Control values were 73 ± 4 nmol ATP/lens, 48 ± 6 nmol GSH/lens, 0.006 ± 0.002 OD units of MTT reduction/mg lens, and 32 ± 1 mg wet weight. $N = 3$–5 lenses per treatment, mean $\pm$ SEM. Values with different letters within a given category are significantly different from each other, $p < 0.05$. Reproduced with permission from Academic Press.[13]

verse changes in lens clarity was progressive, affecting more lenses as a function of concentration.

Since the rat lens responded to DCVC without metabolic activation from an exogenous source, we investigated whether opacity formation was due to DCVC or metabolic activation by the lens to a reactive metabolite. The β-lyase inhibitor AOA (1 mM) almost completely protected lenses from adverse changes in lens clarity and decreases in ATP content and MTT reduction caused by exposure to 1 mM DCVC (FIG. 5). The incidence as well as severity of changes in lens clarity were improved by coincubating AOA with DCVC. Under these conditions, only 50% of the treated lenses were adversely affected visually compared to 100% affected with DCVC treatment alone (clear to slightly cloudy vs. slightly cloudy to cloudy and opaque at the equator, respectively). The dramatic decrease in ATP content and MTT reduction relative to control levels that was observed after treatment with 1 mM DCVC also improved during coincubation with AOA. These results suggest that the explanted lens is capable of metabolizing DCVC to a reactive metabolite and that formation of this metabolite contributes to the cataractogenic potential of DCVC.

Cataract Formation by CJ-12,918 in Vivo

Cataracts were observed upon routine clinical observation of the rats over the course of a 1-month preclinical safety evaluation study with CJ-12,918. Ophthalmic exams performed on day 38 found bilateral cataracts in 10% of males and 70% of females in the 25-mg/kg/day group, and in 100% of males and 100% of females in the 250-mg/kg/day group. The cataracts were characterized by opacification of multiple individual cortical lens fibers with the appearance of a prominent anterior suture line.

While the incidence of cataract formation increased over time with treatment, plasma levels of CJ-12,918 were essentially equivalent across all doses. CJ-12,918 was found to be a potent autoinducer and broad-spectrum microsomal cytochrome P-450 inducer in an earlier 2-week-range finding study (unpublished data). This phenomenon contributed to the dramatic changes in the toxicokinetics of CJ-12,918 observed over time. Within 4 days of treatment, plasma levels dropped substantially to essentially equivalent systemic exposure of the parent drug regardless of administered dose. Since cataract formation was noted earlier and to a greater degree in animals exposed to 250 rather than 25 mg/kg/day, these events strongly suggest that a metabolite(s) was involved in the process of cataract formation caused by CJ-12,918.

CJ-12,918 has at least three metabolically labile sites. If a metabolite(s) was responsible for cataract formation, then blocking metabolism of CJ-12,918 at one or more sites should diminish or prevent cataractogenesis. In order to test whether cataract formation by CJ-12,918 was the result of metabolite formation, CJ-12,918 was modified in an attempt to block one metabolic site. Replacing the 4-methoxy group on the tetrahydropyran structural group with a carboxamide formed the pharmacologically active structural analog, CJ-13,454 (FIG. 1). The cataractogenic potentials of CJ-13,454 (250 mg/kg/day) and another orally active methoxytetrahydropyran, ZD2138 (250 mg/kg/day), were then investigated in a separate 1-month rat study using CJ-12,918 (250 mg/kg/day) as a positive control.

Comparison of Cataractogenic Potential of CJ-12,918, CJ-13,454, and ZD2138 in Vivo

Compared to the same oral dose of CJ-12,918, there was a decrease in the incidence of cataract formation in CJ-13,454-treated rats (2/7 animals affected at 3 weeks and 3/7 animals affected after 5 weeks compared to 7/7 animals affected at 3 weeks with CJ-12,918) (TABLE 1). Although lens exposure to CJ-13,454 was similar to CJ-12,918, there was a decrease in the number of metabolites found in the lens of treated rats from 6 (CJ-12,918) to 4 (CJ-13,454). Similar lens drug levels of parent compound were achieved despite increased systemic exposure as measured by plasma C_{max} and AUC(0–8 h). Systemic exposure to CJ-13,454 was 23- to 38-fold higher during the treatment period compared to CJ-12,918. CJ-13,454 was less metabolically labile (8 metabolites in plasma vs. 12 with CJ-12,918), which no doubt contributed to the higher systemic exposure (C_{max}: 15.4 compared to 0.7 µg/mL with CJ-12,918, day 36) and lower incidence of cataract formation.

In contrast, ZD2138 administration resulted in no evidence of cataract formation. Systemic exposure after 29 days of consecutive daily dosing, based on C_{max} and AUC(0–8 h), was 2- to 6-fold higher than systemic exposure to CJ-12,918. In contrast to either CJ-12,918 and CJ-13,454, ZD2138 was not detected in the lens of treated animals. Equivalent penetration of CJ-12,918 and CJ-13,454 into the lens in light of differences in the incidence of cataract formation further supported a putative role of metabolite(s) involvement in the cataractogenic potential of these two compounds.

TABLE 1. Comparison of effects of 5-lipoxygenase inhibitors on cataract formation and systemic exposure *in vivo*

Compound	Dose (mg/kg/day)	Incidence of cataract formation (Day 31–36)	C_{max} (μg/mL)		AUC_{0-8h} (μg·h/mL)		Parent drug levels in lens (μg/lens)[a]	Number of metabolites in lens
			Day 1	Day 36	Day 1	Day 36		
CJ-12,918	250	7/7	1.3 ± 0.4	0.7 ± 0.3	6.9 ± 1.7	1.7 ± 0.6	<LLOQ–0.016	6
CJ-13,454	250	3/7	30.9 ± 7.6	15.4 ± 2.2	204 ± 46	67.1 ± 21.3	<LLOQ–0.017	4
ZD2138	250	0/6	4.2 ± 0.9	1.9 ± 0.5[b]	26.3 ± 4.6	11.4 ± 2.0[b]	<LLOQ	ND

NOTE: <LLOQ = below lower limit of quantification of 0.012 μg/lens; ND = not determined.
[a]Two hours postdose (C_{max}) after 36 days of consecutive daily dosing.
[b]Determined at day 29.

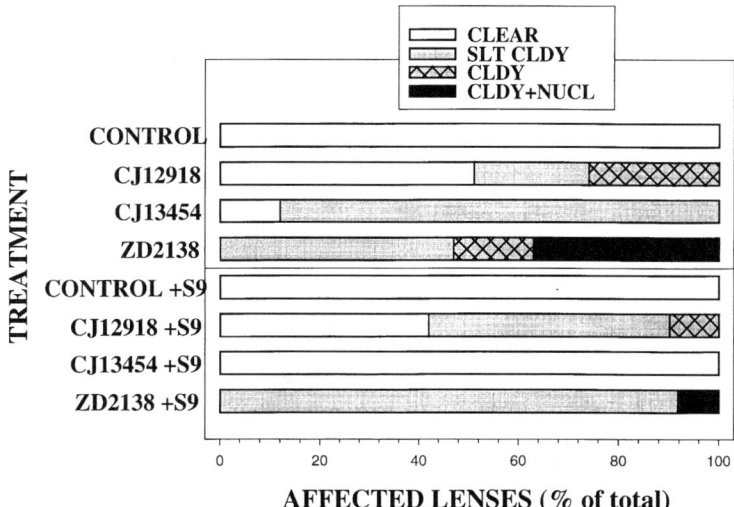

FIGURE 6. Alterations in the clarity of cultured rat lenses that were treated for 48 h with 40 µg/mL of CJ-12,918, CJ-13,454, or ZD2138 in the absence or presence (+S9) of aroclor-induced liver S9 microsomal fraction. Gradation of shading represents percentage of lenses within each treatment group at the various stages of lens clarity indicated. SLT CLDY = slightly cloudy; NUCL = nuclear cataract (cortex SLT CLDY to CLDY). Figure is based on collective results of several independent experiments (8–43 lenses per treatment).

The rank order of cataractogenic potential *in vivo* was therefore CJ-12,918 > CJ-13,454 >> ZD2138, along with evidence to suggest that the toxicities of CJ-12,918 and CJ-13,454 were mediated in some part through metabolite(s) formation.

Comparison of Cataractogenic Potential of CJ-12,918, CJ-13,454, and ZD2138 in Vitro

Lenses were cultured in media containing vehicle, 40 µg/mL of CJ-12,918, CJ-13,454, or ZD2138, with or without an aroclor-induced rat liver S9 for up to 2 days. Concentrations were selected to approximate the highest range of *in vivo* systemic exposure at C_{max} (TABLE 1). After 48 h, all three compounds increased the incidence and severity of lens opacification *in vitro* (FIG. 6). ZD2138 had a noticeably greater impact on the incidence and severity of lenticular opacity formation *in vitro* compared to either CJ-12,918 or CJ-13,454. However, the presence of a liver S9 microsomal fraction in the culture medium only partially predicted the *in vivo* rank-order toxicity of these compounds. When S9 was added to the medium to simulate the type and extent of compound metabolism *in vivo*, the relative toxicity of CJ-12,918 versus CJ-13,454 to the crystalline lens became more distinct. While CJ-12,918 + S9 caused a concentration-dependent increase in the incidence and severity of opacity formation, there were no changes in the clarity of lenses exposed to 40 µg/mL CJ-13,454 + S9 after 48 h. Although CJ-12,918 causes opacification of the lens within 48 h in the presence of S9, CJ-13,454 in the presence of S9 causes opacification after 96 h of exposure. Although the addition of S9 reordered the rank order of toxicity *in vitro* of two compounds (CJ-12,918 and CJ-13,454), the culture system still exaggerated the cataractogenic potential of ZD2138. ZD2138 treatment in the presence of S9 still had the greatest adverse effect on the incidence and severity of lens clarity, while no evidence of cataract formation was observed *in vivo* after 30 days of administration. The lack of predictability may be explained in part by a 10- to 50-fold higher distribution of ZD2138 into the lens after *in vitro* exposure (0.12–0.66 μg/lens at 15 μg/mL for 24–96 h) compared to the lens after *in vivo* exposure (<0.012 μg/lens at 250 mg/kg/day after 29 days).

DISCUSSION

Explanted lenses in organ culture have been effectively used as an *in vitro* model to determine mechanisms of cataract formation caused by several xenobiotics like tamoxifen, naphthalene, and HMG-CoA reductase inhibitors.[7,28,29] This presentation illustrates the simple, yet versatile nature of this model system to rank order compounds within a given structural series with a lower probability of causing cataracts in animal studies or to investigate mechanisms of cataract formation *in vitro*.

The ability to use this model as a predictive tool merits further consideration. When ciglitazone was reported to be cataractogenic in rats, the lens explant model successfully ranked the cataractogenic potential of the thiazolidinediones, ciglitazone, englitazone, and darglitazone, *in vitro*. Unlike ciglitazone, both englitazone and darglitazone were not cataractogenic in 3-month safety assessment studies conducted in rats. However, the retrospective analysis of CJ-12,918, CJ-13,454, and ZD2138 cataractogenic potential *in vitro* was not as predictive. Based on medium concentration alone, ZD2138 was a more potent cataractogen *in vitro* than either CJ-12,918 or CJ-13,454, whether in the presence or absence of an exogenous source of metabolism (an induced S9 microsomal fraction). In contrast to these *in vitro* results, ZD2138 did not produce cataracts in 1-month safety studies compared to CJ-12,918 and CJ-13,454, which both produced cataracts in rats. Although the reason for this discrepancy is unknown, it seems logical to conclude that the differences in cataractogenic potential observed *in vivo* and *in vitro* were most likely related to differences in lens drug content after exposure. In this case, the 10- to 50-fold higher level of ZD2138 in lenses after *in vitro* exposure compared to undetectable levels after *in vivo* exposure may make the *in vitro* model more sensitive and less predictive of the results after *in vivo* exposure. Although CJ-12,918 and CJ-13,454 also appeared to accumulate in the lens to a greater extent after *in vitro* exposure, the major difference here appears to be the potential role that metabolites may also play in the cataractogenic potential of these compounds. Measurements of the actual levels of metabolites in lenses were not feasible at the time of analysis.

Metabolite formation still seems to be an important element in the cataractogenic potential of CJ-12,918 and CJ-13,454. Structural modifications to CJ-12,918 that blocked sites of metabolism made CJ-13,454 less cataractogenic than CJ-12,918 *in vivo*. The decreased ability of CJ-13,454 to produce cataracts *in vivo* in rats was not due to diminished systemic exposure to the parent compound since plasma concentrations of CJ-13,454 were 22- to 38-fold higher than CJ-12,918 throughout the study, while parent drug levels of CJ-12,918 and CJ-13,454 within the lens after

36 days of treatment were essentially equivalent (TABLE 1). In addition, there were fewer metabolites of CJ-13,454 found in the lens than those of CJ-12,918. These factors plus the high degree of metabolic lability of CJ-12,918 strongly suggest that metabolite(s) formation plays a major role in the cataractogenic potential of CJ-12,918. In theory, blocking all three metabolically labile sites on CJ-12,918 should reduce/ameliorate cataract formation *in vivo*. This appears to be the case since a 3-month safety evaluation study with another structural analog did not produce cataracts at equivalent doses and higher systemic exposure (unpublished data). This structural analog was derived from CJ-12,918, but had all three metabolically labile sites modified to reduce metabolite formation. These data, along with the *in vitro* data with lens explants, provide some assurance that the cataractogenic potential of CJ-12,918 and CJ-13,454 will be mediated in part by metabolites.

Another consideration in the utility of this *in vitro* model is the ability to examine mechanisms of cataract formation. The present work briefly illustrates how ciglitazone may cause lenticular opacities through perturbations in mitochondrial Ca^{2+} transport, possibly through the formation of a flaven monooxygenase-derived metabolite(s) within the lens. We were also able to show that cataract formation was not a result of calpain activation, oxidative damage, or osmotic stress. We have further shown the application of this system to investigate mechanisms of DCVC-induced cataract formation, including the role of lenticular metabolism. For more complete information regarding mechanisms of cataract formation by DCVC, see reference 13.

In conclusion, when developing *in vitro* models, it is important to simulate *in vivo* conditions as much as possible. Compounds that induce cataract formation *in vivo* need access to the lens and require penetration into the lens epithelial or fiber cells or a direct interaction with cells located on the lens surface. Therefore, it is important that *in vivo* information, such as differences in metabolism, toxicokinetics, and distribution, be considered before interpreting *in vitro* information. This is especially important when there is no evidence of compound distribution into the lens after *in vivo* exposure. When appropriate, the model can better simulate *in vivo* conditions with the addition of an S9 microsomal fraction. With limitations, the lens explant model can be used to discriminate the rank order of cataractogenic potential of compounds within a given structural class and can also be used to assess mechanisms of toxicity.

ACKNOWLEDGMENTS

We acknowledge Kimberly Holbrook and Suzanne Krueger for their technical assistance; Jim Coutcher for valuable technical advice; the support of Atsushi Nagahisa, Rod Stevens, and Masame Nakane for the synthesis of CJ-12,918, CJ-13,454, and ZD2138; and the support of David Clark for synthesis of the thiazolidinediones.

REFERENCES

1. KIRBY, T.J., R.W.P. ACHOR, H.O. PERRY & R.K. WINKELMANN. 1962. Cataract formation after triparanol therapy. Arch. Ophthalmol. **68:** 486–489.
2. KIRBY, T.J. 1967. Cataracts produced by triparanol (MER/29). Trans. Am. Ophthalmol. Soc. **65:** 493.

3. LAUGHLIN, R.C. & T.F. CAREY. 1962. Cataracts in patients treated with triparanol. J. Am. Med. Assoc. **181:** 129–130.
4. GREINER, J.V. & T. GLONEK. 1988. Effects of the slow calcium-channel blocker verapamil on phosphatic metabolism of crystalline lens. Exp. Eye Res. **46:** 139–148.
5. ISHIDA, H., T. MITAMURA, Y. TAKAHASHI, A. HISATOMI, Y. FUKUHARA, K. MURATO & K. OHARA. 1997. Cataract development induced by repeated oral dosing with FK506 (tacrolimus) in adult rats. Toxicology **123:** 167–175.
6. MACDONALD, J.S., R.J. GERSON, D.J. KORNBRUST, M.W. KLOSS, S. PRAHALADA, P.H. BERRY, A.W. ALBERTS & D.L. BOKERLMAN. 1988. Preclinical evaluation of lovastatin. Am. J. Cardiol. **62:** 16J–27J.
7. MOSLEY, S.T., S.S. KALINOWSKI, B.L. SCHAFER & R.D. TANAKA. 1989. Tissue-selective acute effects of inhibitors of 3-hydroxy-3-methylglutaryl coenzyme A reductase on cholesterol biosynthesis in lens. J. Lipid Res. **30:** 1411–1420.
8. BHUYAN, D.K., K.C. BHUYAN & H.M. KATZIN. 1973. Amizol-induced cataract and inhibition of lens catalase in rabbit. Ophthalmic Res. **5:** 236–247.
9. BHUYAN, D.K. & K.C. BHUYAN. 1979. Mechanism of cataractogenesis induced by 3-amino-1H-1,2,4-triazole II: superoxide dismutase of the eye and its role in protection of the ocular lens from oxidative damage by endogenous O_2^-, H_2O_2, and/or $OH^.$. *In* Biochemical and Clinical Aspects of Oxygen, pp. 797–809. Academic Press. New York.
10. BRON, A.J., J. SPARROW, N.A.P. BROWN, J.J. HARDING & R. BLAKYTNY. 1993. The lens in diabetes. Eye **7:** 260–275.
11. STEVENS, A. 1995. The effectiveness of putative anti-cataract agents in the prevention of protein glycation. J. Am. Optom. Assoc. **66:** 744–749.
12. LUBEK, B.M., P.K. BASU & P.G. WELLS. 1988. Metabolic evidence for the involvement of enzymatic bioactivation in the cataractogenicity of acetaminophen in genetically susceptible (C57BL/6) and resistant (DBA/2) murine strains. Toxicol. Appl. Pharmacol. **94:** 487–495.
13. WALSH CLANG, C.M. & M.D. ALEO. 1997. Mechanistic analysis of S-(1,2-dichlorovinyl)-L-cysteine-induced cataractogenesis *in vitro*. Toxicol. Appl. Pharmacol. **146:** 144–155.
14. SUGIYAMA, K., T-C.L. WANG, J.T. SIMPSON, L. RODRIGUEZ, P.F. KADOR & S. SATO. 1999. Aldose reductase catalyzes the oxidation of naphthalene-1,2-dihydrodiol for the formation of *ortho*-naphthoquinone. Drug Metab. Dispos. **27:** 60–67.
15. STEVENSON, R.W., N.J. HUTSON, M.N. KRUPP, R.A. VOLKMANN, G.F. HOLLAND, J.F. EGGLER, D.A. CLARK, R.K. MCPHERSON, K.L. HALL, B.H. DANBURY, E.M. GIBBS & D.K. KREUTTER. 1990. Actions of novel antidiabetic agent englitazone in hyperglycemic hyperinsulinemic ob/ob mice. Diabetes **39:** 1218–1227.
16. CANTELLO, B.C., M.A. CAWTHORNE, G.P. COTTAM, P.T. DUFF, D. HAIGH, R.M. HINDLEY, C.A. LISTER, S.A. SMITH & P.L. THURLBY. 1994. [[ω-(Heterocyclylamino)alkoxy]benzyl]-2,4-thiazolidinediones as potent antihyperglycemic agents. J. Med. Chem. **37:** 3977–3985.
17. KOBAYASHI, M., M. IWASAKI, S. OHGAKU, H. MAEGAWA, N. WATANABE & Y. SHIGETA. 1983. A new potentiator of insulin action: post-receptor activation *in vitro*. FEBS Lett. **163:** 50–53.
18. KOBAYASHI, M., M. IWANISHI, K. EGAWA & Y. SHIGETA. 1992. Pioglitazone increases insulin sensitivity by activating insulin receptor kinase. Diabetes **41:** 476–483.
19. KIRSCH, D.M., W. BACHMANN & H.U. HARING. 1984. Ciglitazone reverses cAMP-induced post-insulin receptor resistance in rat adipocytes *in vitro*. FEBS Lett. **176:** 49–54.
20. HOFFMANN, C., K. LORENZ & J.R. COLCA. 1991. Glucose transport deficiency in diabetic animals is corrected by treatment with the oral antihyperglycemic agent pioglitazone. Endocrinology **129:** 1915–1925.
21. SALTIEL, A.R. & J.M. OLEFSKY. 1996. Thiazolidinediones in the treatment of insulin resistance and type II diabetes. Diabetes **45:** 1661–1669.
22. PETRIE, J., M. SMALL & J. CONNELL. 1997. "Glitazones", a prospect for non-insulin-dependent diabetes. Lancet **349:** 70–71.
23. KRAEGEN, E.W., D.E. JAMES, A.B. JENKINS, D.J. CHISHOLM & L.H. STORLIEN. 1989. A potent *in vivo* effect of ciglitazone on muscle insulin resistance induced by high fat feeding of rats. Metab. Clin. Exp. **38:** 1089–1093.

24. ALEO, M.D. & C.M. WALSH CLANG. 1997. Mechanisms of ciglitazone-induced cataractogenesis [abstract]. Fundam. Appl. Toxicol. (Suppl.) **36:** 45.
25. JAFFE, D.R., A.J. GANDOLFI & R.B. NAGLE. 1984. Chronic toxicity of S-($trans$-1,2-dichlorovinyl)-L-cysteine in mice. J. Appl. Toxicol. **4**(6): 315–319.
26. STEVENS, J.L., P. HAYDEN & G. TAYLOR. 1986. The role of glutathione conjugate metabolism and cysteine conjugate beta-lyase in the mechanism of S-cysteine conjugate toxicity in LLC-PK$_1$ cells. J. Biol. Chem. **261:** 3325–3332.
27. HOTTENDORF, G.H., D.A. LASKA, P.D. WILLIAMS & S.M. FORD. 1987. Role of desacetylation in the detoxification of cephalothin in renal cells in culture. J. Toxicol. Environ. Health **22:** 101–111.
28. XU, G-T., J.S. ZIGLER, JR. & M.F. LOU. 1992. The possible mechanism of naphthalene cataract in rat and its prevention by an aldose reductase inhibitor (AL01576). Exp. Eye Res. **54:** 63–72.
29. ZHANG, J.J., T.J.C. JACOB, M.A. VALVERDE, S.P. HARDY, G.M. MINTENIG, F.V. SEPULVEDA, D.R. GILL, S.C. HYDE, A.E.O. TREZISE & C.F. HIGGINS. 1994. Tamoxifen blocks chloride channels: a possible mechanism for cataract formation. J. Clin. Invest. **94:** 1690–1697.

In Vitro Percutaneous Absorption Models

ROBERT L. BRONAUGH[a]

*Office of Cosmetics and Colors, Food and Drug Administration,
Laurel, Maryland 20708, USA*

ABSTRACT: *In vitro* **skin absorption studies are commonly used to estimate** *in vivo* **skin absorption in topical safety and efficacy evaluations.** *In vitro* **studies are more economical and result in minimization or elimination of the use of animals.**

INTRODUCTION

In vitro skin absorption studies are commonly used to estimate *in vivo* skin absorption in topical safety and efficacy evaluations. A major reason is the ability to test potentially toxic chemicals in human skin without the inherent risk of clinical studies. Another advantage of *in vitro* studies is the ability to directly measure material absorbed into and through the skin, in contrast to *in vivo* human studies that require estimations of absorption based on excretion of the test compound in body fluids. Skin metabolism of topically absorbed chemicals without systemic interference can only be measured by *in vitro* methods. *In vitro* studies are more economical and result in minimization or elimination of the use of animals. If animals need to be used, fewer animals are required for *in vitro* studies.

DEFINITION

Skin absorption is a process in which a chemical passes into the skin. The amount of test compound that passes through the skin during an absorption study should clearly be considered as systemically absorbed. For safety evaluations, absorbed material remaining in the skin should also be included as systemically absorbed unless additional studies are conducted to demonstrate that the material will remain in the skin, presumably because of solubility or binding considerations.

SOURCE OF SKIN

Human skin is generally recommended over animal skin for the most relevant data. When human skin is not available, animal skin is used for absorption studies. Animal skin is usually more permeable than human skin, so it gives conservative estimates of skin absorption for safety evaluations.

---

[a]Address for correspondence: Office of Cosmetics and Colors, Food and Drug Administration, 8301 Muirkirk Road, Laurel, MD 20708. Voice: 301-594-5813; fax: 301-594-0517.
rbronaug@CFSAN.fda.gov

PREPARATION OF THE BARRIER LAYER OF SKIN

A split-thickness piece of skin is prepared for *in vitro* studies to simulate the barrier layer of skin. Frequently, this preparation is made with a dermatome to include the whole epidermis and the upper, papillary dermis.[1] This results in a section of skin of approximately 200 to 300 µm. It is important to remove the bulk of the dermal tissue, particularly with the thicker skin of humans and larger animals. The dermal tissue can serve as an artificial reservoir of absorbed material confounding the accurate determination of systemic absorption from measurements of the receptor fluid beneath the skin.

The stratum corneum is generally recognized as the primary barrier to absorption for most chemicals.[2] However, the absorption of water-insoluble chemicals is significantly influenced by the more aqueous viable tissue of the epidermis and dermis. The viable tissue also contains most of the enzyme activity in skin responsible for biotransformation of absorbed compounds.

DIFFUSION CELLS

Diffusion cells support the skin above a receptor fluid that is either continuously replaced (flow-through cell) or not replaced (static cell).[3] A flow-through cell is used in studies that maintain the viability of skin with a physiological receptor fluid and temperature. The test material is applied to the surface of the skin to simulate exposure conditions. Similar absorption results can generally be obtained with either type of diffusion cell.

RECEPTOR FLUID

In vitro absorption studies commonly use either a physiological buffer to maintain viability of skin or an isotonic buffer when metabolism studies are not desired or cannot be done (such as when cadaver skin or previously frozen skin is used). An antibacterial agent is often added to the receptor fluid to prevent bacterial growth during the diffusion experiments. This is particularly important in skin metabolism studies to prevent confounding of results by bacterial metabolism.

MAINTENANCE OF VIABILITY

Viability of skin can be maintained in diffusion cells for at least 24 hours by perfusion with a physiological buffer such as Hanks' balanced salt solution or minimum essential medium.[4] The metabolism of chemicals during absorption through skin can then be assessed in a percutaneous absorption study. Skin viability has frequently been assessed by measuring glucose utilization.[4] Recently, viable cells in skin have also been determined by measuring the reduction of MTT by skin.[5] A color change is formed that can be readily quantitated spectrophotometrically. Unlike the glucose utilization assay, the MTT assay was not adversely affected by the presence of bovine serum albumin in the diffusion cell receptor fluid.[5]

Enzymes such as esterase,[6] alcohol dehydrogenase,[7] and acetyltransferase[8,9] are responsible for significant metabolism of absorbed compounds. In general, compounds do not seem to be metabolized extensively in skin by P450 microsomal enzymes. Presumably, this reduced metabolism from P450 enzymes is due to the levels of these enzymes found in skin, which are much lower than corresponding levels in the liver.[10]

RECOVERY

Determination of the recovery of test compound lends credibility to the study results. Normally, recovery in experiments with radiolabeled materials exceeds 80%. High recovery values are often not obtained for volatile compounds unless a trap is used to capture the evaporating material.

EXPRESSION OF RESULTS

Total percutaneous absorption is the sum of the test compound appearing in the receptor fluid during the study plus material absorbed—but remaining—in the skin. A prolonged study conducted for an additional few days can show whether *in vitro* skin levels of test compound would be available for systemic absorption *in vivo*.[11] Absorption is usually expressed in terms of the percent of the applied dose absorbed or as an absorption rate.

REFERENCES

1. BRONAUGH, R.L. & R.F. STEWART. 1986. Methods for *in vitro* percutaneous absorption studies. VI. Preparation of the barrier layer. J. Pharm. Sci. **75:** 487–491.
2. BRONAUGH, R.L., R.F. STEWART, E.R. CONGDON & A.R. GILES, JR. 1982. Methods for *in vitro* percutaneous absorption studies. I. Comparison of *in vivo* results. Toxicol. Appl. Pharmacol. **62:** 474–480.
3. BRONAUGH, R.L. & R.F. STEWART. 1985. Methods for *in vitro* percutaneous absorption studies. IV. The flow-through cell. J. Pharm. Sci. **74:** 64–67.
4. COLLIER, S.W., N.M. SHEIKH, A. SAKR, J.L. LICHTIN, R.F. STEWART & R.L. BRONAUGH. 1989. Maintenance of skin viability during *in vitro* percutaneous absorption/metabolism studies. Toxicol. Appl. Pharmacol. **99:** 522–533.
5. HOOD, H.L. & R.L. BRONAUGH. 1999. A comparison of skin viability assays for *in vitro* skin absorption/metabolism studies. In Vitro Mol. Toxicol. **12:** 3–9.
6. KENNEY, G.R., A. SAKR, J.L. LICHTIN, H. CHOU & R.L. BRONAUGH. 1995. *In vitro* skin absorption and metabolism of padimate-O and a nitrosamine (NMPABAO) formed in padimate-O-containing cosmetic products. J. Soc. Cosmet. Chem. **46:** 117–127.
7. BOEHNLEIN, J., A. SAKR, J.L. LICHTIN & R.L. BRONAUGH. 1994. Metabolism of retinyl palmitate to retinol (vitamin A) in skin during percutaneous absorption. Pharm. Res. **11:** 1155–1159.
8. NATHAN, D., A. SAKR, J.L. LICHTIN & R.L. BRONAUGH. 1990. *In vitro* skin absorption and metabolism of benzoic acid, *p*-aminobenzoic acid, and benzocaine in the hairless guinea pig. Pharm. Res. **7:** 1147–1151.
9. KRAELING, M.E.K., R.J. LIPICKY & R.L. BRONAUGH. 1996. Metabolism of benzocaine during percutaneous absorption in the hairless guinea pig: acetylbenzocaine formation and activity. Skin Pharmacol. **9:** 221–230.

10. MUKHTAR, H. & D. BICKERS. 1981. Drug metabolism in skin. Drug Metab. Dispos. **9:** 311–314.
11. HOOD, H.L., R.R. WICKETT & R.L. BRONAUGH. 1996. The *in vitro* percutaneous absorption of the fragrance ingredient musk xylol. Food Chem. Toxicol. **34:** 483–488.

In Vitro and Human Testing Strategies for Skin Irritation

MICHAEL K. ROBINSON,[a] ROSEMARIE OSBORNE, AND MARY A. PERKINS

The Procter & Gamble Company, Miami Valley Laboratories, Cincinnati, Ohio, USA

ABSTRACT: Prior to the manufacture, transport, and marketing of chemicals or products, it is critical to assess their potential for skin toxicity (corrosion or irritation), thereby protecting the worker and consumer from adverse skin effects due to intended or accidental skin exposure. Traditionally, animal testing procedures have provided the data needed to assess the more severe forms of skin toxicity, and current regulations may require animal test data before permission can be obtained to manufacture, transport, or market chemicals or the products that contain them. In recent years, the use of animals to assess skin safety has been opposed by some as inhumane and unnecessary. The conflicting needs of the industrial toxicologist to (1) protect human safety, (2) comply with regulations, and (3) reduce animal testing have led to major efforts to develop alternative, yet predictive, test methods. A variety of *in vitro* skin corrosion test methods have been developed and several have successfully passed initial international validation. These have included skin or epidermal equivalent assays that have been shown to distinguish corrosive from noncorrosive chemicals. These skin/epidermal equivalent assays have also been modified and used to assess skin irritation potential relative to existing human exposure test data. The data show a good correlation between *in vitro* assay data and different types of human skin irritation data for both chemicals and consumer products. The effort to eliminate animal tests has also led to the development of a novel human patch test for assessment of acute skin irritation potential. A case study shows the benefits of *in vitro* and human skin irritation tests compared to the animal tests they seek to replace, and strategies now exist to adequately assess human skin irritation potential without the need to rely on animal test methods.

INTRODUCTION

The assessment of the skin corrosion and skin irritation potential of chemicals and finished products is an essential part of the toxicological evaluation prior to manufacture, transport, or marketing. The intent is to protect workers from any toxicities associated with normal or accidental chemical or product exposures in the workplace and to protect consumers from any toxicities associated with normal product use and reasonably foreseeable misuse exposures in the marketplace. The assessment process for skin toxicities requires an understanding of potential exposures and a determination (via appropriate test methods) of the actual toxicity potential, generally under exaggerated exposure conditions. Factoring the two elements together, and bench marking against similar chemicals or products with known safe

[a]Address for correspondence: The Procter & Gamble Company, P.O. Box 538707, Cincinnati, OH 45253-8707. Voice: 513-627-2192; fax: 513-627-0400.
robinson.mk@pg.com

or unsafe pedigrees, will allow for the assessment of risk. Application of this process for allergic skin sensitization has been described.[1–4]

The evaluation of skin corrosion/irritation potential has traditionally been conducted in animals (rabbits) following the original method of Draize.[5] The procedure involves direct application of a test material to the skin of albino rabbits under an occlusive dressing and the subsequent assessment of induced skin damage (erythema, edema, necrotic changes). Various modifications of this basic method are currently required by regulatory authorities worldwide and form the basis for classification of skin corrosion or irritation hazard to humans.[6] The modifications relate to the number of animals tested, the duration of test material exposure, the application on intact versus abraded skin, and the number and frequency of skin evaluations.[7] Depending on the nature and severity of the skin reactions, their speed of onset, and their persistence or reversibility, classifications are made regarding corrosion or irritation hazard. Labeling requirements and/or transport restrictions imposed upon chemicals and products are based upon the length of time required to develop a proscribed level of skin response.

Over the past several years, this testing approach has been the focus of a concerted effort among government, academic, and industrial scientists to develop alternative methods. Part of this effort has been driven by the animal rights movement to eliminate animal testing altogether.[8] There has also been concern that the Draize test is not adequately predictive of skin corrosion or irritation potential in humans.[9–11] The primary focus of this development of alternative methods has been on evaluation of various *in vitro* techniques for both skin corrosion and irritation testing and, more recently, on the development of a clinical test method for assessment of skin irritation potential.

Presented below is a brief description of our work in the area of *in vitro* skin corrosion and skin irritation test method development and human skin irritation test method development, as well as a summary of the development and validation status of different test methods. It provides a schematic approach to the use of *in vitro* and human test methods for the skin safety assessment of new materials and a case study exemplifying the utility of this approach.

IN VITRO SKIN CORROSION

Our efforts to develop *in vitro* skin corrosion tests have focused on the use of so-called skin or epidermal "equivalent" culture systems. Originally developed as skin replacement therapy for burn patients, these systems found a unique niche for skin toxicology testing as well. While clearly not the same as intact skin, these cultures, particularly cornified versions, provided a three-dimensional model of skin with major structural components intact. Our development efforts centered on two such constructs, the Skin^{2TM} culture system (originally produced by Advanced Tissue Sciences, but no longer commercially available) and the EpiDerm™ culture system (produced by MatTek). These two systems are shown in FIGURE 1.

Test materials, either chemicals or product formulations, were directly applied to the surface of these cultures for various periods of time, and cell culture viability was assessed by inhibition of metabolic conversion of the yellow tetrazolium salt 3-[4,5-dimethylthiazol-2-yl] 2,5-diphenyl tetrazolium bromide to a purple formazan dye,

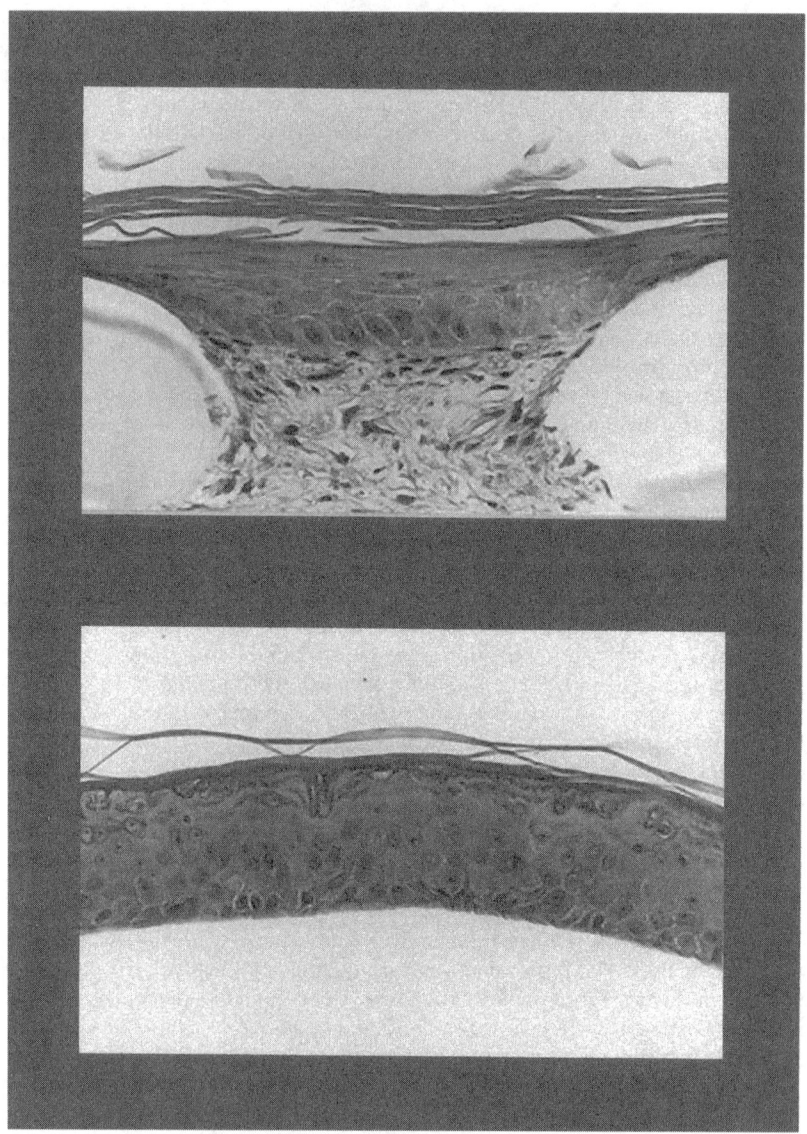

FIGURE 1. The Skin^{2TM} (**top**) and EpiDerm™ (**bottom**) culture constructs. Skin^{2TM} comprises a stromal (dermal fibroblast) component and multilayered epidermis consisting of a basal layer of keratinocytes and a stratum corneum grown on a nylon mesh. EpiDerm™ cultures consist of human keratinocytes grown into a multilayered epidermis with a basal layer and stratum corneum on a culture filter insert.

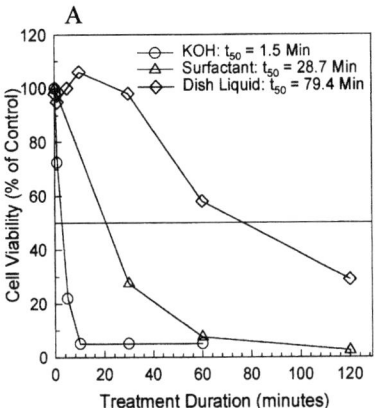

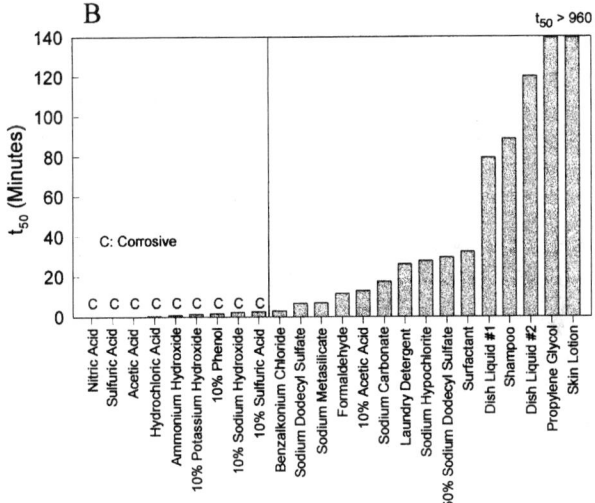

FIGURE 2. (A) Time course of decrease in cell viability in human skin cultures treated with selected substances. Cell viability in Skin^2 (ZS1300) cultures was measured as MTT (3-[4,5-dimethylthiazol-2-yl] 2,5-diphenyl tetrazolium bromide) metabolism and is expressed as a percentage of control values for each experiment. Three test substances are shown to illustrate the calculation of the T_{50} values, which are interpolated at the 50% level along a straight line between the two points spanning the 50% response level (horizontal line). **(B)** T_{50} response times of Skin^2 (ZS1300) cultures to test substances in a range from corrosive to mild. Test substances are rank-ordered based on increasing T_{50} values (ordinate), that is, exposure times required to produce a 50% reduction of cell viability (MTT uptake), calculated from time-course data as shown in part A. The data indicate that corrosive substances ("C") had T_{50} values of less than 3 min. From reference 13.

the MTT assay.[12] A time-response profile was developed for each test material (FIG. 2A) and a prediction model established. Under the prediction model, materials that caused >50% reduction in viability in ≤3 min of exposure were considered corrosive. Histopathology was used to confirm the MTT assay results and the model was successful in discriminating among a test set of 24 corrosive and noncorrosive test materials (FIG. 2B).[13] Similar results were obtained with both culture systems.

The Skin2^{TM} culture system, along with two nonculture systems, the transcutaneous electrical resistance (TER) assay and the Corrositex™ assay system (a noncellular biobarrier system), underwent initial prevalidation testing for skin corrosion. All three assays performed well in terms of overall consistency, sensitivity, and specificity. However, each assay encountered specific problems in one of those areas or with chemical incompatibility issues.[14] It was recommended that studies be conducted to address these concerns and the assays further evaluated in a full validation study.

The validation study began in 1995 under the auspices of the European Center for the Validation of Alternative Methods (ECVAM) and ended two years later.[15] Along with the 3 assays listed above, the validation study included a second commercial skin equivalent construct, EpiSkin™. Twelve labs participated in the validation exercise, with each assay evaluated by 3 independent labs. A total of 60 corrosive and noncorrosive chemicals were included in the validation set. Two of the assays, TER and EpiSkin™, met the first study objective of distinguishing corrosive from noncorrosive chemicals with adequate sensitivity and specificity. The Corrositex™ assay was incompatible with 40% of the test set chemicals, and the Skin2^{TM} culture system showed low sensitivity. The EpiSkin™ system also met a second study objective by distinguishing stronger (R35, packing group I) from weaker (R34, packing group II/III) corrosive chemicals. For the Skin2^{TM} system, the results had little relevance since the cultures were withdrawn from the market in 1996. The Corrositex™ assay did not meet the study criteria for a validated replacement test; however, that did not preclude its utility for certain chemical classes. Recently, the U.S. Interagency Coordinating Committee on the Validation of Alternative Methods (ICCVAM) concluded that Corrositex™ is equivalent to the rabbit skin corrosion test for predicting corrosivity and noncorrosivity for specified chemical classes.[16a] Also, the EpiDerm™ culture system, following a modification of the published skin corrosion protocol,[13] has completed successful prevalidation[16b] and has recently been accepted as an additional skin culture system appropriate for assessment of skin corrosivity.[16c]

IN VITRO SKIN IRRITATION

Unlike corrosion, skin irritation encompasses a vast range of severity, from near corrosive at one extreme to cumulative or only sensory irritation at the other. As a result, systems developed initially to examine more severe degrees of irritation have needed to be optimized for prediction of more subtle effects. Ultimately, any response generated *in vitro* has had to be correlated to the relevant clinical response patterns in order to establish predictive value. Over the years, a variety of cell culture systems have been developed and evaluated for prediction of skin irritation potential. The first systems investigated were simple monolayer keratinocyte cultures submerged in culture medium. Using cell viability assay endpoints, certain predictions

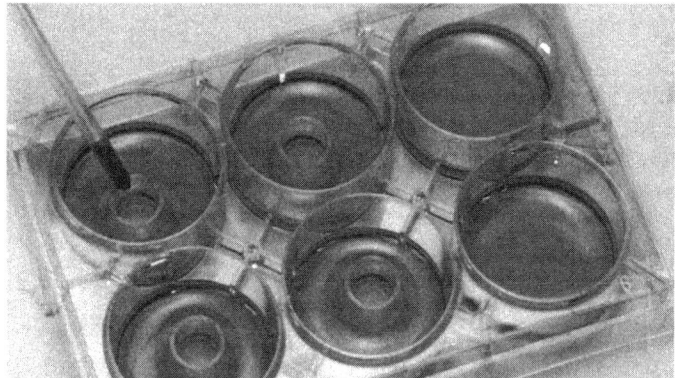

FIGURE 3. Test materials are applied topically to the stratum corneum surface of the EpiDerm™ cultures using a positive displacement pipette. From reference 20.

of skin irritation potential could be made, but the utility was limited to test materials that were compatible with the aqueous cell culture medium environment.[17–19]

As with skin corrosion assays, the evolution of this field has led to a focus on the use of skin or epidermal "equivalent" culture systems for prediction of skin irritation. Our laboratory has used the EpiDerm™ culture system for this purpose and we have evaluated its utility for prediction of the skin irritation potential of both chemicals and finished products.[18–20] Test materials are applied directly to the surface of the skin cultures (FIG. 3) and the cultures are incubated for up to 24 h. After washing the cultures free of test material, the cells are assayed for residual viability (MTT assay) and the surrounding culture medium is assayed for content of cytoplasmic enzymes (indication of membrane integrity) and the cytokine, interleukin-1α (IL-1α; indication of inflammation).

An example of the application of this method to finished product testing (antiperspirants and deodorants) is shown in FIGURE 4. In this study, the clinical data were based solely on a reported incidence (in subject diaries) of adverse skin effects from a product use study. While such data are admittedly soft, they do provide a semiquantitative index of consumer irritation (based on the percent incidence of adverse responses). In spite of this limitation, we saw remarkable correlation between the various *in vitro* endpoints and the human skin irritation data. The inflammation endpoint (IL-1α) was best able to predict human skin irritation across the entire range of clinical responses.

Many other laboratories worldwide have been active in the development of skin equivalent culture methods for chemical and/or product irritation testing. The EpiDerm™ system has been used to study surfactants and surfactant-containing products,[21,22] compare skin irritants and allergens,[23] and examine mixed surfactant antagonism.[24] Others, using their own laboratory-generated skin constructs, have examined a variety of chemical irritants *in vitro*.[25–27] Recently, several laboratories have used various skin equivalent constructs to examine the skin irritation properties of cosmetic formulations.[20,28–30] All of the groups listed have shown good correlations between their *in vitro* data and corresponding clinical skin irritation response

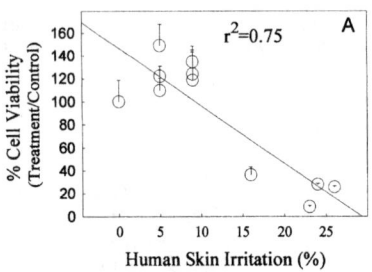
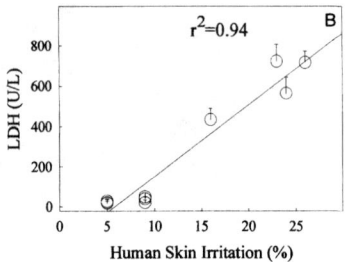
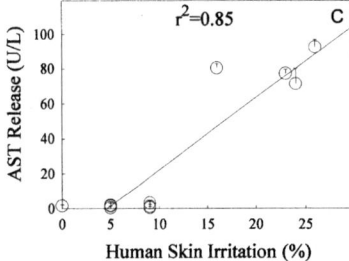
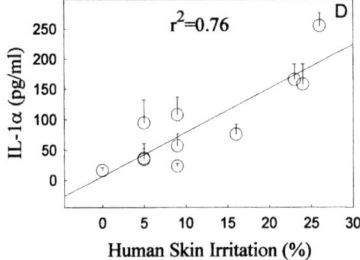

FIGURE 4. Antiperspirant/deodorant study: The percent of human subjects reporting either subjective or objective skin irritation for 11 products is plotted versus each *in vitro* endpoint. The *in vitro* endpoints evaluated include **(A)** cell viability (MTT assay), **(B)** enzyme release (lactic dehydrogenase [LDH]), **(C)** aspartate aminotransferase [AST], and **(D)** extracellular IL-1α. Symbols and error bars represent the mean ± SD across four replicate cultures. To compare the *in vitro* endpoints to the human skin irritation % response, a simple linear regression analysis was used (r^2 = 0.75–0.94). From reference 20.

data. Currently, ECVAM is sponsoring a prevalidation program to examine different human skin culture constructs and a nonhuman skin system (pig ear perfusion system) for prediction of acute skin irritation potential.[31]

CLINICAL SKIN IRRITATION

For acute skin irritation prediction, one is not limited to testing in animals or *in vitro* culture systems. The testing can be easily and ethically conducted in volunteer human subjects following a graduated exposure acute irritation patch test procedure recently developed and applied to the irritation screening of chemicals.[32–34] All that is necessary is that the chemicals lack other toxicities (e.g., mutagenicity, sensitization, corrosivity, etc.) that would preclude testing in humans at the desired exposure levels. In this procedure, approximately 30 test subjects are exposed each week to the test materials under occluded patch and the skin sites are graded for irritation at

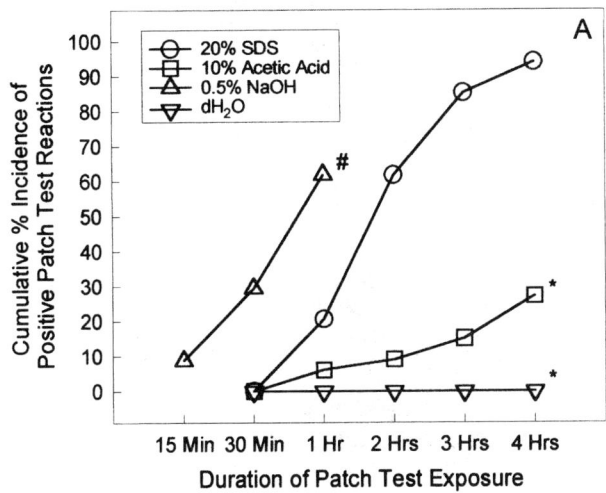

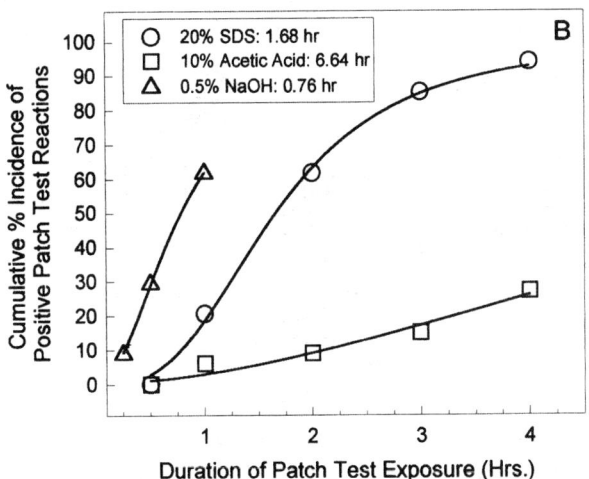

FIGURE 5. (A) Patches containing the indicated test materials were applied for 0.25 to 1 h (0.05% NaOH) or 0.5 to 4 h (other materials), increasing the duration of exposure until a positive response was seen. The asterisk (*) and pound (#) symbols designate a statistically significant difference (Fisher's exact test) at $p < 0.05$ relative to the response to 20% SDS at the same time point. (B) The data from part A were regraphed using logistic curve-fitting procedures and a TR_{50} value (time for 50% of test subjects to respond) was determined for each test material. From reference 41.

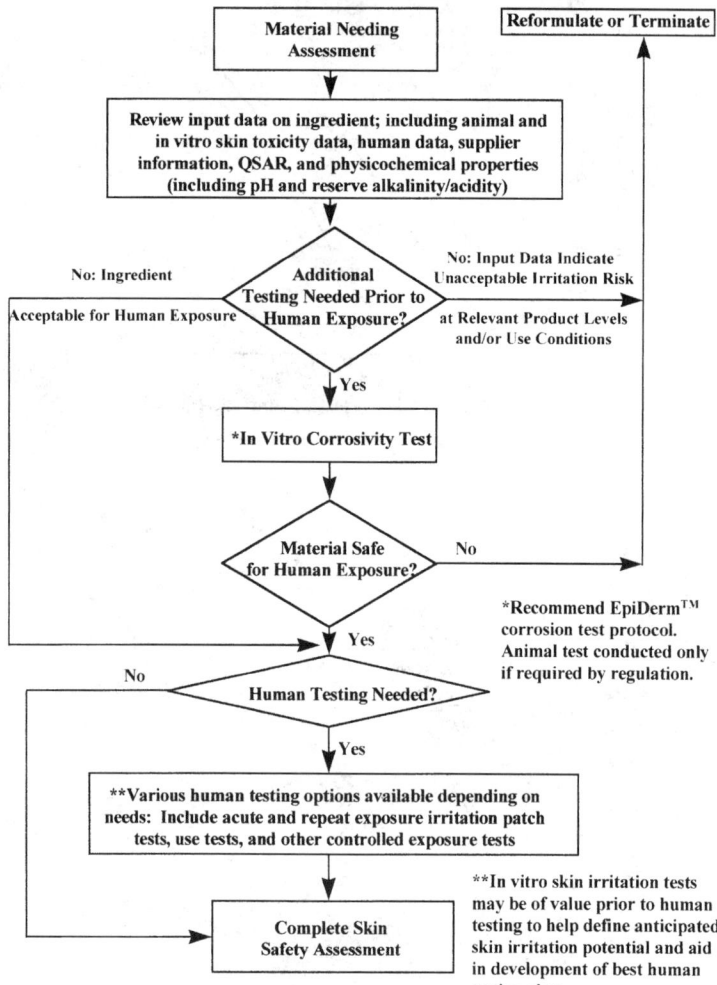

FIGURE 6. A skin safety testing and risk assessment process for human skin irritation.

24, 48, and 72 h after patch removal. The time of exposure is increased from 30 min or 1 h to 2, 3, and 4 h. Once a skin reaction develops, there are no further exposures to that test material. The cumulative incidence of positive skin reactions to any test material is compared to that of a positive control material (20% SDS) to determine whether the test material should be classified as irritant or nonirritant.

TABLE 1. Case study: Draize, *in vitro*, and clinical skin irritation data on chemical X

Test method[a]	Positive control[b]	Chemical X
Draize rabbit test	ND	PII:[c] 7.17/8 (R34)
In vitro: MTT	5% viability	96% viability
Human 4-h patch	90% responders	13% responders[d]

[a]Chemical X was tested for skin corrosion and irritation potential using three test methods: the Draize rabbit irritation test, *in vitro* skin corrosion using MTT metabolism as an indicator of cellular cytotoxicity, and the human 4-h patch test.

[b]No positive control chemical was tested in the Draize test (ND); 100% acetic acid was used as the positive control in the *in vitro* skin corrosion test and 20% SDS was the positive control for the human patch test.

[c]PII: Primary irritation index and EU hazard designation.

[d]Significantly fewer responders than positive control, suggesting designation as nonclassified.[33]

Multiple chemicals have been tested by this procedure and discrepancies noted in comparison to current European dangerous substances directive classifications.[33,34] In addition, the procedure has undergone extensive interlaboratory evaluation and has been found to be robust in intralaboratory and interlaboratory comparisons.[35–37] The procedure has also been used to study the basic characteristics of clinical skin irritation.[38–41]

Typical results from this method are shown in FIGURE 5. The response patterns are shown for both statistical comparisons and time-response comparisons. Efforts have been ongoing to have this method accepted as an alternative test under European Union (EU) directive. As such, it would be a useful adjunct to *in vitro* and other clinical test methods used in the skin irritation testing and risk assessment process (FIG. 6).

CASE STUDY

A case study example of the utility of *in vitro* skin corrosion and acute human skin irritation patch testing in assessment of new chemicals is depicted in TABLE 1. A novel chemical structure was proposed for a product upgrade and submitted for skin corrosion testing in rabbits as required under European regulation for base set notification on new chemicals. An unexpected positive skin corrosion result was obtained—unexpected because of the close chemical similarity of this material to the nonirritating ingredient that it was replacing in the product formulation. A follow-up *in vitro* skin corrosion study showed no evidence of skin corrosivity. A series of 4-h human patch tests were conducted in both Europe and the United States. The results of these studies supported the conclusion that the material was nonirritating to human subjects. The data from each of the three test types are summarized in TABLE 1. Under EU directive requirements, only the rabbit test results were admissible for skin safety evaluation and the new chemical was withdrawn from development. However, these data provide compelling evidence for the utility of both *in vitro* and clinical test methods in the overall risk assessment process.

REFERENCES

1. ROBINSON, M.K., J. STOTTS, P.J. DANNEMAN, T.L. NUSAIR & P.H. BAY. 1989. A risk assessment process for allergic contact sensitization. Food Chem. Toxicol. **27:** 479–489.
2. GERBERICK, G.F., M.K. ROBINSON & J. STOTTS. 1993. An approach to allergic contact sensitization risk assessment of new chemicals and product ingredients. Am. J. Contact Dermatitis **4:** 205–211.
3. BASKETTER, D.A., G.F. GERBERICK & M.K. ROBINSON. 1996. Risk assessment. *In* Toxicology of Contact Hypersensitivity, pp. 152–164. Taylor & Francis. London.
4. BASKETTER, D.A. 1998. Skin sensitization: risk assessment. Int. J. Cosmet. Sci. **20:** 141–150.
5. DRAIZE, J.H., G. WOODARD & H.O. CALVERY. 1944. Methods for the study of irritation and toxicity of substances applied topically to the skin and mucous membranes. J. Pharmacol. Exp. Ther. **82:** 377–390.
6. EC. 1992. Annex to Commission Directive 92/69/EEC of 31 July 1992 adapting to technical progress for the seventeenth time Council Directive 67/548/EEC on the approximation of laws, regulations, and administrative provisions relating to the classification, packaging, and labelling of dangerous substances. Off. J. Eur. Comm. **L84:** 36.
7. PATIL, S.M., E. PATRICK & H.I. MAIBACH. 1998. Animal, human, and *in vitro* test methods for predicting skin irritation. *In* Dermatotoxicology Methods, pp. 89–113. Taylor & Francis. Washington, D.C.
8. EEC. 1993. Council Directive 93/35/EEC of 14 June 1993 amending for the sixth time Directive 76/768/EEC on the approximation of the laws of the Member States relating to cosmetic products. Off. J. Eur. Comm. **L15:** 32.
9. PHILLIPS, L., M. STEINBERG, H.I. MAIBACH & W.A. AKERS. 1972. A comparison of rabbit and human skin response to certain irritants. Toxicol. Appl. Pharmacol. **21:** 369–382.
10. NIXON, G.A., C.A. TYSON & W.C. WERTZ. 1975. Interspecies comparisons of skin irritancy. Toxicol. Appl. Pharmacol. **31:** 481–490.
11. CAMPBELL, R.L. & R.D. BRUCE. 1981. Comparative dermatotoxicology. I. Direct comparison of rabbit and human primary skin irritation responses to isopropyl myristate. Toxicol. Appl. Pharmacol. **59:** 555–563.
12. MOSSMAN, T. 1983. Rapid colorimetric assay for cellular growth and survival: applications to proliferation and cytotoxicity assays. J. Immunol. Methods **65:** 55–63.
13. PERKINS, M.A., R. OSBORNE & G.R. JOHNSON. 1996. Development of an *in vitro* method for skin corrosion testing. Fundam. Appl. Toxicol. **31:** 9–18.
14. BOTHAM, P.A., M. CHAMBERLAIN, M.D. BARRATT, R.D. CURREN, D.J. ESDAILE, J.R. GARDNER, V.C. GORDON, B. HILDEBRAND, R.W. LEWIS, M. LIEBSCH, P. LOGEMANN, R. OSBORNE, M. PONEC, J.F. REGNIER, W. STEILING, A.P. WALKER & M. BALLS. 1995. A prevalidation study on *in vitro* skin corrosivity testing: the report and recommendations of ECVAM workshop 6. ATLA-Altern. Lab. Anim. **23:** 219–255.
15. FENTEM, J.H., G.E.B. ARCHER, M. BALLS, P.A. BOTHAM, R.D. CURREN, L.K. EARL, D.J. ESDAILE, H.G. HOLZHÜTTER & M. LIEBSCH. 1998. The ECVAM international validation study on *in vitro* tests for skin corrosivity. 2. Results and evaluation by the management team. Toxicol. In Vitro **12:** 483–524.
16. (a) SCALA, R., J.H. FENTEM, J. CHEN, M.J. DERELANKO, S. GREEN, J. HARBELL, K.A. KOHRMAN, D.N. SAUDER & J. STEGEMAN. 1999. Corrositex®: an *in vitro* test method for assessing dermal corrosivity potential of chemicals. Internet URL: http://www.iccvam.niehs.nih.gov/corprrep.htm//. (b) LIEBSCH, M., D. TRAUE, C. BARRABAS, H. SPIELMANN, P. UPHILL, S. WILKINS, C. WIEMANN, T. KAUFMANN, M. REMMELE & H.G. HOLZHÜTTER. 2000. The ECVAM prevalidation study on the use of EpiDerm for skin corrosivity testing. ATLA-Altern. Lab. Anim. **28:** 371–401. (c) BALLS, M. & E. HELLSTEN. 2000. Statement on the application of the EpiDerm™ human skin model for skin corrosivity testing. ATLA-Altern. Lab. Anim. **28:** 365–366.
17. OSBORNE, R. & M.A. PERKINS. 1994. An approach for development of alternative test methods based on mechanisms of skin irritation. Food Chem. Toxicol. **32:** 133–142.
18. ROBINSON, M.K., M.A. PERKINS & R. OSBORNE. 1997. Comparative studies on cultured human skin models for irritation testing. *In* Animal Alternatives, Welfare, and Ethics, pp. 1123–1134. Elsevier. Amsterdam/New York.

19. PERKINS, M.A., M.K. ROBINSON & R. OSBORNE. 1998. Alternative methods in dermatotoxicology. *In* Dermatotoxicology Methods, pp. 319–336. Taylor & Francis. Washington, D.C.
20. PERKINS, M.A., R. OSBORNE, F. RANA, A. GHASSEMI & M.K. ROBINSON. 1999. Comparison of *in vitro* and *in vivo* human skin responses to consumer products and ingredients with a range of irritancy potential. Toxicol. Sci. **48:** 218–229.
21. CANNON, C.L., P.J. NEAL, J.A. SOUTHEE, J. KUBILUS & M. KLAUSNER. 1994. New epidermal model for dermal irritancy testing. Toxicol. In Vitro **8:** 889–891.
22. BERNHOFER, L.P., S. BARKOVIC, Y. APPA & K.M. MARTIN. 1999. IL-1a and IL-1ra secretion from epidermal equivalents and the prediction of the irritation potential of mild soap and surfactant-based consumer products. Toxicol. In Vitro **13:** 231–239.
23. KUBILUS, J., C. CANNON, P. NEAL, H. SENNOTT & M. KLAUSNER. 1996. Response of the EpiDerm skin model to topically applied irritants and allergens. In Vitro Toxicol. **9:** 157–166.
24. HOLLAND, G., L.K. EARL & T.J. HALL-MANNING. 1998. Assessment of the skin irritation effect of mixed surfactants using the 4 hour human patch test and EpiDerm™ EPI-100 *in vitro* skin model. *In* Proceedings of the 38th International Detergency Conference, pp. 81–85.
25. PONEC, M. 1994. The use of *in vitro* skin recombinants to evaluate cutaneous toxicity. *In* In Vitro Skin Toxicology, pp. 107–116. Mary Ann Liebert, Inc. New York.
26. PONEC, M. & J. KEMPENAAR. 1995. Use of human skin recombinants as an *in vitro* model for testing the irritation potential of cutaneous irritants. Skin Pharmacol. **8:** 49–59.
27. BOELSMA, E., H. TANOJO, H.E. BODDE & M. PONEC. 1996. Assessment of the potential irritancy of oleic acid on human skin: evaluation *in vitro* and *in vivo*. Toxicol. In Vitro **10:** 729–742.
28. AUGUSTIN, C., C. COLLOMBEL & O. DAMOUR. 1997. Use of dermal equivalent and skin equivalent models for identifying phototoxic compounds *in vitro*. Photodermatol. Photoimmunol. Photomed. **13:** 27–36.
29. AUGUSTIN, C., C. COLLOMBEL & O. DAMOUR. 1998. Use of dermal equivalent and skin equivalent models for *in vitro* cutaneous irritation testing of cosmetic products: comparison with *in vivo* human data. J. Toxicol. Cutaneous Ocul. Toxicol. **17:** 5–17.
30. ROGUET, R., C. COHEN, C. ROBLES, P. COURTELLEMONT, M. TOLLE, J.P. GUILLOT & X.P. DUTEIL. 1998. An interlaboratory study of the reproducibility and relevance of episkin, reconstructed human epidermis, in the assessment of cosmetics irritancy. Toxicol. In Vitro **12:** 295–304.
31. ECVAM. 1999. Prevalidation of *in vitro* tests for acute skin irritation. ATLA-Altern. Lab. Anim. **27:** 221–223.
32. YORK, M., D.A. BASKETTER, J.A. CUTHBERT & L. NEILSON. 1995. Skin irritation testing in man for hazard assessment—evaluation of four patch systems. Hum. Exp. Toxicol. **14:** 729–734.
33. YORK, M., H.A. GRIFFITHS, E. WHITTLE & D.A. BASKETTER. 1996. Evaluation of a human patch test for the identification and classification of skin irritation potential. Contact Dermatitis **34:** 204–212.
34. BASKETTER, D.A., M. CHAMBERLAIN, H.A. GRIFFITHS, M. ROWSON, E. WHITTLE & M. YORK. 1997. The classification of skin irritants by human patch test. Food Chem. Toxicol. **35:** 845–852.
35. BASKETTER, D.A., H.A. GRIFFITHS, X.M. WANG, K.P. WILHELM & J. MCFADDEN. 1996. Individual, ethnic, and seasonal variability in irritant susceptibility of skin: the implications for a predictive human patch test. Contact Dermatitis **35:** 208–213.
36. GRIFFITHS, H.A., K.P. WILHELM, M.K. ROBINSON, X.M. WANG, J. MCFADDEN, M. YORK & D.A. BASKETTER. 1997. Interlaboratory evaluation of a human patch test for the identification of skin irritation potential/hazard. Food Chem. Toxicol. **35:** 255–260.
37. ROBINSON, M.K., E. WHITTLE & D.A. BASKETTER. 1999. A two center study of the development of acute irritation responses to fatty acids. Am. J. Contact Dermatitis **10:** 136–145.
38. BASKETTER, D., L. BLAIKIE & F. REYNOLDS. 1996. The impact of atopic status on a predictive human test of skin irritation potential. Contact Dermatitis **35:** 33–39.

39. JUDGE, M.R., H.A. GRIFFITHS, D.A. BASKETTER, I.R. WHITE, R.J.G. RYCROFT & J.P. MCFADDEN. 1996. Variation in response of human skin to irritant challenge. Contact Dermatitis **34:** 115–117.
40. MCFADDEN, J.P., S.H. WAKELIN & D.A. BASKETTER. 1998. Acute irritation thresholds in subjects with type I–type VI skin. Contact Dermatitis **38:** 147–149.
41. ROBINSON, M.K., M.A. PERKINS & D.A. BASKETTER. 1998. Application of a 4-h human patch test method for comparative and investigative assessment of skin irritation. Contact Dermatitis **38:** 194–202.

New Technologies to Prevent and Treat Contact Hypersensitivity Responses

AKIRA TAKASHIMA,[a,b] MARK MUMMERT,[a] TOSHIYUKI KITAJIMA,[c] AND HIROYUKI MATSUE[a]

[a]*Department of Dermatology, University of Texas Southwestern Medical Center, Dallas, Texas 75235, USA*

[c]*Yamanashi Medical University, Yamanashi, Japan 409-3815*

ABSTRACT: Allergic contact dermatitis is a common inflammatory skin disease caused by T cells that recognize environmental and industrial allergens (i.e., haptens). Langerhans' cells (LC), which are skin-specific and "immature" members of the dendritic cell (DC) family of antigen-presenting cells, play crucial roles in the induction of contact hypersensitivity (CH) responses. Upon exposure to haptens, LC migrate from the epidermis to draining lymph nodes, mature into T cell–stimulatory DC, and activate hapten-reactive T cells. Therefore, CH responses should be preventable at the sensitization phase by interfering with one of these changes that occur in LC. Our objective is to develop new technologies for the prevention and treatment of allergic contact dermatitis. In this article, we will introduce three technologies that we have recently developed. First, using a phage display strategy, we have identified a 12-mer peptide (termed "peptide 1") that binds and blocks the function of hyaluronan (HA), which is known to serve as an adhesive substrate for LC migration. Local injection of peptide 1 in mice before topical application of DNFB blocked almost completely the emigration of LC from the epidermis to the draining lymph node, where antigen presentation takes place. Peptide 1 represents a new strategy that is designed to inhibit the initial event of CH. Second, we have established an *in vitro* experimental system to study the terminal maturation of LC during antigen-specific interaction with T cells. This experimental system, which employs a long-term LC line and T cell clones, should provide a unique tool for the identification of new immunosuppressive agents that block LC terminal maturation selectively. Finally, under the hypothesis that LC, which are engineered to overexpress a death ligand, would deliver apoptotic signals instead of activation signals to T cells, we created a "killer" LC clone by introducing CD95L cDNA into our long-term LC line XS106. *In vivo* administration of DNFB-pulsed killer LC into mice, either before or after sensitization, resulted in marked suppression of CH responses to DNFB. The killer LC technology represents an entirely new immunosuppressive therapy that is designed to eliminate only the pathogenic T cells.

[b]Address for correspondence: Department of Dermatology, University of Texas Southwestern Medical Center, 5323 Harry Hines Boulevard, Dallas, TX 75390-9069. Voice: 214-648-3419; fax: 214-648-3472.

atakas@mednet.swmed.edu

OVERVIEW OF ALLERGIC CONTACT HYPERSENSITIVITY RESPONSES

Effector Leukocytes

Contact hypersensitivity (CH) responses are clinically manifested as allergic contact dermatitis, a common skin disease caused by skin exposure to environmental or industrial allergens. Immunologically, CH responses are defined as T cell–mediated inflammatory responses to reactive haptens and are experimentally inducible in mice by topical sensitization, followed by topical challenge onto ear skin with the same hapten. This CH model has been used by many investigators to study pathogenic mechanisms underlying allergic contact dermatitis. According to textbook knowledge, CH responses are classified as one of the conventional delayed-type hypersensitivity (DTH) responses. However, CH responses appear to be unique in many respects, as pointed out in the recent review article by Grabbe and Schwarz.[1]

Most importantly, conventional DTH responses to foreign protein antigens are mediated primarily by MHC class II–restricted $CD4^+$ T cells,[1,2] whereas the CH responses appear to be mediated predominantly by MHC class I–restricted $CD8^+$ T cells. Gocinski and Tigelaar reported that depletion of $CD4^+$ T cells by iv injection of anti-CD4 monoclonal antibody (mAb) resulted in striking enhancement of ear swelling responses, whereas depletion of $CD8^+$ T cells diminished ear swelling.[3] Subsequently, Bour et al. observed that MHC class I–deficient mice were unable to mount significant CH responses. By contrast, MHC class II–deficient mice, which were unable to mount the conventional DTH responses, exhibited exaggerated CH responses.[4] More recently, Bouloc et al. extended these observations by showing that ear swelling responses in MHC class II–deficient mice can be abrogated by depleting $CD8^+$ T cells with anti-CD8 mAb.[5] Taken together, these findings indicate that $CD8^+$ T cells alone are sufficient to express CH responses. On the other hand, we know that $CD4^+$ T cells are also functionally involved in CH responses. For example, $CD4^+$ T cells are known to play a downregulatory role and they may even play an effector role depending upon experimental conditions (e.g., different haptens, different doses of haptens, and different strains of mice).[1]

Langerhans' Cells in CH Responses

Langerhans' cells (LC), which are members of the dendritic cell (DC) family of antigen-presenting cells, reside normally at the environmental interface (i.e., epidermis), extending their characteristic long dendrites.[6–8] Upon skin exposure to reactive haptens, LC begin to migrate to draining lymph nodes, where antigen presentation takes place. At the same time, they change their morphology and phenotype, thus acquiring characteristic features of "mature" DC. These features include (a) elevated surface expression of MHC class II molecules, (b) induced expression of costimulatory molecules (e.g., CD80, CD86, and CD40), (c) altered expression of adhesion molecules (e.g., E-cadherin, CD44, and CD54), and (d) production of a wide variety of inflammatory cytokines (e.g., IL-1β, IL-6, and TNFα). These maturational changes are considered to represent the critical transition of LC from DC that are specialized for antigen uptake and processing into DC that are specialized for delivering T cell–stimulatory signals.

With respect to the ability of LC to present haptens to T cells, Tamaki *et al.* demonstrated that subcutaneous (sc) injection of trinitrophenyl (TNP)–conjugated epidermal cells (containing LC) into mice leads to successful sensitization as measured by subsequent ear swelling responses to dinitrochlorobenzene (DNCB).[9] Sullivan *et al.* subsequently reported that CH responses are inducible by FACS-purified, TNP-conjugated I-A$^+$ epidermal cells (i.e., LC).[10] More recently, we observed that sc injection of dinitrofluorobenzene (DNFB)–pulsed XS106 cells, one of the long-term LC lines established from mouse epidermis,[11] was sufficient for full sensitization, thus excluding formally the potential contribution of contaminating other epidermal cell populations.[12] These observations together illustrate the ability of LC to present reactive haptens to T cells.

Working with an immature LC line XS52, which we developed several years ago from the epidermis of newborn BALB/c mice,[13] we have observed a unique phenomenon: LC undergo maturational changes upon antigen-specific interaction with T cells. Briefly, when cocultured with antigen-reactive T cell clones in the presence of relevant antigens, XS52 LC begin to secrete proinflammatory cytokines, alter their surface phenotype, and lose their adhesive and phagocytotic capacities, thus acquiring the characteristic features of mature LC (see below). During antigen presentation, it is evident that not only do LC deliver activation signals to T cells (leading to T cell activation), but they also receive signals back from T cells (leading to LC terminal maturation).

In summary, in response to topical application of reactive haptens, a sequential series of events take place in LC (FIG. 1). First, LC leave the epidermis to migrate to the draining lymph node. Second, LC begin to mature during this migration. Third, LC interact with hapten-reactive T cells in a bidirectional manner, delivering activation signals and receiving terminal maturation signals. From these observations, we reason that CH responses should be preventable by interfering with any one of these events.

LANGERHANS' CELL–BASED IMMUNOSUPPRESSIVE PROTOCOLS

Currently Available Protocols for the Induction of Immunological Tolerance

Use of immunosuppressive reagents, such as glucocorticoids, is the most common approach in treating patients with allergic contact dermatitis. On the other hand, this approach is not always effective, especially for those patients with unavoidable (e.g., occupational) exposure to the same sensitizers. Several attempts have been made to induce antigen-specific immunological tolerance. For example, hapten-specific tolerance has been induced experimentally by sensitization through ultraviolet (UV)–irradiated skin sites[14] or by sensitization through the nonirradiated skin after exposure elsewhere to relatively high UV doses.[15] Tolerance against foreign protein antigens has been induced by administering antigens via unconventional routes, such as oral administration,[16] intravenous injection,[17] or intrathymic injection before or at birth.[18]

Molecular interaction between MHC-associated antigenic peptides (expressed on antigen-presenting cells) and the T cell receptor complex (expressed on effector T cells) underlies antigen specificity in cellular immunity. This rationalizes the use of antigen-presenting cells to initiate antigen-specific tolerance. Examples of success-

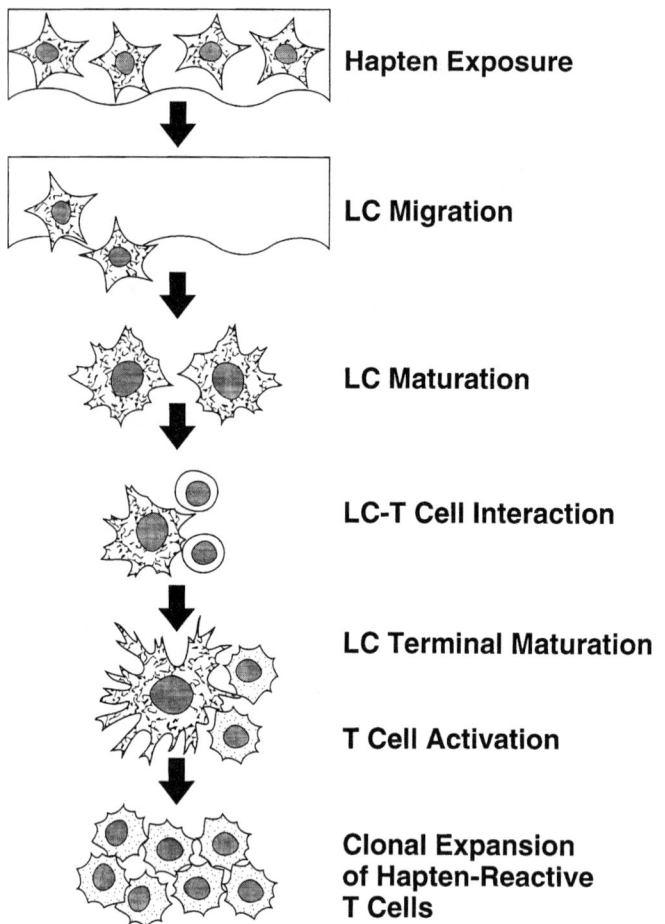

FIGURE 1. The diagram illustrates a series of cellular events that are known to take place during the sensitization phase of CH responses. Briefly, in response to exposure to reactive haptens, LC that normally reside within the epidermal compartment begin to emigrate from the epidermis. At the same time, LC begin to exhibit phenotypic and functional features of mature DC. Upon arrival to the T cell area in the draining lymph node, the hapten-carrying LC achieve the initial contact with hapten-reactive T cells. During the antigen-specific interaction with T cells, not only do LC deliver activation signals to T cells, but they also receive signals back from T cells; the bidirectional signaling triggers the terminal maturation of LC as well as the activation and subsequent clonal expansion of hapten-reactive T cells.

ful applications include (a) iv injection of antigen-pulsed B cells, splenic DC, or epidermal LC,[19–21] (b) administration of UV-irradiated LC or IL-10-treated LC,[22–24] (c) prevention of experimentally induced autoimmunity by administering DC that express autoantigen-derived peptides,[25] and (d) use of CD95L-transduced macrophages.[26,27] These observations validate our central hypothesis that CH responses should be preventable by manipulating LC function experimentally.

Blocking of LC Emigration from Epidermis

A fundamental aspect of the function of LC is their highly migratory capacity.[28] LC precursors that are generated in bone marrow must first migrate into the epidermis, most likely through the bloodstream. Upon exposure to reactive haptens, LC must then exit the epidermis and enter the lymphatic vessels to reach the draining lymph node. Price *et al.* reported that α_6 integrins are expressed by epidermal LC and that anti-α_6 monoclonal antibodies (mAb) inhibit hapten-triggered LC emigration from epidermis, with the implication that α_6 integrins mediate LC migration across the epidermal basement membrane.[29] Weiss *et al.* documented that, upon activation, LC elevate the surface expression of CD44 variant isoforms and that mAb against selected CD44 isoforms (v4 and v6) inhibit LC emigration from the epidermis as well as the onset of CH responses at the elicitation phase.[30] This observation is in complete agreement with the theory that molecular interaction between CD44 (on leukocytes) and hyaluronan (HA), a glycosaminoglycan that is expressed on endothelial cells and epithelial cells, mediates leukocyte homing.[31,32] In summary, LC migration can be blocked by interfering with the molecular interaction of LC-associated adhesive receptors (e.g., $\alpha_6\beta_4$ integrin and CD44 isoforms) with their respective ligands (e.g., laminin and HA).

As an initial step to translate this knowledge into a clinically applicable form, we developed small peptide inhibitors of HA. By using the phage display strategy, we have identified a peptide inhibitor of HA (Mummert and Takashima, manuscript in preparation). Briefly, we started from a phage display library consisting of random 12-mer peptides fused to the gIII protein of M13 phage, with a complexity of about 10^9. After four rounds of panning on HA-coated plates, we isolated a phage clone that encodes a unique 12-mer peptide motif, termed "peptide 1". A synthetic peptide containing this motif showed significant binding to HA-coated beads, as well as to the HA expressed on keratinocytes. None of the control 12-mer peptides showed significant binding to either substrate. Local injection of synthetic peptide 1 into the ears of mice significantly reduced hapten-triggered LC migration, validating its biological activity in mice and suggesting its clinical utility for the prevention of allergic contact dermatitis at the sensitization phase. Interaction between CD44 (expressed on inflammatory T cells) and HA (expressed on endothelial cells and present abundantly in the extracellular matrix) also plays a crucial role in the elicitation phase by mediating skin-directed homing of hapten-reactive effector T cells. Ear swelling responses to DNFB in sensitized mice was suppressed markedly by local injection of peptide 1, but not by any of the control peptides, immediately before challenge (Mummert and Takashima, manuscript in preparation). Thus, peptide 1 and its derivatives appear to represent an entirely new strategy for the prevention and treatment of allergic contact dermatitis. The strategy is designed to prevent both the emigration of epidermal LC from skin and the immigration of effector leukocytes into skin.

Prevention of Terminal Maturation of LC

During antigen presentation, not only do DC deliver activation signals to T cells, but they also receive signals back from T cells. For example, ligation of CD40 on DC with CD40L expressed on T cells triggers the secretion of IL-12 by DC.[33,34]

Working with the immature LC line, XS52, established from the epidermis of newborn mice,[13] we have observed that XS52 LC undergo rapid and profound changes upon antigen-specific interaction with T cells *in vitro*. Briefly, when cultured with HDK-1 T cells, which are a keyhole limpet hemocyanin (KLH)–specific CD4$^+$ T cell clone, in the presence of antigen (KLH), the XS52 cells (a) secreted relatively large amounts of IL-1β, IL-6, and TNFα, (b) elevated surface expression of CD86, (c) diminished surface expression of CD115 (CSF-1 receptor), and (d) lost their adhesive and phagocytotic capacities.[35–39] None of these changes were detectable when XS52 cells were incubated with HDK-1 T cells alone or KLH alone. On the other hand, virtually all of the changes were inducible by culturing XS52 cells in the presence of bacterial lipopolysaccharide (LPS), consistent with the theory that LPS and other bacterial products function as an immunological adjuvant by promoting the maturation of DC.[40,41] Importantly, these changes that occur in XS52 cells during antigen presentation (or following LPS treatment) duplicate the changes that are known to accompany LC maturation during short-term culture and in response to topical application of reactive haptens. Hence, we have postulated that LC undergo a critical transition, termed "T cell–mediated terminal maturation", into fully competent DC upon antigen-specific interaction with T cells (or exposure to bacterial products).

Glucocorticoids (GCs) have been used effectively for several decades as potent immunosuppressive agents in treating T cell–mediated inflammatory skin diseases, including allergic contact dermatitis. With respect to pharmacological mechanisms of action, GCs have been shown to inhibit several immunologically relevant activities of monocytes/macrophages and T cells. We have identified a new mechanism in which GCs modulate LC maturation. Briefly, dexamethasone (DEX) at relatively low concentrations (10^{-9}–10^{-7} M) inhibited, substantially or completely, T cell–mediated, as well as LPS-triggered, terminal maturation of XS52 cells. By contrast, the changes that accompany DC-mediated T cell activation were much more resistant to DEX at the same concentrations.[36] Although the *in vivo* relevance of these observations remains to be determined, they form the basis for a new concept that GCs suppress T cell–mediated immune responses by interfering with terminal maturation of DC. Moreover, our experimental system will provide a technical platform for the development of new immunosuppressive agents for allergic contact dermatitis, which are designed to prevent LC terminal maturation.

Depletion of Hapten-Reactive T Cells by "Killer" LC

Hapten-pulsed LC, when administered into experimental animals, activate hapten-reactive T cells, thus leading to successful sensitization.[10] We reasoned that "killer" LC, that is, LC that are engineered to overexpress "death ligands" CD95L, would deliver death signals, instead of activation signals, to T cells upon antigen-specific interaction, thus leading to the depletion of hapten-reactive T cells. To test this hypothesis, we introduced the gene encoding a prototypic death ligand CD95L (or Fas ligand) into the XS106 LC line, which differs from the XS52 line by showing mature features,[11] and selected a permanently transfected LC clone. The resulting clone, termed XS106-CD95L, expressed functionally active CD95L on the surface, as assessed by its ability to kill the Jurkat target cells (expressing CD95 constitutively). Killer LC pulsed with a protein antigen, ovalbumin (OVA), induced apoptosis of OVA-reactive T cells efficiently. By contrast, no cytotoxic potential was observed with the parental XS106 cells or the control XS106 clone transfected with the vector alone, neither of which expressed detectable CD95L on their surfaces. Anti-CD95L mAb reverted the killer LC clone into conventional T cell–stimulatory LC, indicating that the induced expression of CD95L alone was responsible for its cytotoxic potential. These *in vitro* observations suggested that antigen-specific immunosuppression might be inducible by killer LC.[12]

In vivo administration of killer LC pulsed with OVA, before standard sensitization with OVA in complete Freund's adjuvant, prevented the induction of DTH responses to OVA as measured by footpad swelling. Nonpulsed killer LC showed no effect, indicating antigen requirement. Moreover, OVA-pulsed killer LC suppressed OVA responsiveness without affecting immunoreactivity to a second protein antigen, hen egg lysosome (HEL), whereas HEL-pulsed killer LC inhibited only HEL responses, validating antigen specificity. Antigen-pulsed killer LC also reversed the ongoing OVA-specific immune responses in previously immunized mice. Administration of DNFB-pulsed killer LC before standard sensitization presented the onset of CH responses to DNFB as measured by ear swelling. DNFB-pulsed killer LC also suppressed ear swelling responses to DNFB even in previously sensitized animals, documenting the therapeutic potential of this protocol.[12] These results demonstrate that one can convert LC from ordinary antigen-presenting cells (that deliver T cell–stimulatory signals during antigen presentation) into unique antigen-presenting cells (that deliver apoptotic signals to responding T cells) by introduction of cDNA encoding CD95L. Our killer LC technology, which is designed to eliminate only pathogenic T cells recognizing a given antigen, may be clinically applicable for the prevention and treatment of allergic contact dermatitis and perhaps other T cell–mediated inflammatory disorders.

CONCLUDING REMARKS

Using CH responses as a model, we have developed and tested new strategies for the prevention and treatment of T cell–mediated inflammatory skin disorders. In summary, we have observed that (a) LC emigration from epidermis and T cell immigration into skin can be inhibited by a small peptide designed to block HA function, (b) the immunosuppressive activity of GCs is attributable, at least partially, to their capacity to prevent terminal maturation of LC, and (c) CD95L-transduced killer LC can be used to eliminate the pathogenic T cells of CH. Not only do these observations suggest potential benefits of the technologies per se, but they also reaffirm the concept that LC play critical roles in the initiation and regulation of T cell–mediated cutaneous immune responses. We believe that this line of investigation will, ultimately, lead to the development of new therapies for allergic contact dermatitis.

ACKNOWLEDGMENTS

This work was supported by NIH (Grant Nos. RO1-AR35068, RO1-AR43777, and RO1-AI43262) and by a CE.R.I.E.S. Award (to A. Takashima).

REFERENCES

1. GRABBE, S. & T. SCHWARZ. 1998. Immunoregulatory mechanisms involved in elicitation of allergic contact hypersensitivity. Immunol. Today **19:** 37–44.
2. FONG, T.A.T. & T.R. MOSMANN. 1989. The role of IFN-gamma in delayed-type hypersensitivity mediated by Th1 clones. J. Immunol. **143:** 2887–2893.
3. GOCINSKI, B.L. & R.E. TIGELAAR. 1990. Roles of $CD4^+$ and $CD8^+$ T cells in murine contact sensitivity revealed by *in vivo* monoclonal antibody depletion. J. Immunol. **144:** 4121–4128.
4. BOUR, H., E. PEYRON, M. GAUCHERAND et al. 1995. Major histocompatibility complex class I–restricted CD8+ T cells and class II restricted CD4+ T cells, respectively, mediate and regulate contact sensitivity to dinitrofluorobenzene. Eur. J. Immunol. **25:** 3006–3010.
5. BOULOC, A., A. CAVANI & S.I. KATZ. 1998. Contact hypersensitivity in MHC class II–deficient mice depends on CD8 T lymphocytes primed by immunostimulating Langerhans' cells. J. Invest. Dermatol. **111:** 44–49.
6. BANCHEREAU, J. & R.M. STEINMAN. 1998. Dendritic cells and the control of immunity. Nature **392:** 245–252.
7. STEINMAN, R.M. 1991. The dendritic cell system and its role in immunogenicity. Annu. Rev. Immunol. **9:** 271–296.
8. STINGL, G., C. HAUSER & K. WOLFF. 1993. The epidermis: an immunologic microenvironment. *In* Dermatology in General Medicine, pp. 172–197. McGraw-Hill. New York.
9. TAMAKI, K., H. FUJIWARA & S.I. KATZ. 1999. The role of epidermal cells in the induction and suppression of contact sensitivity. J. Invest. Dermatol. **76:** 275–278.
10. SULLIVAN, S., P.R. BERGSTRESSER, R.E. TIGELAAR et al. 1986. Induction and regulation of contact hypersensitivity by resident, bone-marrow derived, dendritic epidermal cells: Langerhans' cells and Thy-1+ epidermal cells. J. Immunol. **137:** 2460–2467.
11. TIMARES, L., A. TAKASHIMA & S.A. JOHNSTON. 1998. Quantitative analysis of the immunopotency of genetically transfected dendritic cells. Proc. Natl. Acad. Sci. U.S.A. **95:** 13147–13152.
12. MATSUE, H., K. MATSUE, M. WALTERS et al. 1999. Induction of antigen-specific immunosuppression by CD95L cDNA-transfected "killer" dendritic cells. Nat. Med. In press.
13. XU, S., K. ARIIZUMI, G. CACERES-DITTMAR et al. 1995. Successive generation of antigen-presenting, dendritic cell lines from murine epidermis. J. Immunol. **154:** 2697–2705.
14. TOEWS, G.B., P.R. BERGSTRESSER & J.W. STREILEIN. 1980. Epidermal Langerhans' cell density determines whether contact hypersensitivity or unresponsiveness follows skin painting with DNFB. J. Immunol. **124:** 445–453.
15. NOONAN, F.P., M.L. KRIPKE, G.M. PEDERSEN et al. 1981. Suppression of contact hypersensitivity in mice by ultraviolet irradiation is associated with defective antigen presentation. Immunology **43:** 527–534.
16. WEINER, H.L. 1997. Oral tolerance: immune mechanisms and treatment of autoimmune diseases. Immunol. Today **18:** 335–343.
17. LIBLAU, R., R. TISCH, N. BERCOVICI et al. 1997. Systemic antigen in the treatment of T-cell-mediated autoimmune diseases. Immunol. Today **18:** 599–603.
18. POSSELT, A.M., C.F. BARKER, A.L. FRIEDMAN et al. 1992. Prevention of autoimmune diabetes in the BB rat by intrathymic islet transplantation at birth. Science **256:** 1321–1324.
19. BENNETT, S.R.M., F.R. CARBONE, T. TOY et al. 1998. B cells directly tolerize $CD8^+$ T cells. J. Exp. Med. **188:** 1977–1983.
20. MORIKAWA, Y., M. FUROTANI, K. KURIBAYASHI et al. 1992. The role of antigen-presenting cells in the regulation of delayed-type hypersensitivity. Immunology **77:** 81–87.
21. MORIKAWA, Y., M. FUROTANI, K. KURIBAYASHI et al. 1993. The role of antigen-presenting cells in the regulation of delayed-type hypersensitivity. Cell. Immunol. **152:** 200–210.

22. CRUZ, P.D., JR., J. NIXON-FULTON, R.E. TIGELAAR et al. 1989. Disparate effects of *in vitro* UVB irradiation on intravenous immunization with epidermal cell subpopulations for the induction of contact hypersensitivity. J. Invest. Dermatol. **92:** 160–165.
23. ENK, A.H., J. SALOGA, D. BECKER et al. 1994. Induction of hapten-specific tolerance by interleukin-10 *in vivo*. J. Exp. Med. **179:** 1397–1402.
24. ENK, A.H., V.L. ANGELONI, M.C. UDEY et al. 1993. Inhibition of Langerhans' cell antigen-presenting function by IL-10. J. Immunol. **151:** 2390–2398.
25. CLARE-SALZLER, M., J. BROOKS, A. CHAI et al. 1992. Prevention of diabetes in nonobese diabetic mice by dendritic cell transfer. J. Clin. Invest. **90:** 741–748.
26. ZHANG, H-G., D. LIU, Y. HEIKE et al. 1998. Induction of specific T-cell tolerance by adenovirus-transfected, Fas ligand–producing antigen presenting cells. Nat. Biotechnol. **16:** 1045–1049.
27. ZHANG, H., X. SU, D. LIU et al. 1999. Induction of specific T cell tolerance by Fas ligand–expressing antigen-presenting cells. J. Immunol. **162:** 1423–1430.
28. SALLUSTO, F. & A. LANZAVECCHIA. 1999. Mobilizing dendritic cells for tolerance, priming, and chronic inflammation. J. Exp. Med. **189:** 611–614.
29. PRICE, A.A., M. CUMBERBATCH, I. KIMBER et al. 1997. a_6 integrins are required for Langerhans' cell migration from the epidermis. J. Exp. Med. **186:** 1725–1735.
30. WEISS, J.M., J. SLEEMAN, A.C. RENKL et al. 1997. An essential role for CD44 variant isoforms in epidermal Langerhans' cell and blood dendritic cell function. J. Cell Biol. **137:** 1137–1147.
31. DEGRENDELE, H., P. ESTESS, L.J. PICKER et al. 1996. CD44 and its ligand hyaluronate mediate rolling under physiologic flow: a novel lymphocyte–endothelial cell primary adhesion pathway. J. Exp. Med. **183:** 1119–1130.
32. CLARK, R.A., R. ALON & T.A. SPRINGER. 1996. CD44 and hyaluronan-dependent rolling interactions of lymphocytes on tonsillar stroma. J. Cell Biol. **134:** 1075–1087.
33. KOCH, F., U. STANZL, P. JENNEWEIN et al. 1996. High level IL-12 production by murine dendritic cells: upregulation via MHC class II and CD40 molecules and downregulation by IL-4 and IL-10. J. Exp. Med. **184:** 741–746.
34. CELLA, M., D. SCHEIDEGGER, K. PALMER-LEHMANN et al. 1996. Ligation of CD40 on dendritic cells triggers production of high levels of interleukin-12 and enhances T cell stimulatory capacity: T-T help via APC activation. J. Exp. Med. **184:** 747–752.
35. KITAJIMA, T., K. ARIIZUMI, P.R. BERGSTRESSER et al. 1995. T cell–dependent loss of proliferative responsiveness to colony-stimulating factor-1 by a murine epidermal-derived dendritic cell line, XS52. J. Immunol. **155:** 5190–5197.
36. KITAJIMA, T., K. ARIIZUMI, P.R. BERGSTRESSER et al. 1996. A novel mechanism of glucocorticoid-induced immune suppression: the inhibition of T cell–mediated terminal maturation of a murine dendritic cell line. J. Clin. Invest. **98:** 142–147.
37. KITAJIMA, T., K. ARIIZUMI, P.R. BERGSTRESSER et al. 1996. UVB radiation sensitizes a murine epidermal dendritic cell line (XS52) to undergo apoptosis upon antigen presentation to T cells. J. Immunol. **157:** 3312–3316.
38. KITAJIMA, T., K. ARIIZUMI, M. MOHAMADZADEH et al. 1995. T cell–dependent secretion of IL-1b by a dendritic cell line (XS52) derived from murine epidermis. J. Immunol. **155:** 3794–3800.
39. KITAJIMA, T., G. CACERES-DITTMAR, F.J. TAPIA et al. 1996. T cell–mediated terminal maturation of dendritic cells: loss of adhesive and phagocytotic capacities. J. Immunol. **157:** 2340–2347.
40. SALLUSTO, F., M. CELLA, C. DANIELI et al. 1995. Dendritic cells use macropinocytosis and the mannose receptor to concentrate macromolecules in the major histocompatibility complex class II compartment: downregulation by cytokines and bacterial products. J. Exp. Med. **182:** 389–400.
41. ROAKE, J.A., A.S. RAO, P.J. MORRIS et al. 1995. Dendritic cell loss from nonlymphoid tissues after systemic administration of lipopolysaccharide, tumor necrosis factor, and interleukin 1. J. Exp. Med. **181:** 2237–2247.

The Role of Tumor Necrosis Factor α in Chemical-Induced Hepatotoxicity

MICHAEL I. LUSTER,[a,b] PETIA P. SIMEONOVA,[a] RANDLE M. GALLUCCI,[a] ALEX BRUCCOLERI,[c] MARK E. BLAZKA,[d] BERRAN YUCESOY,[a] AND JOANNA M. MATHESON[a]

[a]Toxicology and Molecular Biology Branch, Health Effects Laboratory Division, National Institute for Occupational Safety and Health, Morgantown, West Virginia 26505, USA

[c]Department of Microbiology, University of Milan, Milan, Italy

[d]Product Safety Assurance, Colgate-Palmolive Company, Piscataway, New Jersey 08855, USA

ABSTRACT: Only recently have toxicologists come to understand the role of inflammation, and TNFα specifically, in classical toxicological processes. This relationship appears fairly complex, as inflammation and proliferation may well be only one facet of a time- and dose-dependent continuum of toxicological and repair processes. Not surprisingly, considerable efforts are being undertaken using our newly found understanding of molecular control to develop specific and safe chemical, biological, and molecular regulators of TNFα for potential therapeutic use. Their effectiveness in controlling environmental or occupational diseases has yet to be established.

INTRODUCTION

Increasing evidence suggests that inflammation plays a role in many classical chemical toxicities including, among others, hepatotoxicity induced by carbon tetrachloride or acetaminophen, pulmonary toxicity from asbestos and silica, and even neurotoxicity from organotins.[1,2] The overarching hypothesis that links these toxicities is illustrated in FIGURE 1 and can be summarized as follows: initial toxic injury produces focal tissue damage and necrosis in a target organ. As a result of this damage, tissue-fixed macrophages, along with adjacent endothelial cells and epithelial cells, are activated and secrete inflammatory products. These products include the proinflammatory cytokine tumor necrosis factor (TNF) α, which is a central regulator that aids in tissue repair by stimulating apoptosis and cell proliferation as well as exacerbates cell damage by initiating an overly aggressive inflammatory process. The latter ultimately results in the recruitment and activation of neutrophils and monocytes into the damaged site and the release of reactive oxygen species and the nitrogen-centered radical, nitric oxide, producing cell damage. Support for this path-

[b]Address for correspondence: Toxicology and Molecular Biology Branch, Health Effects Laboratory Division, National Institute for Occupational Safety and Health, 1095 Willowdale Drive, Morgantown, WV 26505. Voice: 304-285-5940; fax: 304-285-6038.
myl6@cdc.gov

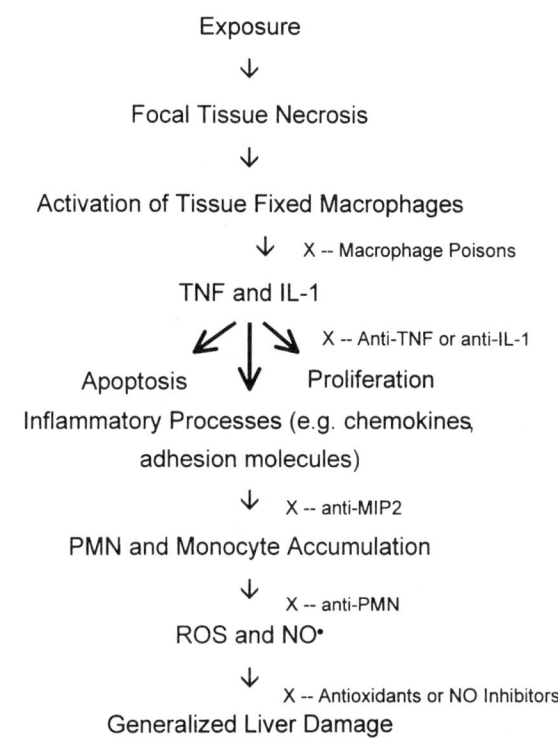

FIGURE 1. Hypothesis of chemical-induced liver injury. Increasing evidence has suggested that inflammation plays a major role in chemical-induced hepatotoxicity and repair. Initial damage is thought to produce focal tissue necrosis resulting in activation of tissue-fixed macrophages. These activated macrophages secrete primary cytokines, including IL-1 and TNFα, which may induce apoptosis, stimulate cell growth, or initiate inflammatory processes. The inflammatory process ultimately results in the recruitment of activated neutrophils and the release of toxic products such as reactive oxygen species (ROS) and nitric oxide. The strongest evidence for this hypothesis originates from the use of different classes of inhibitors.

way and that TNFα is a central mediator stems from several observations: (1) elevated levels of inflammatory mediators, including TNFα, chemokines, and reactive oxygen and nitrogen species, are found in target organs following exposure to many toxic agents; (2) inhibitors of this pathway (see FIG. 1), such as antioxidants, cytokine antagonists, and macrophage poisons, prevent many of the pathophysiological or repair processes from occurring; and (3) direct administration of these mediators, such as TNFα, in experimental animals mimics many of the pathophysiological responses observed in the chemical response.[3–11]

RESULTS AND DISCUSSION

Work in our laboratory has focused on the role of TNFα in this process as it is a central regulator for many bioactive molecules including those responsible for

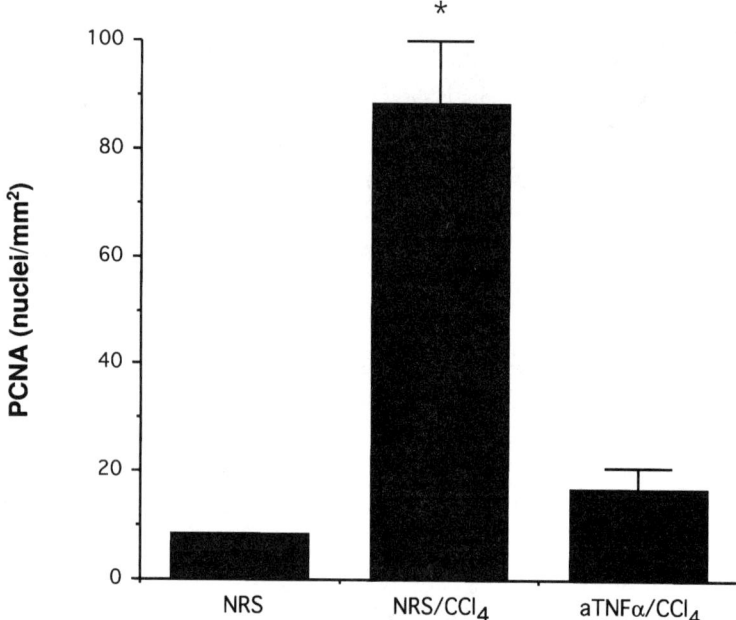

FIGURE 2. PCNA immunostaining. Mice were administered either normal rabbit serum (NRS), CCl_4 (0.1 mL/kg body weight), or CCl_4 plus neutralizing antibodies to TNFα (aTNF).[13] Livers were collected at 48 h later and the number of nuclei in the S-phase of the cell cycle (per square millimeter) determined using standard methodology.[13]

chronic inflammation, induction of acute phase proteins, cell proliferation, and cytotoxicity. Evidence that proinflammatory cytokines are involved in hepatotoxic responses was first provided from studies by Blazka et al.,[12] who demonstrated that neutralizing antibodies to TNFα or IL-1 partially prevented liver damage in mice initiated by hepatotoxic doses of acetaminophen. These studies were stimulated by observations that hepatocytes treated with acetaminophen release factors that activate Kupffer cells, which in turn are associated with areas of the liver that subsequently become necrotic.[5] In later studies, we demonstrated that increased TNFα expression in the liver is also associated with carbon tetrachloride (CCl_4) exposure in mice. Surprisingly, however, TNFα neutralization was not associated with decreased hepatotoxicity, but rather delayed normal repair processes.[13] Subsequent studies using this model for chemical liver injury indicated that TNFα was involved in liver repair through its ability to support hepatocyte proliferation following chemical injury. This is illustrated in FIGURE 2 using proliferating cell nuclear antigen (PCNA) staining, a measurement of hepatocyte proliferation. Forty-eight hours following exposure of mice to 0.1 mL/kg body weight of CCl_4, a marked increase in the percent of cells in S-phase was detected in the livers of treated mice compared to controls. Nuclear PCNA staining was reduced nearly to control levels in mice pretreated with neutralizing antibodies to TNFα, indicating its importance in hepatocyte proliferation. As with chemical-induced hepatic damage, it had been demonstrated that

TNFα is expressed in the liver of rats following partial hepatectomy[14] and administration of neutralizing antibodies to TNFα before partial hepatectomy significantly impairs liver regeneration.[15] In this respect, the ability of TNFα to serve as a mitogen for human and rodent hepatocytes has recently been demonstrated *in vitro*.[15] Thus, TNFα is both mitogenic for hepatocytes, being implicated in liver repair following chemical damage and in regeneration following partial hepatectomy, as well as capable of causing cell damage by inducing an overzealous inflammatory response.

Cell proliferation is a complex and tightly controlled process that is modulated by cell-to-cell contact and bioactive macromolecules such as hepatocyte growth fac-

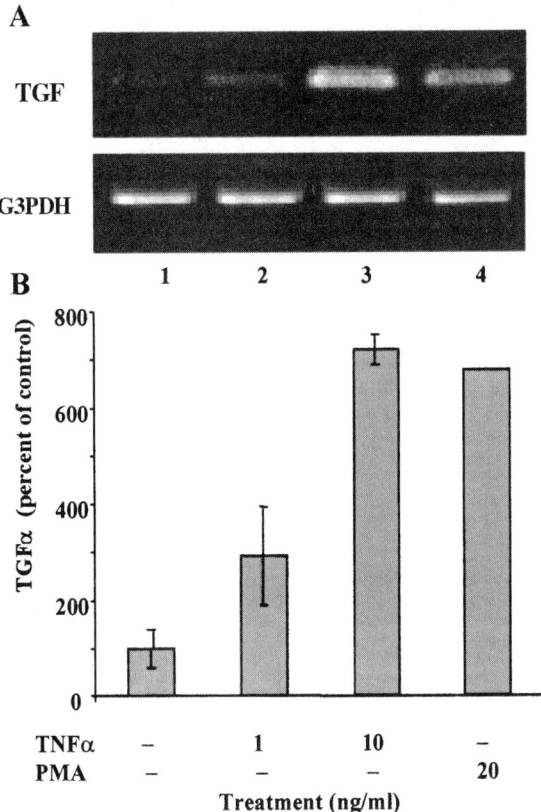

FIGURE 3. TGFα expression in isolated murine hepatocytes. Following a 2-h incubation of mouse hepatocytes with murine recombinant TNFα (R & D Systems, Minneapolis, MN) or PMA, RNA was isolated and RT-PCR performed using mouse commercial TGFα and G3PDH specific primers as described previously.[18] (**A**) Ethidium bromide–stained 1.5% agarose gels representative of three experiments. Lane 1, saline; lane 2, 1 ng/mL TNFα; lane 3, 10 ng/mL TNFα; lane 4, 20 ng/mL TPA. (**B**) Gels were scanned with a digital image analysis system. The PCR products were quantified and data are expressed as a percent of control values ($n = 3$, ±SE).

tor (HGF), transforming growth factor (TGF) α, and epidermal growth factor (EGF).[16] Evidence exists that TNFα may influence the expression of several of these growth factors in certain cell lines such as TGFα in pancreatic cells.[17] To determine whether TNFα could influence the expression of TGFα in the liver, isolated mouse hepatocytes were cultured on a growth factor–depleted extracellular matrix and treated with either TPA, as a positive control, or recombinant murine TNFα for up to 2 h.[18] RT-PCR indicated that a 7-fold increase in TGFα mRNA occurred following treatment with 10 ng/mL of TNFα (FIG. 3). Although TNFα also increased the expression of IL-6 in hepatocytes (data not shown) and IL-6 has been implicated as a hepatocyte mitogen,[19] studies using IL-6 antagonists, recombinant IL-6, or protein inhibitors clearly demonstrated that TNFα directly stimulates TGFα induction and is independent of IL-6.[18] These studies have subsequently been confirmed *in vivo* following injections of TNFα or CCl_4 in mice where increased hepatic TGFα expression was observed. As TNFα is mitogenic for hepatocytes *in vitro*,[14] we determined whether its mitogenic activity is ultimately due to TGFα by stimulating hepatocytes with TNFα in the presence of antibodies to TGFα and monitoring ^{3}H-TdR incorporation.[18] The addition of neutralizing antibodies to TGFα prevented the increase in DNA synthesis, suggesting that the stimulatory effect of TNFα is due primarily to its ability to stimulate TGFα.

To help discern the factors that determine whether TNFα will participate in a proliferative or inflammatory process in the liver, TNFα receptor transgenic mice were studied. Like other cytokines, TNFα confers its signals through binding to specific cell surface membrane receptors found on most nucleated cells. Two distinct receptors mediate the biological activities of TNFα, one of molecular mass of 55 kDa (p55, R1) and the other of 75 kDa (p75, R2). R1 is constitutively expressed and historically has been considered the primary mediator for TNFα responses, while R2 is inducible and provides for ligand passing as well as limited responses such as cyto-

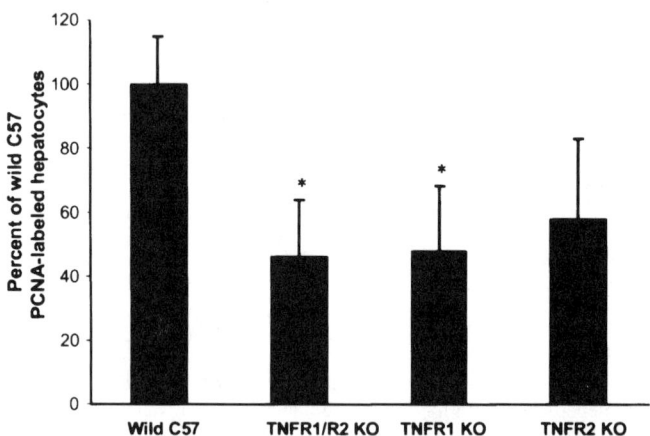

FIGURE 4. Wild-type C57 black mice or TNFα receptor–deficient mice (TNFR1/R2, TNFR1, TNFR2), originally obtained from L. Schook (University of Minnesota), were intraperitoneally injected with CCl_4 as described in the legend to FIGURE 2. After 48 h, the livers were collected, prepared histologically, and stained for PCNA as described previously[13] ($n = 5$, ±SE).

toxicity. In FIGURE 4, the percentages of PCNA positive nuclear stained cells are shown from livers of transgenic mice in which the R1, R2, or R1/R2 genes have been deleted. All mice, including the wild type, were administered 0.1 mL/kg body weight of CCl_4 at 48 h prior to examination. Although the percent of PCNA stained cells was reduced to a slightly greater degree in TNFR1 knockout mice, compared to the TNFR2, both transgenics demonstrated significant effects. A similar pattern emerged when the vigor of the inflammatory response was measured in these knockout mice following chemical exposure (Simeonova *et al.*, in preparation). Taken together, these results indicate that both receptors are involved in the TNFα induction of proliferation and inflammation, although R1 may play a more dominant role.

CONCLUDING REMARKS

In summary, only recently have toxicologists come to understand the role of inflammation, and TNFα specifically, in classical toxicological processes. This relationship appears fairly complex, as inflammation and proliferation may well be only one facet of a time- and dose-dependent continuum of toxicological and repair processes. Not surprisingly, considerable efforts are being undertaken using our newly found understanding of molecular control to develop specific and safe chemical, biological, and molecular regulators of TNFα for potential therapeutic use. Their effectiveness in controlling environmental or occupational diseases has yet to be established.

The gene for TNFα is located within the class III region of the MHC, between HLA-B and DR. Polymorphisms in the promoter region have been described that are associated with both quantitative responses and severity of certain inflammatory diseases. Studies in our laboratory are currently under way to examine the influence of TNFα genetic polymorphisms in populations with environmental diseases such as silicosis and occupational asthma.

REFERENCES

1. LUSTER, M.I. *et al.* 1999. Tumor necrosis factor α and toxicology. Crit. Rev. Toxicol. **29:** 491–511.
2. SCHOOK, L.B. *et al.* 1994. Xenobiotics and inflammation. Academic Press. San Diego.
3. ROTH, R.A. *et al.* 1997. Is exposure to bacterial endotoxin a detriment of susceptibility to intoxication from xenobiotic agents? Toxicol. Appl. Pharmacol. **147:** 300–311.
4. CZAJA, M.J. *et al.* 1994. Lipopolysaccharide-neutralizing antibody reduces hepatocyte injury from acute hepatotoxin administration. Hepatology **21:** 294–302.
5. LASKIN, D.L. *et al.* 1995. Modulation of macrophage functioning abrogates the acute hepatotoxicity of acetaminophen. Hepatology **23:** 1045–1050.
6. KAYAMA, F. *et al.* 1995. Role of tumor necrosis factor-α in cadmium-induced hepatotoxicity. Toxicol. Appl. Pharmacol. **131:** 224–234.
7. IIMURO, Y. *et al.* 1997. Antibodies to tumor necrosis factor attenuate hepatic necrosis and inflammation caused by chronic exposure to ethanol in the rat. Hepatology **26:** 1530–1537.
8. MAIER, W.E. *et al.* 1995. Trimethyltin increases interleukin (IL)–1α, IL-6, and tumor necrosis factor-α mRNA levels in rat hippocampus. J. Neuroimmunol. **59:** 65–75.

9. PIGUET, P.F. *et al.* 1990. Subcutaneous perfusion of tumor necrosis factor induces local proliferation of fibroblasts, capillaries, and epidermal cells, or massive tissue necrosis. Am. J. Pathol. **136:** 103–113.
10. PIGUET, P.F. *et al.* 1990. Requirement of tumor necrosis factor for development of silica-induced pulmonary fibrosis. Nature **344:** 245–247.
11. CORSINI, E. *et al.* 1997. Induction of TNF *in vivo* by a skin irritant, tributyltin, through activation of transcription factors: its pharmacological modulation by anti-inflammatory drugs. J. Invest. Dermatol. **108:** 892–896.
12. BLAZKA, M.E. *et al.* 1995. Role of proinflammatory cytokines in acetaminophen hepatotoxicity. Toxicol. Appl. Pharmacol. **133:** 224–234.
13. BRUCCOLERI, A. *et al.* 1997. Induction of early-immediate genes by tumor necrosis factor contribute to liver repair following chemical-induced hepatotoxicity. Hepatology **25:** 133–141.
14. SATOH, M. *et al.* 1992. Tumor necrosis factor stimulates DNA synthesis of mouse hepatocytes in primary culture and is suppressed by transforming growth factor-β and interleukin-6. Cell. Physiol. **150:** 134–139.
15. AKERMAN, P. *et al.* 1992. Antibodies to tumor necrosis factor-α inhibit liver regeneration after partial hepatectomy. Am. J. Physiol. **263:** G579–G585.
16. MICHALOPOULOS, G.K. *et al.* 1997. Liver regeneration. Science **276:** 60–66.
17. KALTHOFF, H. *et al.* 1993. Tumor necrosis factor (TNF) up-regulates the expression of p75, but not p55 TNF receptors, and both receptors mediate, independently of each other, up-regulation of transforming growth factor alpha and epidermal growth factor receptor mRNA. J. Biol. Chem. **268:** 2762–2766.
18. GALLUCCI, R.M. *et al.* 1999. Tumor necrosis factor-α modulates transforming growth factor-alpha in murine regenerating liver and isolated hepatocytes. J. Immunol. In press.
19. YAMADA, Y. *et al.* 1998. Deficient liver regeneration after carbon tetrachloride injury in mice lacking type 1, but not type 2 tumor necrosis factor receptor. Am. J. Pathol. **152:** 1577–1589.

Aging and Resistance to *Trichinella spiralis* Infection following Xenobiotic Exposure

ROBERT W. LUEBKE,[a] CAREY B. COPELAND, AND DEBORA L. ANDREWS

Immunotoxicology Branch, Experimental Toxicology Division, United States Environmental Protection Agency, Research Triangle Park, North Carolina, USA

ABSTRACT: Aging is accompanied by well-documented physiological changes, including alterations in the immune system that can lead to reduced resistance to a variety of infectious agents. We tested the hypothesis that immunosenescence exacerbates the immunosuppressive effect of xenobiotics. If proven true, a given dose of an immunosuppressive xenobiotic would cause greater suppression of host resistance in an aged population.

INTRODUCTION

Aging is accompanied by well-documented physiological changes, including alterations in the immune system that can lead to reduced resistance to a variety of infectious agents. Because age-related immunosuppression increases the risk of functional immunodeficiency and subsequent disease development, the elderly may constitute an immunologically sensitive subpopulation, just as the very young do. From a public health perspective, regulatory agencies, including the EPA, consider susceptible subpopulations when addressing research needs and when performing risk assessments.[1] However, research efforts to determine the potential interactions between age- and xenobiotic-induced immunotoxicity have been minimal. Increased sensitivity to chemical immunosuppression has been reported in advanced age,[2] whereas others[3] found no interaction.

TCDD is a well-known environmental contaminant that suppresses both humoral and cellular immunity. Antibody production to sheep red blood cells (SRBC) in adult mice is very sensitive to TCDD exposure; the ID_{50} for this response has been calculated to be 0.7 µg TCDD/kg.[4] T cell–mediated immunity is particularly sensitive to *in utero* TCDD exposure,[5,6] although the effects of TCDD exposure on adult T cell immunity are not as clear-cut.[7] Resistance to certain infectious agents, including *Listeria monocytogenes*,[5,8] mouse-adapted influenza virus,[9,10] and malaria,[11] is suppressed in exposed rodents.

In these experiments, we tested the hypothesis that immunosenescence exacerbates the immunosuppressive effect of xenobiotics. If this is correct, then a given dose of an immunosuppressive xenobiotic would cause greater suppression of host resistance in an aged population. To test the hypothesis, animals were exposed to 2,3,7,8-tetrachlorodibenzo-*p*-dioxin (TCDD, dioxin) as a model xenobiotic and then

---

[a]Address for correspondence: Bob Luebke, Ph.D., MD-92, U.S. EPA, Research Triangle Park, NC 27711. Voice: 919-541-3672; fax: 919-541-4284.
luebke.robert@epamail.epa.gov

challenged with *Trichinella spiralis* (Ts), a parasitic nematode of carnivores and omnivores, including humans. Distinct phases of the parasite life cycle engender host-protective responses mediated by T cells or by a combination of T cell–dependent antibodies and accessory cells.[12] Furthermore, either advanced age[13] or TCDD exposure suppresses resistance to Ts infection in adult mice[14] and rats,[15] thus providing an appropriate model to test the hypothesis.

MATERIALS AND METHODS

Female B6C3F1 mice were obtained from Charles River Labs (Portage, MI) at 9 weeks of age and were allowed to acclimate to the animal facility for a minimum of 1 week before use in experiments. Old animals were obtained from the same vendor and housed in our facility until they reached 76 weeks of age. Aged male F344 rats were obtained from an EPA colony maintained by Charles River Labs and arrived at 74–78 weeks of age. Young rats were obtained from the same vendor. Chemical exposure, infection, parasite counts, and lymphocyte proliferation were performed as described previously,[14,15] except that adult parasite counts were done on day 11 of infection. All procedures employed in these studies were reviewed and approved by the Institutional Animal Care and Use Committee before the initiation of experiments.

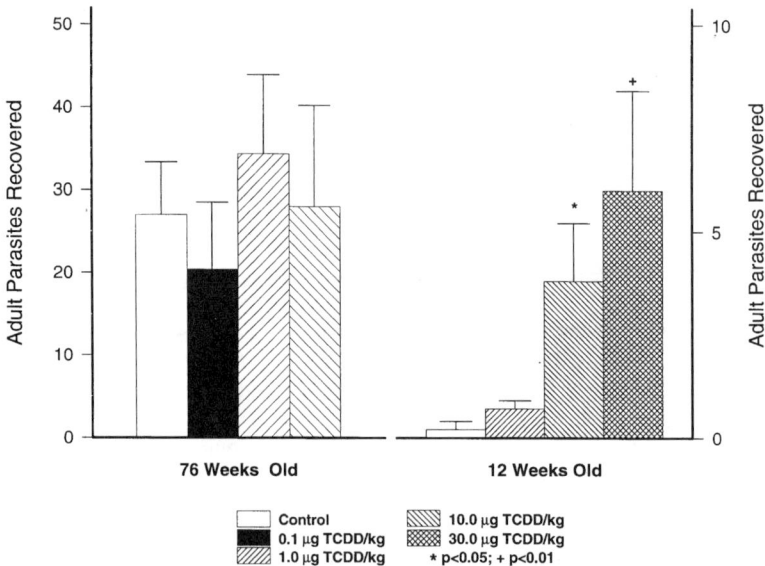

FIGURE 1. Adult parasite counts in mice on day 11 of infection. Aged and young mice were infected with 200 Ts larvae by gavage at 7 days after a single oral exposure to TCDD. Values are the mean ± SEM. (Note different scales for y-axes.) Statistical significance (*p* value) is indicated for comparisons between TCDD-exposed and a vehicle-only control group of the same age.

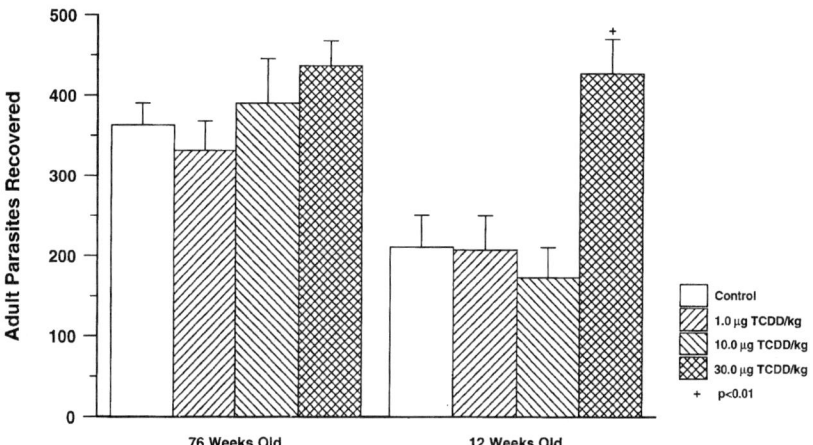

FIGURE 2. Adult parasite counts in rats on day 11 of infection. Rats were infected with 1000 Ts larvae by gavage at 7 days after a single oral exposure to TCDD. Values are the mean ± SEM. Statistical significance (p value) is indicated for comparisons between TCDD-exposed and a vehicle-only control group of the same age.

RESULTS

Effects of Age and TCDD Exposure on Resistance to Infection

As a group, older mice were much less resistant to infection than were young mice; an average of 27 parasites was recovered from aged controls versus 1 parasite recovered from 1 of the 6 young controls (FIG. 1). Exposure to TCDD decreased parasite elimination by young mice at doses of 10 or 30 μg/kg, but did not exacerbate the age-related suppression of parasite elimination in old animals (FIG. 1).

Parasite expulsion by aged rats was not affected by TCDD exposure, in contrast to the decreased elimination observed in young rats exposed to 30 μg TCDD/kg (FIG. 2). The number of larvae/g of muscle was significantly lower in old control rats than in young controls (FIG. 3). Aged rats exposed to either 10 or 30 μg TCDD/kg had significantly more larvae/g of muscle than age-matched controls, whereas in younger rats only the highest dose increased the number of encysted larvae (FIG. 3).

Effects of Age and TCDD Exposure on Parasite-Specific Lymphocyte Proliferation

Proliferative responses to parasite antigen were suppressed in spleen cells of aged and young mice by exposure to ≥1 μg TCDD/kg (FIG. 4). Mesenteric lymph node cell (MLNC) responses to parasite antigen in aged mice were similar, regardless of TCDD dose, whereas doses of 10 or 30 μg TCDD/kg significantly suppressed proliferation by MLNCs of young animals. It is also noteworthy that lymphocyte responses to stimulation with either TsE or mitogen were less vigorous (i.e., 4- to 5-fold less ^{3}H-TdR incorporation) in aged mice than in younger animals.

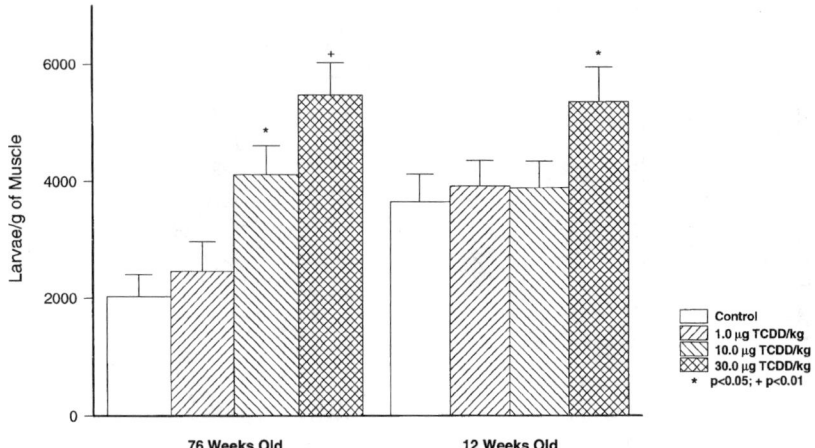

FIGURE 3. Recovery of encysted muscle larvae from rats on day 28 of infection. Rats were infected with 1000 Ts larvae by gavage at 7 days after a single oral exposure to TCDD. Values are the mean ± SEM. Statistical significance (p value) is indicated for comparisons between TCDD-exposed and a vehicle-only control group of the same age. Two-way ANOVA indicated a significantly greater burden of encysted larvae in young, compared to old, controls.

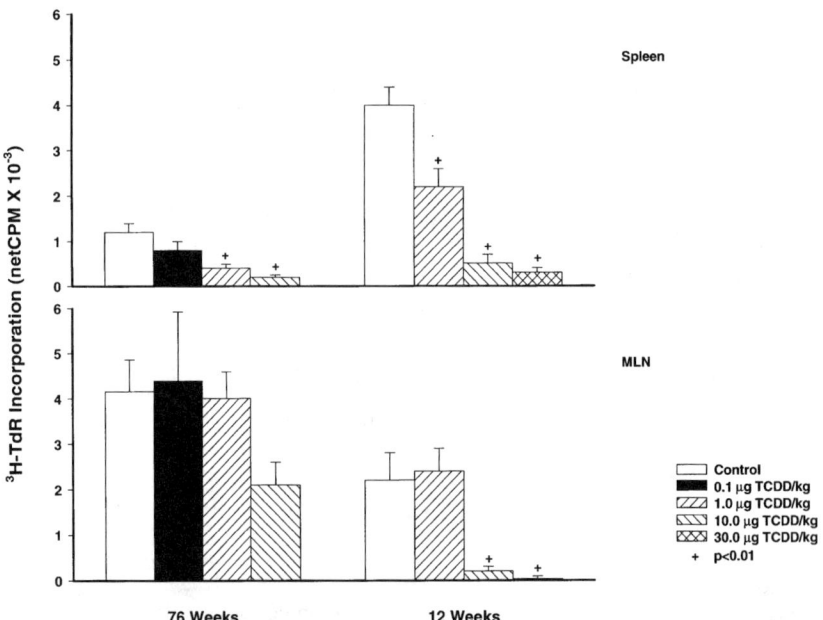

FIGURE 4. Parasite-specific lymphoproliferative responses in aged and young adult mice killed for counts of adult parasites. Values are the mean ± SEM. (Note different scales for x-axes.) Statistical significance (p value) is indicated for comparisons between TCDD-exposed and a vehicle-only control group of the same age.

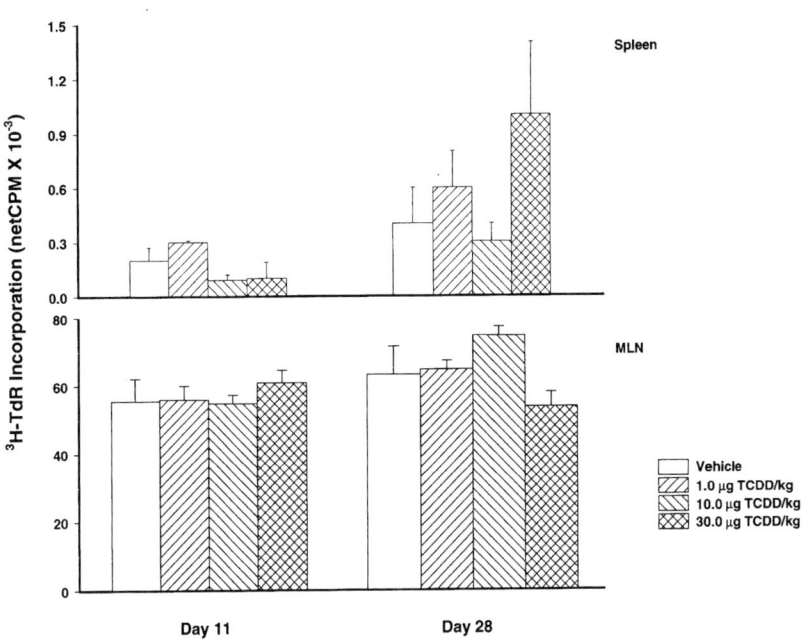

FIGURE 5. Parasite-specific lymphoproliferative responses in aged rats killed for counts of adult parasites (day 11) or encysted muscle larvae (day 28). Values are the mean ± SEM.

In contrast to responses in aged mice, proliferation of aged rat lymphocytes was in the same range that we observed for TCDD-exposed 10-week-old male (unpublished data) and female rats at 7, 14, and 28 days after infection.[15] Aged rat splenocytes made minimal responses to *T. spiralis* antigen at 11 and 28 days after infection, compared to MLNCs, and no exposure-related effects were noted in either cell population (FIG. 5). These data are in contrast to enhanced splenic responses to TsE observed in young male (unpublished results) and female rats at 7 and 14 days after infection.[15]

DISCUSSION

In aged individuals, immune system dysfunction may be the result of altered activity at the level of the cell, changes in the relative proportion of cell types, or the loss of normal homeostatic control.[16] The qualitative and quantitative changes associated with increased age often lead to depressed or inappropriate antibody production in response to infection or immunization,[17] as well as decreased T cell[18] and accessory cell activity. These alterations are often cited as contributing to the greater incidence of infections and cancer in older individuals. Following this line of reasoning, we tested the hypothesis that an age-related decrease in constitutive resistance to Ts infection[13] would exacerbate the suppressive effects of TCDD exposure and therefore decrease resistance to Ts infection at lower dioxin doses in aged rodents.

Contrary to our expectations, TCDD exposure did not exacerbate age-related suppression of parasite expulsion from the intestine of rats and mice. This outcome is not unprecedented, however. Similar results were reported by Vos et al.[19] for rats that were 1 year old at the start of a 5-month exposure to bis(tri-n-butyltin) oxide (TBTO); resistance to Ts infection was suppressed at a lower dose in young adult rats than in the 17-month-old animals. Data from Vos et al.[19] and the current studies suggest that advanced age may actually provide some degree of protection from the effects of xenobiotics on the T cell response to Ts infection since parasite elimination was decreased by both TCDD and TBTO in young rodents at doses that had no effect on resistance in older animals.

Age-related differences in the quantity of TCDD reaching lymphoid target tissues might explain the apparent age-related "protection" from the effects of dioxin exposure in aged animals. However, absorption of TCDD from the intestine is similar in old and young rats.[20] Pegram et al.[21] determined that advanced age did not affect induction of p4501A1 and 1A2 in mice, although age-related changes in body composition did tend to alter the pharmacokinetics and pharmacodynamics of TCDD at 1 week after dosing. Nevertheless, blood levels of TCDD were similar in aged and young animals;[21] therefore, essentially equivalent amounts of TCDD were available for tissue uptake in young and old animals. In a separate study by the same group (J. Diliberto, personal communication), age did not affect the percentage of TCDD dose localizing in the spleen of old and young mice, supporting the concept that age-related differences in the quantity of TCDD reaching lymphoid target tissue do not explain the differences observed between aged and young animals.

In contrast to effects on parasite expulsion, exposure to TCDD increased burdens of muscle larvae in both young and aged rats. The effect of TCDD exposure on muscle burdens of larvae was apparently exacerbated by age in rats since increased larvae burdens were observed at both 10 and 30 μg TCDD/kg in aged rats, but only at the higher dose in young animals. Thus, old rats may control the numbers of encysting larvae better than young rats, but old age makes the resistance process more susceptible to suppression by TCDD exposure. The number of larvae encysted in host muscle is influenced by the residence time of adult parasites in the gut, the fecundity of female parasites, and the number of larvae that survive the migratory phase.[12] Dioxin exposure did not affect parasite expulsion in old rats; thus, increased residence time is not responsible for increased larvae burdens in treated animals. Since parasite-specific antibodies have been shown to damage the reproductive structures of the female parasite,[22] and to sensitize migrating newborn larvae for attack by granulocytes and macrophages,[23–25] suppression of antibody synthesis or bone marrow function could potentially increase the burdens of muscle larvae. TCDD is myelotoxic[26] and has been reported to decrease granulocyte colony formation,[27] effects that could limit required cellular components of resistance. Furthermore, control of female parasite fecundity is suppressed in young rats exposed to TCDD as exposure increases the number of offspring produced per female parasite.[15] The limited number of aged rats available for these studies precluded evaluating parasite fecundity in aged, TCDD-exposed animals, making it impossible to judge whether increased larvae production was solely responsible for increased larvae burdens. Nevertheless, exposure reduced the ability of aged animals to control burdens of encysted larvae, at a dose lower than that required to have the same effect in young animals.

At the cellular level, proliferative responses to parasite antigen by spleen cells from both ages of mice were equally sensitive to TCDD exposure; that is, reductions in thymidine incorporation at the 1 and 10 µg TCDD/kg exposures were similar in young and aged mice on a percent of control basis. Thymidine incorporation following TsE stimulation of cells from aged animals was less than half of that of cells from young animals, although identical numbers of viable spleen cells were cultured, and even larger differences in label incorporation between aged and young cells stimulated with Con A (data not shown) were observed. These results suggest that, in aged mice, either a smaller proportion of spleen cells are capable of responding to specific and nonspecific stimulation or the magnitude of the per cell response is dramatically decreased by aging. Age-related differences in proliferative responses in mice and humans have been reported and attributed to a variety of mechanisms including alterations in signal transduction[28–30] and lipid metabolism.[31] Regardless of the underlying mechanism, it is clear that aging attenuates the response to parasite antigen in mice, but age is not related to the magnitude of suppression induced by a particular dose of TCDD.

In these experiments, both aging and TCDD exposure suppressed aspects of resistance to Ts infection. Older rodents were found to be less susceptible to TCDD-induced suppression of T cell–mediated adult parasite elimination as TCDD exposure had no apparent effect on parasite expulsion. Conversely, the ability to control body burdens of encysted larvae, in which humoral immunity has a significant role, was suppressed at a lower dose of TCDD in aged versus young animals, suggesting that age increased the sensitivity of humoral immunity to TCDD exposure in rats. Thus, the hypothesis that TCDD-mediated suppression of resistance to Ts infection is exacerbated by the effects of aging on immune function can be neither accepted nor rejected for the rat model. In humans, both T cell– and B cell–mediated resistance to infection can be compromised by age;[32] thus, if TCDD has similar effects in aged humans as it does in aged rats, elevated TCDD levels in aged humans may put them at greater risk of infections in which resistance is mediated by antibodies. It remains to be determined whether resistance to other infectious agents is affected similarly in aged, TCDD-exposed animals.

DISCLAIMER

This report has been reviewed by the Environmental Protection Agency's Office of Research and Development and approved for publication. Approval does not signify that the contents necessarily reflect the views of the Agency nor does mention of trade names or commercial products constitute endorsement or recommendation for use.

ACKNOWLEDGMENTS

We thank Wanda Williams and Marie Riddle for excellent technical support, and Ralph Smialowicz, Robert House, and Linda Birnbaum for their comments and suggestions.

REFERENCES

1. U.S. EPA. 1997 (November). Research plan for microbial pathogens and disinfection by-products in drinking water. Office of Research and Development, Office of Water. EPA/600/R-97/122.
2. LYTE, M. & P.H. BICK. 1985. Differential immunotoxic effects of the environmental chemical benzo[α]pyrene in young and aged mice. Mech. Ageing Dev. **30:** 333–341.
3. LUBET, R.A., B.N. LEMAIRE, D. AVERY & R.E. KOURI. 1986. Induction of immunotoxicity by polyhalogenated biphenyls. Arch. Toxicol. **59:** 71–77.
4. SMIALOWICZ, R.J., M.M. RIDDLE, W.C. WILLIAMS & J.J. DILIBERTO. 1994. Effects of 2,3,7,8-tetrachlorodibenzo-p-dioxin (TCDD) on humoral immunity and lymphocyte subpopulations: differences between mice and rats. Toxicol. Appl. Pharmacol. **124:** 248–256.
5. LUSTER, M.I., G.A. BOORMAN, J.H. DEAN, M.W. HARRIS, R.W. LUEBKE, M.L. PADARATHSINGH & J.A. MOORE. 1980. Examination of bone marrow, immunologic parameters, and host susceptibility following pre- and postnatal exposure to 2,3,7,8-tetrachlorodibenzo-p-dioxin (TCDD). Int. J. Immunopharmacol. **2:** 301–310.
6. GEHRS, B.C., M.M. RIDDLE, W.C. WILLIAMS & R.J. SMIALOWICZ. 1997. Alterations in the developing immune system of the F344 rat after perinatal exposure to 2,3,7,8-tetrachlorodibenzo-p-dioxin. II. Effects on the pup and the adult. Toxicology **122:** 229–240.
7. HOLSAPPLE, M.P., N.K. SNYDER, S.C. WOOD & D.L. MORRIS. 1991. A review of 2,3,7,8-tetrachlorodibenzo-p-dioxin-induced changes in immunocompetence: 1991 update. Toxicology **69:** 219–255.
8. HINSDILL, R.D., D.L. COUCH & R.S. SPEIRS. 1980. Immunosuppression in mice induced by dioxin (TCDD) in feed. J. Environ. Pathol. Toxicol. **4:** 401–425.
9. HOUSE, R.V., L.D. LAUER, M.J. MURRAY, P.T. THOMAS, J.P. EHRLICH, G.R. BURLESON & J.H. DEAN. 1990. Examination of immune parameters and host resistance mechanisms in B6C3F1 mice following adult exposure to 2,3,7,8-tetrachlorodibenzo-p-dioxin. J. Toxicol. Environ. Health **31:** 203–215.
10. BURLESON, G.R., H. LEBREC, Y.G. YANG, J.D. IBANES, K.N. PENNINGTON & L.S. BIRNBAUM. 1996. Effect of 2,3,7,8-tetrachlorodibenzo-p-dioxin (TCDD) on influenza virus host resistance in mice. Fundam. Appl. Toxicol. **29:** 40–47.
11. TUCKER, A.N., S.J. VORE & M.I. LUSTER. 1986. Suppression of B cell differentiation by 2,3,7,8-tetrachlorodibenzo-p-dioxin. Mol. Pharmacol. **29:** 372–377.
12. VAN LOVEREN, H., R.W. LUEBKE & J.G. VOS. 1995. Assessment of immunotoxicity with the parasitic infection model *Trichinella spiralis*. *In* Methods in Immunotoxicology. Volume 2, pp. 243–271. Wiley–Liss. New York.
13. CRANDALL, R.B. 1975. Decreased resistance to *Trichinella spiralis* in aged mice. J. Parasitol. **63:** 566–567.
14. LUEBKE, R.W., C.B. COPELAND, J.J. DILIBERTO, P.I. AKUBUE, D.L. ANDREWS, M.M. RIDDLE, W.C. WILLIAMS & L.S. BIRNBAUM. 1994. Assessment of host resistance to *Trichinella spiralis* in mice following pre-infection exposure to 2,3,7,8-TCDD. Toxicol. Appl. Pharmacol. **125:** 7–16.
15. LUEBKE, R.W., C.B. COPELAND & D.L. ANDREWS. 1995. Host resistance to *T. spiralis* infection in rats exposed to 2,3,7,8-tetrachlorodibenzo-p-dioxin. Fundam. Appl. Toxicol. **24:** 285–289.
16. EFFROS, R.B. 1993. Immunosenescence-related diseases in the elderly. Immunol. Allergy Clin. North Am. **13:** 695–712.
17. RICHMOND, G.W. & H.J. ZEITZ. 1993. B-cell and immunoglobulin immunodeficiency in the elderly. Immunol. Allergy Clin. North Am. **13:** 517–533.
18. MILLER, R.A., 1994. Aging and immune function: cellular and biochemical analyses. Exp. Gerontol. **29:** 21–35.
19. VOS, J.G., A. DE KLERK, E.I. KRAJNC, W. KRUIZINGA, H. VAN LOVEREN & J. ROZING. 1990. Immunotoxicity of bis(tri-n-butyltin)oxide in the rat: effects on thymus-dependent immunity and on nonspecific resistance following long-term exposure in young versus aged rats. Toxicol. Appl. Pharmacol. **105:** 144–155.

20. HERBERT, C.D. & L.S. BIRNBAUM. 1987. The influence of aging on intestinal absorption of TCDD in rats. Toxicol. Lett. **37:** 47–55.
21. PEGRAM, R.A., J.J. DILIBERTO, T.C. MOORE, P. GAO & L.S. BIRNBAUM. 1995. 2,3,7,8-Tetrachlorodibenzo-p-dioxin (TCDD) distribution and cytochrome P4501A induction in young adult and senescent male mice. Toxicol. Lett. **76:** 119–126.
22. LOVE, R.J., B.M. OGILVIE & D.J. MCLAREN. 1976. The immune mechanism which expels the intestinal stage of *Trichinella spiralis* from rats. Immunology **30:** 7–15.
23. KAZURA, J.W. & M. AIKAWA. 1980. Host defense mechanisms against *Trichinella spiralis* infection in the mouse: eosinophil-mediated destruction of newborn larvae *in vitro*. J. Immunol. **124:** 355–361.
24. RUITENBERG, E.J., J. BUYS, J.S. TEPPEMA & A. ELGERSMA. 1983. Rat mononuclear cells and neutrophils are more efficient than eosinophils in antibody-mediated stage-specific killing of *Trichinella spiralis in vitro*. Z. Parasitenkd. **69:** 807–815.
25. BUYS, J., R. WEVER & E.J. RUITENBERG. 1984. Myeloperoxidase is more efficient than eosinophil peroxidase in the *in vitro* killing of newborn larvae of *Trichinella spiralis*. Immunology **51:** 601–607.
26. LUSTER, M.I., L.H. HONG, G.A. BOORMAN, G. CLARK, H.T. HAYES, W.F. GREENLEE, K. DOLD & A.N. TUCKER. 1985. Acute myelotoxic responses in mice exposed to 2,3,7,8-tetrachlorodibenzo-p-dioxin (TCDD). Toxicol. Appl. Pharmacol. **81:** 156–165.
27. ACKERMANN, M.F., T.A. GASIEWICZ, K.R. LAMM, D.R. GERMOLEC & M.I. LUSTER. 1989. Selective inhibition of polymorphonuclear neutrophil activity by 2,3,7,8-tetrachlorodibenzo-p-dioxin. Toxicol. Appl. Pharmacol. **101:** 470–480.
28. PROUST, J.J., C.R. FILBURN, S.A. GARRUSIB, M.A. BUCHHOLZ & A.A. NORDIN. 1987. Age-related defect in signal transduction during lectin activation of murine T lymphocytes. J. Immunol. **139:** 1472–1478.
29. UTSUYAMA, M., Z. VARGA, K. FUKAMI, Y. HOMA, T. TAKENAWA & K. HIROKAWA. 1993. Influence of age on the signal transduction of T cells in mice. Int. Immunol. **5:** 1177–1182.
30. FÜLÖP, T. 1994. Signal transduction changes in granulocytes and lymphocytes with ageing. Immunol. Lett. **40:** 259–268.
31. STULING, T.M., E. BÜHLER, G. BÖCK, C. KIRCHEBNER, D. SCHÖNITZER & G. WICK. 1995. Altered switch in lipid composition during T cell blast transformation in the healthy elderly. J. Gerontol. **50A:** B383–B390.
32. BEN-YEHUDA, A. & M.E. WEKSLER. 1992. Host resistance and the immune system. Infect. Dis. **8:** 701–711.

Animal Models to Assess the Effects of Air Pollutants on Allergic Lung Disease

MARYJANE K. SELGRADE,[a,b] AMY L. LAMBERT,[c] MARSHA D. W. WARD,[a] AND M. IAN GILMOUR[a]

[a]National Health and Environmental Effects Research Laboratory, United States Environmental Protection Agency, Research Triangle Park, North Carolina, USA

[c]Curriculum in Toxicology, University of North Carolina, Chapel Hill, North Carolina, USA

ABSTRACT: Animal models provide toxicologists with useful tools for assessing risks associated with respiratory allergy. Both the mouse and BN rat models described exhibit many of the features of human allergic asthma. It is clear that environmental contaminants can exacerbate the expression of these features. Work is under way to explore underlying mechanisms and to develop methods for applying these data to human health risk assessment.

ALLERGY AND ASTHMA: ISSUES FOR IMMUNOTOXICOLOGY

The incidence of respiratory allergies and asthma has increased worldwide (especially in Western societies) over the past 20 years. About 75% of asthmatics are atopic and have respiratory allergies that may act as stimuli for asthma attacks.[1] Allergic asthma will be the focus of this paper. The prevalence of asthma in the United States has increased linearly from about 3% in 1980 to 5.5% in 1994, an increase of 83%. It is estimated that there are now about 13 million people in this country with allergic asthma.[2] The incidence of asthma has increased among all age groups; however, the greatest increases have occurred in young children, where the disease is almost always associated with allergy. Since the early 1980s, the prevalence of asthma among children 0–4 years has increased by 160% and among children 5–14 years by 74%. These statistics make it clear that asthma will be a significant public health concern in the next millennium.

It is uncertain to what extent increased asthma prevalence reflects improved diagnosis of the disease versus an actual increase in the number of sensitized individuals as a result of some change(s) in the environment and/or lifestyle. Genetic predisposition is clearly a risk factor for asthma; however, it is unlikely that changes in the gene pool account for the rapid increase in asthma prevalence. Changes in air quality, both indoors and outdoors, may be one of the factors contributing to the increased incidence of asthma. This increase coincides with efforts to make buildings more airtight in the interest of energy conservation, resulting in increased exposure to indoor air pollutants, both chemical and biologic.[3] Dust mite and molds are com-

[b]Address for correspondence: Dr. MaryJane Selgrade, MD-92, U.S. Environmental Protection Agency, Research Triangle Park, NC 27711. Voice: 919-541-1821; fax: 919-541-4284.
Selgrade.MaryJane@EPA.Gov

mon indoor air contaminants, which contain allergens frequently associated with asthma. Asthma is most prevalent in urban areas,[4,5] where air pollution is highest. It is well documented that hospital visits for asthma increase following episodes of high air pollution.[6,7] Exposure to sulfur dioxide causes bronchoconstriction and asthma-like symptoms,[8] nitrogen dioxide from wood stoves has been associated with increased asthma morbidity,[9] and ozone exposure elicits bronchial reactivity and pulmonary inflammation in asthmatics.[10] In animal models, O_3, NO_2, SO_2, residual oil fly ash (ROFA), and diesel exhaust have all been shown to exacerbate pulmonary allergic responses.[11–15] Conversely, a study of the incidence of asthma in East and West Germany shortly after reunification did not support the hypothesis that asthma is more prevalent in areas of high air pollution.[16] It is clear that one of the challenges for toxicologists in the next millennium will be to determine the extent to which air pollutants contribute to morbidity and mortality associated with allergic asthma.

Proteins and certain low-molecular-weight (<3000) compounds have the potential to cause allergic sensitization. Here, we will focus on protein allergens in our environment. These allergens come from a number of sources, including dust mite, cockroach, animal dander, plants, and a variety of microbes. Adverse effects of hypersensitivity (allergy) develop in two stages: (1) induction (sensitization) requires a sufficient or cumulative exposure dose of the sensitizing agent to induce immune responses that cause no obvious symptoms; (2) elicitation occurs in sensitized individuals upon subsequent exposure to the allergen (immunogen) and results in adverse, antigen-specific responses that include inflammation and reduced lung function. The dose of allergen required to achieve sensitization is generally higher than that required to elicit a response in a previously sensitized individual. Air pollutants may be involved in allergic reactions in the lung either directly as the allergen or indirectly by enhancing allergic sensitization (induction) to common allergens and/or by exacerbating the symptoms that are associated with subsequent exposure (elicitation).

With respect to allergy and asthma, toxicologists are faced with several issues. All proteins are not allergenic. However, no characteristic amino acid sequences specific for allergenicity have been identified thus far. Hence, one of the challenges to toxicologists in the new millennium is to develop test methods to readily assess the potential allergenicity and rank the relative potency of various contaminants in our environment. Toxicologists also need the tools to determine whether (and under what conditions) other environmental contaminants, particularly air pollutants, can act as adjuvants to enhance allergic sensitization, thus contributing potentially to the development of allergic respiratory diseases such as asthma. In addition, there is a need to determine whether these pollutants exacerbate the symptoms of allergic disease in previously sensitized individuals.

We have developed two animal models of allergic lung disease that are useful in addressing these issues. The Brown Norway (BN) rat model of house dust mite (HDM) allergy has been used primarily to assess the effects of air pollutants on allergic sensitization.[12,13,17] We have used the BALB/c mouse model and the microbial pesticide, *Metarhizium anisopliae*, as a prototype to develop methods to assess environmental contaminants for allergenic potential.[18,19] Either model could be adapted to address the other issue. Presented below are the essential features of the models, as well as examples of model applications.

TABLE 1. Endpoints characteristic of allergic asthma assessed in animal models

- Immediate responses
    Antigen-induced bronchoconstriction
    IgE (serum and BALF)
    IL-4, IL-10
- General
    Lymphocyte proliferation
    Protein and LDH in BALF
- Late phase
    Hyperresponsiveness to nonspecific stimuli (methacholine)
    Eosinophilic inflammation
    IL-5, IL-6, IL-13, TNFα

CHARACTERISTICS OF ALLERGIC ASTHMA PROVIDE THE BASIS FOR ENDPOINTS ASSESSED IN ANIMAL MODELS

Endpoints that are characteristic of allergic asthma were assessed in both animal models (TABLE 1). A major determinant in occupationally and environmentally induced respiratory diseases is immediate (type I) bronchial hypersensitivity to specific allergens, often referred to as atopy.[1] Atopy is the presence of cytotropic, antigen-specific immunoglobulin (Ig) E. In sensitized asthmatic individuals, antigen challenge causes an immediate hypersensitivity response by cross-linking of IgE molecules on mast cells and subsequent release of mediators responsible for bronchoconstriction.[20,21] Therefore, in our rodent models, we assess IgE levels (total and antigen-specific) in both serum and bronchoalveolar lavage fluid (BALF) using an enzyme-linked immunoabsorbent assay (ELISA). Interleukin-4 (IL-4), a cytokine important in B cell class switching from IgM to IgE,[22] is also measured in mouse BALF by ELISA. We have not been able to detect IL-4 in our rat model, but have found that IL-10 appears in BALF soon after sensitization and may, in rats, play a role in the immediate response. Others have made similar observations.[23,24] In rats, we are also able to measure immediate bronchoconstriction responses to HDM using a whole body plethysmograph (Buxco Electronic, Troy, NY). Using this rat model, we adoptively transferred serum or lymphocytes from HDM-sensitized rats to naive rats. Three days after, the transfer recipients were challenged with HDM. Immediate bronchoconstriction responses were observed in rats that received serum, but not in those that received cells, thereby suggesting that the immediate response in this model is antibody-mediated.[25]

Between 2 and 8 hours after the immediate response, asthmatics experience a more severe and prolonged (late phase) reaction that is characterized by mucus hypersecretion, bronchoconstriction, airway hyperresponsiveness to a variety of nonspecific stimuli (e.g., histamine, methacholine), and airway inflammation characterized by eosinophils.[26] The number of lymphocytes in the airway is also increased. Late phase responses may last up to 12 hours and do not appear to be mediated by IgE. The mechanisms for the late phase response are not fully understood. However, Th2 lymphocytes and associated cytokines (particularly IL-5 and

IL-13), as well as eosinophils, are thought to play a significant role.[27,28] In order to detect late phase responses in our models, we assess eosinophils, IL-5, and inflammatory cytokines IL-6 and TNFα (by ELISA) in BALF, IL-5 mRNA expression in lung tissue, and more recently IL-13 mRNA. Finally, we assess bronchial hyperresponsiveness to a nonspecific agonist (e.g., acetylcholine). In the adoptive transfer studies mentioned above, naive rats that received lymphocytes experienced immune-mediated inflammatory responses characterized by eosinophils and increased hyperresponsiveness to acetylcholine at 2–3 days after HDM challenge. Those that received serum did not display these responses, suggesting that the late phase response in this model is cell-mediated.

Because both the immediate and late phase responses depend on activation of lymphocytes, we test for antigen-specific lymphocyte proliferation by removing lung-associated lymph nodes, culturing cells with HDM antigen, and measuring [^{3}H]-thymidine incorporation. Finally, we assess BALF for protein and lactate dehydrogenase, indicators of pulmonary edema and cell damage, respectively, using assays adapted for automated analysis by a Cobas Fara II centrifugal spectrophotometer.

EFFECTS OF RESIDUAL OIL FLY ASH (ROFA) ON DUST MITE SENSITIZATION

In order to assess the effects of ROFA on HDM sensitization,[13] BN rats were instilled intratracheally (IT) with saline or 200 or 1000 μg ROFA (suspended in saline) that had been collected on Teflon-coated glass fiber filters downstream of the cyclone of a power plant burning low sulfur number 6 residual oil. Three and 5 days later, rats were sensitized with 10 μg HDM IT. Two weeks after the second sensitization, rats were challenged IT with 10 μg HDM. Endpoints were examined at 2, 7, and 14 days after sensitization and at 2 and 7 days after challenge. Data are summarized in TABLE 2. In rats treated with 1000 μg ROFA, IgE levels were increased just prior to and 2 and 7 days after challenge. IL-10 levels in BALF were increased 2 days postsensitization. Immediate bronchoconstriction assessed at the time of challenge in a separate group of animals was significantly enhanced in those that had been pretreated with ROFA. The data indicate that both the immunologic and physiologic responses associated with the immediate response were enhanced in rats treated prior to sensitization with ROFA. Eosinophil numbers in BALF were also increased after challenge, suggesting that late phase responses were enhanced as well. Lymphocyte proliferation was enhanced at 7 days after sensitization and again at 7 days after challenge, indicating enhanced immune responses to dust mite in ROFA-exposed animals. In rats treated with 200 μg ROFA, significant increases were observed for IL-10 levels at 2 days postsensitization and for lymphocyte proliferation at 7 days postsensitization, and specific IgE increased at 7 days postchallenge. For all other endpoints and times, there were no significant differences between the 200 μg ROFA group and saline controls.

In a later study[17] using a similar design, additional cytokine responses were assessed at 16 days postsensitization (2 days postchallenge). IL-10 was not present in BALF at this time point; however, the inflammatory cytokines IL-6 and TNFα were

TABLE 2. Effects of 1000 μg residual oil fly ash on HDM sensitization

	Days Postsensitization				
	2	7	14 (c)	16	21
Lymphocyte proliferation	=	+	=	=	+
HDM-specific IgE	=	=	+	+	+
BALF IL-10	+	ND	ND	ND	ND
Eosinophils in BALF	+	=	=	+	+
BALF protein	+	+	=	=	=
BALF LDH	+	=	=	+	=

NOTE: Rats were treated with ROFA or saline; all were sensitized with HDM at 3 and 5 days later and challenged with HDM at 14 days after the last sensitization. Days indicate the time after the last sensitization; hence, 16 and 21 days are 2 and 7 days after challenge (c). Terms: =, not significantly different from saline control; +, significantly increased over saline control; ND, not done.

TABLE 3. Summary of residual oil fly ash effects on cytokines

	mRNA	Protein in BALF
2 days postsensitization 1000 & 200 μg ROFA	ND	IL-10 ↑
16 days postsensitization (2 days postchallenge) 1000 μg ROFA	IL-5 ↑ IL-13 =	IL-6 ↑ IL-10 (none) TNFα ↑

NOTE: Rats were treated with ROFA or saline; all were sensitized with HDM at 3 and 5 days later and challenged with HDM at 14 days after the last sensitization. Terms: =, not significantly different from saline control; ↑, significantly increased over saline control; ND, not done.

both present and significantly higher in rats treated with ROFA (TABLE 3). Expression of IL-5 mRNA was enhanced in lung tissue at this time point, but expression of IL-13 mRNA was not different from the saline control. This same study demonstrated that the metallic constituents (nickel, iron, and vanadium) of ROFA appear to mediate the enhanced sensitization, although different metals enhanced different components of the response (data not shown).

In the example just described, we used the BN rat HDM model to assess the effects of an air pollutant (ROFA) on allergic sensitization and began to determine the dose response. In addition, we explored the underlying mechanisms and determined the active components of the particulate. The model has also been used to assess the effects of NO_2 exposure at the time of HDM sensitization and/or at the time of HMD challenge.[12] Effects of ingestion of the pesticide carbaryl on allergic sensitization have also been examined.[29] The model is well characterized and provides the means to assess the effects of other pollutants on allergic sensitization and/or expression of allergic responses, as well as approaches for studying the underlying mechanisms.

TABLE 4. Responses in mice sensitized with *Metarhizium anisopliae* by local or systemic routes

	Days postchallenge					
	1		3		8	
	IP	IT	IP	IT	IP	IT
Serum IgE	+	=	+	=	+	=
BALF IgE	=	=	=	+	=	+
BALF IL-4	+	++	=	=	=	=
BALF eosinophils	+	++	+	++	+	+
Airway pressure	+	++	+	++	+	+
Compliance	+	+	+	++	+	+
BALF protein	+	+	=	+	=	=
BALF LDH	+	+	=	+	=	=

NOTE: IP, mice were injected IP with MACA and adjuvant, challenged IT at 14 days later, and tested at 1, 3, and 8 days postchallenge; IT, mice received 4 exposures over 2 weeks and were tested at 1, 3, and 8 days after the last exposure; =, not significantly different from saline control; +, significantly increased over saline control; ++, significantly increased over saline control and greater than IP group.

ASSESSING THE ALLERGENICITY OF *METARHIZIUM ANISOPLIAE*

M. anisopliae is one of a number of microorganisms used as pesticides. Because these organisms are known to be nontoxic and nonpathogenic for humans, they are considered desirable alternatives to chemical pesticides. However, little is known about the allergenicity of these agents. Because some microbial products are known allergens, there is a need to develop test methods to screen such agents for the potential to induce respiratory hypersensitivity. Use of *M. anisopliae* against cockroaches results in its introduction into the indoor environment. Unlike the HDM model, specific antigens have not been identified. Thus, we created a crude antigen from the extracts of both mycelia and spores and the filtrate from fungal cultures grown under conditions known to favor the induction of enzymes (proteases and chitinases) needed to penetrate the cockroach exoskeleton. In order to deal with microbial pesticides, methods are needed to determine the potential of the organisms to induce respiratory allergy, to determine the potency relative to other known allergens, and to identify the components of the organism that act as allergens.

Initially, we sensitized mice with a single intraperitoneal (IP) inoculation of *M. anisopliae* crude antigen (MACA) in 1.3% alhydrogel (aluminum hydroxide adjuvant).[18] Mice were challenged 2 weeks later IT with MACA in saline, and endpoints were assessed before and 1, 3, and 7 days after challenge. Although this systemic sensitization with alhydrogel is not a "natural" route of exposure, this initial approach was designed to determine whether the organisms had any potential to induce respiratory allergy and to generate enough antibody to begin to identify which of the protein components induced IgE. Significant IgE and eosinophil responses were observed, and a midrange sensitization dose of 25 μg MACA and a challenge dose of 10 μg MACA were selected for future studies. In a subsequent study,[19] significant hyperresponsiveness to methacholine was observed in MACA-sensitized mice. Hence, responses typical of both immediate and late phase reactions were observed. Using serum from these studies, we have begun to identify the allergenic components in MACA and believe there may be up to 4 proteins (representing about 7% of the MACA proteins) that elicit IgE responses (unpublished data).

Most recently,[30] we have compared the IP (systemic sensitization) protocol with a local sensitization protocol in which mice received 4 IT treatments with 10 μg MACA over a 4-week period and were assessed for responses at 1, 3, and 8 days after the last exposure. Systemically sensitized mice were assessed at the same time points after IT challenge. Results from this study are summarized in TABLE 4. Higher total serum IgE levels were observed in the systemically sensitized mice; however, the local lung effects, including BALF IgE, IL-4, and eosinophils, as well as increases in airway pressure and decreases in compliance (indicators of airway hyperresponsiveness) in methacholine-challenged mice were greater following local sensitization. Because we do not know the actual antigen involved, we have not assessed MACA-specific IgE, which may provide a better indicator of sensitization. We also have not assessed antigen-specific lymphocyte proliferation with the crude antigen preparation. The present data suggest that it would be prudent to monitor more than one endpoint when assessing the potential allergenicity and relative potency of an organism. IgE alone may not be sufficient.

The mouse model is currently limited by our inability to assess immediate hyperresponsiveness following antigen challenge. An advantage to the mouse model is the availability of antibodies to a large number of mouse cytokines such that the model may be readily expanded to assess relevant cytokines as the need arises. Once the relevant antigens are identified, it should be possible to develop dose response and relative potency information needed to facilitate risk assessment.

The approach that we used here was designed to assess potential allergenicity in a microbial extract of unknown potency. Our particular application involved assessing the safety of microbial pesticides. However, a number of molds contaminate indoor environments for a variety of reasons and there is growing concern that some of these may represent health hazards. When trying to determine whether molds present in any particular indoor environment pose a risk as respiratory allergens, the issues are similar to those posed by *M. anisopliae*. Thus, the approach described here has applicability beyond microbial pesticides.

SUMMARY

In summary, animal models provide toxicologists with useful tools for assessing risks associated with respiratory allergy. Both the mouse and BN rat models described here exhibit many of the features of human allergic asthma. It is clear that environmental contaminants can exacerbate the expression of these features. Work is under way to explore underlying mechanisms and to develop methods for applying these data to human health risk assessment.[31]

DISCLAIMER

This paper has been reviewed by the National Health and Environmental Effects Research Laboratory, U.S. Environmental Protection Agency, and approved for publication. Approval does not signify that the contents necessarily reflect the views and policies of the Agency, nor does mention of trade names or commercial products constitute endorsement or recommendation for use.

REFERENCES

1. BOCHNER, B.S., B.J. UNDEM & L.M. LICHTENSTEIN. 1994. Immunological aspects of allergic asthma. Annu. Rev. Immunol. **12:** 295–335.
2. MANNINO, D.M., D.M. HOMA, C.A. PERTIOWSHI, A. ASHIZAWA, L.L. NIXON, C.A. JOHNSON, L.B. BALL, E. JACK & D.S. KANG. 1998. Surveillance for asthma—United States, 1960–1995. Morb. Mortal. Wkly. Rep. **47:** 1–27.
3. PLATTS-MILLS, T.A. 1994. How environment affects patients with allergic disease: indoor allergens and asthma. Ann. Allergy **72:** 381–384.
4. WEISS, K.B., P.J. GERGEN & E.F. CRAIN. 1992. Inner-city asthma. Chest **101:** 363S–367S.
5. EVANS, R., III. 1992. Asthma among minority children. Chest **101:** 368S–371S.
6. SCHWARTZ, J., D. SLATER, T.V. LARSON, W.E. PIERSON & J.Q. KOENIG. 1993. Particulate air pollution and hospital emergency room visits for asthma in Seattle. Am. Rev. Respir. Dis. **147:** 826–831.
7. LIPSETT, M., S. HURLEY & B. OSTRO. 1997. Air pollution and emergency room visits for asthma in Santa Clara County, California. Environ. Health Perspect. **105:** 216–222.
8. BALMES, J.R., J.M. FINE & D. SHEPPARD. 1987. Symptomatic bronchoconstriction after short-term inhalation of sulfur dioxide. Am. Rev. Respir. Dis. **136:** 1117–1121.
9. OSTRO, B.D., M.J. LIPSETT, J.K. MANN, M.B. WIENER & J. SELNER. 1994. Indoor air pollution and asthma: results from a panel study. Am. J. Respir. Crit. Care Med. **149:** 1400–1406.
10. KREIT, J.W., K.B. GROSS, T.B. MOORE, T.J. LORENZEN, J. D'ARCY & W.L. ESCHENBACHER. 1989. Ozone-induced changes in pulmonary function and bronchial responsiveness in asthmatics. J. Appl. Physiol. **66:** 217–222.
11. MATSAMURA, Y. 1970. The effects of ozone, nitrogen dioxide, and sulfur dioxide on the experimentally induced allergic respiratory disorder in guinea pigs. Am. Rev. Respir. Dis. **102:** 430–443.
12. GILMOUR, M.I., P. PARK & M.J.K. SELGRADE. 1996. Increased immune and inflammatory responses to dust mite antigen in rats exposed to 5 ppm NO_2. Fundam. Appl. Toxicol. **31:** 65–70.
13. LAMBERT, A.L., W. DONG, D.W. WINSETT, M.J.K. SELGRADE & M.I. GILMOUR. 1999. Residual oil fly ash exposure enhances allergic sensitization to house dust mite. Toxicol. Appl. Pharmacol. **158:** 269–277.
14. MIYABARA, Y., H. TAKANO, T. ICHINOSE, H-B. LIM & M. SAGAI. 1998. Diesel exhaust enhances allergic airway inflammation and hyperresponsiveness in mice. Am. J. Respir. Crit. Care Med. **157:** 1138–1144.
15. TAKANO, H., T. YOSHIKAWA, T. ICHINOSE, Y. MIYABARA, K. IMAOKA & M. SAGAI. 1997. Diesel exhaust particles enhance antigen-induced airway inflammation and local cytokine expression in mice. Am. J. Respir. Crit. Care Med. **156:** 36–42.
16. VON MUTIUS, E., F.D. MARTINEZ, C. FRITZSCH, T. MICOLAI, G. ROELL & H.H. THIEMANN. 1994. Prevalence of asthma and atopy in two areas of West and East Germany. Am. J. Respir. Crit. Care Med. **149:** 358–364.
17. LAMBERT, A.L., W. DONG, M.J.K. SELGRADE & M.I. GILMOUR. 2000. Enhanced allergic sensitization by residual oil fly ash particles is mediated by soluble metal constituents. Toxicol. Appl. Pharmacol. **165:** 84–93.

18. WARD, M.D.W., D.M. SAILSTAD & M.J.K. SELGRADE. 1998. Allergic responses to the biopesticide *Metarhizium anisopliae* in BALB/c mice. Toxicol. Sci. **45:** 195–203.
19. WARD, M.D.W., S.L. MADISON, D.L. ANDREWS, D.M. SAILSTAD, S.H. GAVETT & M.J.K. SELGRADE. 2000. Allergen-triggered airway hyperresponsiveness and lung pathology in mice sensitized with the biopesticide *Metarhizium anisopliae*. Toxicology. In press.
20. GRAMMAR, L.C. & P.A. GREENBERGER. 1992. Diagnosis and classification of asthma. Chest **101:** 393S–395S.
21. PLAUT, M. 1993. Cytokines and modulation of diseases of immediate hypersensitivity. Ann. N.Y. Acad. Sci. **685:** 512–520.
22. KAY, A.B. 1991. T lymphocytes and their products in atopic allergy and asthma. Int. Arch. Allergy Appl. Immunol. **94:** 189–193.
23. MOSMANN, T.R. 1994. Properties and functions of interleukin-10. Adv. Immunol. **56:** 1–26.
24. VAN LOVEREN, H., C. MEREDITH, M.P. SCOTT, M.E.A. VAN DIJK & R.J. VANDERBRIEL. 1999. Effects of *in vivo* exposure to hexachlorobenzene and *Trichinella spiralis* infection on cytokine expression and production by cultured splenocytes from Lewis and Brown Norway rats. Toxicol. Sci. **48:** 5.
25. LAMBERT, A.L., D.W. WINSETT, D.L. COSTA, M.J.K. SELGRADE & M.I. GILMOUR. 1998. Differential transfer of allergic airway responses with serum and lymphocytes from house dust mite sensitized rats. Am. J. Respir. Crit. Care Med. **157:** 1991–1999.
26. LARSEN, G.L. 1985. Hypersensitivity lung disease. Annu. Rev. Immunol. **3:** 59–85.
27. NAKAJIMA, H., I. IWAMOTO, S. TOMOE, R. MAATSUMARA, H. TOMIOKA, K. TAKATSU & S. YOSHIDA. 1992. $CD4^+$ T-lymphocytes and interleukin-5 mediate antigen-induced eosinophil infiltration into the mouse trachea. Am. Rev. Respir. Dis. **146:** 374–377.
28. WILLS-KARP, M., J. LUYIMBAZI, X. XU, B. SCHOFIELD, T. NEBEN, C. KARP & D. DONALDSON. 1998. Interleukin-13: central mediator of allergic asthma. Science **282:** 2258–2260.
29. DONG, D., M.I. GILMOUR, A.L. LAMBERT & M.J.K. SELGRADE. 1998. Enhanced allergic responses to house dust mite by oral exposure to carbaryl in rats. Toxicol. Sci. **44:** 63–69.
30. WARD, M.D.W., S.L. MADISON, D.L. ANDREWS, D.M. SAILSTAD, S.H. GAVETT & M.J.K. SELGRADE. 1999. Comparison of respiratory responses to *Metarhizium anisopliae* following local and systemic sensitization. Toxicology. In press.
31. SELGRADE, M.J.K. 2000. Applying pulmonary immunotoxicity data to risk assessment. *In* Pulmonary Immunotoxicology, pp. 411–432. Kluwer Academic Pub. Norwell, MA.

From Developmental Biology to Developmental Toxicology

RUDI BALLING[a] AND MARTIN HRABÉ DE ANGELIS

Institute of Mammalian Genetics, GSF-Research Center for Environment and Health, 85758 Neuherberg, Germany

ABSTRACT: Progress derived from the human genome project will have tremendous impact on toxicology. Questions concerning genetic susceptibility or resistance to toxic compound exposure and the dissection of the molecular mechanisms involved will be at the forefront of future toxicological research. In recent years, it was recognized that many of the molecular control mechanisms of embryogenesis have been conserved during evolution. The relevance of these observations for toxicology and the application of genetic approaches using mouse mutants as a tool for functional genome analysis are discussed.

INTRODUCTION

It is now 20 years since Christiane Nüsslein-Volhard and Eric Wieschaus published their paper about a large-scale mutagenesis screen in fruit flies.[1] The authors described the isolation of a wide range of *Drosophila* mutants representing at least 15 loci with defects in the segmentation of the insect body pattern. It took less than 10 years to clone the genes responsible for most of these mutants and to develop a conceptual framework of how positional information is specified during insect embryogenesis. The biggest surprise from all of this work was the discovery that similar developmental control genes, with a high degree of DNA sequence conservation, could also be found in other organisms, including mice and humans. We now know that not only the DNA sequence, but also entire regulatory networks are conserved throughout the animal kingdom.

GENETIC APPROACHES TO DEVELOPMENTAL QUESTIONS

Applying a genetic approach to a developmental biology problem turned out to be an incredibly powerful strategy. By first looking for mutants with a specific phenotype and then trying to find the responsible genes, one was not dependent on preconceived ideas of which pathway or molecular mechanism would be involved. Needless to say, this approach resulted in many surprises. Despite their large number, the *Drosophila* mutants could be grouped into a reasonable number of classes based on phenotypic criteria. These included gap, segmentation, segment polarity, and homeotic mutations. Other criteria were based on whether the affected genes act maternally or zygotically, or are transcription factors, secreted factors, ligands, or re-

[a]balling@gsf.de

ceptors.[2] Elegant molecular embryological, cell biological, and biochemical experiments led to the recognition of a few major signal transduction pathways that seem to play a role in almost every process during embryogenesis.[3–5] Segmentation of the insect embryo was thereby used as a first entry point into the general mechanisms of how cells become different from each other, how they proliferate or differentiate, and how they know where to do what and for how long.[6,7] We now know, for example, that the "Sonic hedgehog signaling pathway" not only determines whether the surface of a *Drosophila* cuticle is covered by bristles or not. We also know that this pathway is essential for other aspects of *Drosophila* development, as well as for vertebrate organogenesis, such as eye, kidney, lung, heart, limb, and brain development.[8–11] The famous statement from J. Monod, "what is true for *E. coli* is true for the elephant", turned out to be equally true for developmental biologists 20 years later.

However, it was not only the field of developmental biology that was revolutionized by the recognition of evolutionary conservation as the integrative element in biology. Cancer biologists now have plenty of examples demonstrating that developmental control genes can be synonymous with oncogenes or tumor suppressor genes.[12–17] The same genes that are important for development of an organ are often involved in maintaining integrity and homeostasis of this organ during the entire life of an organism. By studying embryogenesis and organogenesis, we often get important insight into the pathogenesis of diseases in adults. On a molecular basis, this translates into the discovery that genes can play many roles during the life of an organism.[18,19] A gene that is essential for gastrulation might also play a role in blood pressure regulation, memory, or wound repair.

What does this all have to do with toxicology? Toxicologists try to explore which compounds at which concentration and through which mechanisms are toxic to humans and other organisms. Molecular biology has given us the tools to dissect the responses of a cell or an entire organism after exposure to a toxic compound in terms of the molecules involved. Toxicologists will therefore need to study the genes and proteins that are induced, repressed, or modified after toxic exposure. Developmental biology provides us with the concepts of how these genes are connected with each other and what their functional significance might be during the development of an organism. Signal transduction pathways recognized by toxicologists as responses after toxic exposure turn out to be the same as those that developmental biologists have identified as regulators of embryonic processes.[20] Recognizing these similarities helps tremendously in the interpretation not only of the molecular data, but also of associated pathophysiological phenotypes. The relevance of developmental biology is particularly obvious in the field of teratology. It is known for quite some time that certain drugs or chemicals can induce phenocopies of congenital developmental defects. Drugs or toxic compound exposure can lead to the same phenotype as the effect of a mutation in a specific developmental control gene.

One of the most convincing examples of the convergence of developmental biology and teratology is the pathogenesis of retinoic acid embryopathy. Retinoic acid has been identified as a teratogen in the 1980s.[21] However, the molecular basis of how retinoic acid exerts its effects (i.e., when taken by pregnant women for the treatment of acne) remained unknown. Two independent observations solved this question. One of these was the discovery by the group of Eduardo Boncinelli that adding retinoic acid to human embryonic carcinoma cells cultured *in vitro* led to the induction of the expression of Hox genes.[22,23] Which of the 38 Hox genes were turned on depended on the position within one of the four chromosomal Hox gene clusters. Genes located more 5′ in a cluster were turned on later than those located more 3′. The second important observation involved the production of transgenic mice that overexpressed the homeobox gene Hox 1.1, now called Hox A7.[24,25] Ectopic expression through a ubiquitous chicken β-actin promoter resulted in a phenotype that was very reminiscent to that seen in retinoic acid embryopathy. It turned out that the application of retinoic acid during embryogenesis led to ectopic expression of Hox genes and thereby resulted in the same phenotype as when Hox genes were expressed at the wrong time or in the wrong place. The fields of developmental biology and teratology thus met at the level of gene regulation and gene deregulation.

In the meantime, we know of many more examples in which developmental pathways turn out to be the target of a teratogen. *Shh* mutations cause holoprosencephaly in humans[26] and so does exposure to cholesterol inhibitors.[27,28] Homeotic mutations are induced in mice after exposure to valproic acid, which is a commonly used anticonvulsant.[29] A very similar phenotype can be observed in mice with loss-of-function mutations in Hox genes or retinoic acid receptor genes.[30,31] One of the exciting challenges for the future is the question of how mutations in human genes, which alone do not lead to developmental defects, might lead to an increased risk of toxicological or teratological side effects when these carriers are exposed to toxicological compounds. The field of toxicogenetics and toxicogenomics will move into the center stage of tomorrow's toxicology research. This, of course, triggers the question of whether the genetic tools that were so successful for developmental biology could also be applied to the field of toxicology.

PHENOTYPE-DRIVEN VERSUS GENOTYPE-DRIVEN MUTAGENESIS

As described earlier, one of the most successful strategies for dissecting the mechanisms of embryogenesis in *Drosophila* was the use of large-scale mutagenesis screens. Thousands of *Drosophila* embryos derived from mutagenized flies were scored for abnormal segmentation phenotypes.[1] Recently, this kind of large-scale phenotype-driven mutagenesis has also been applied to mice.[32–35] The mouse has developed into the most important model organism to investigate the genetics and pathogenesis of human disease.[36] Mice are 2000- to 3000-fold lighter than humans. Their generation time is 10 weeks and, with a litter size of 5–10, there is no other mammal that can be kept and studied as cost-efficiently as the mouse. Mouse embryonic stem cell technology and homologous recombination have opened the possibility to produce mutants for any gene that is cloned. In a few years, the entire human and mouse genome will be sequenced, making this approach even more powerful and efficient.

The majority of mutants that are produced by gene targeting will be insertional mutations that interrupt gene function. In most cases, these mutations will be null alleles. Complementary to such a gene-driven approach is a phenotype-driven approach, in which a gene is inactivated and then the resulting mice are analyzed for the phenotypic consequences. Mutants are produced by chemical mutagenesis or other means and mice with a desired phenotype are isolated from a large number of mutagenized animals. In these phenotype-oriented screens, there is no need to have any knowledge about the underlying genes or molecular mechanisms. Once a mutant has been found, genomic strategies, such as candidate or positional cloning, will allow the identification of the genes underlying the phenotype of interest. While this can take some time, the researcher starts from a phenotype in which he has a strong interest. Gene knockouts often do not result in a detectable phenotype or give rise to phenotypes that lie outside the expertise of the researcher. Furthermore, many abnormalities of knockout mice are missed due to inappropriate phenotypic characterization of the mutants. Having access to a large collection of mutant mice with specific inherited abnormalities would be an enormous tool not only as a model to study the pathogenesis of human diseases, but also for the analysis of basic biological mechanisms.

ENU MUTAGENESIS

One of the strategies to produce a large number of mouse mutants is the use of chemical mutagenesis. ENU is an alkylating reagent and currently the most powerful mutagen in mice.[37] ENU induces mainly A-T substitutions and, if given at the most efficient dose, a mutation frequency of more than 1 in 1000 can be achieved.[18,38–40] Male mice are injected with ENU and then mated to normal wild-type females. The first generation of offspring, the F1 animals, are then analyzed for dominant traits or bred further to identify mutations that lead to recessive phenotypes. Large numbers of mice can be easily scored for dominant visible abnormalities. A genome-wide scan for recessive phenotypes is much more labor-intensive, but other strategies (e.g., region-specific screens with mice that already carry a deletion) provide interesting alternatives.[41] Currently, two large-scale ENU mutagenesis screens are being carried out[32,34]—one at the GSF Research Center in Munich and the other at the MRC Mammalian Genetics Unit in Harwell (United Kingdom). Additional screens are in preparation in Japan, the United States, and Australia. In the meantime, the labs in Harwell and the GSF have produced about 200 new mouse mutants each, providing a rich source of mutants and a wide range of phenotypes. Whereas the screen in Harwell focuses on the isolation of neurodegenerative and behavior mutants, the GSF screen is primarily targeted towards the isolation of congenital malformations, biochemical alterations of clinical relevance, and immunological and hematological defects. Unlike gene targeting or insertional mutagenesis, mutations produced by ENU are not molecularly tagged. In order to identify the genes affected, positional or candidate cloning is required. A prerequisite for this is the determination of the chromosomal localization of the mutation. This is achieved by backcross strategies and genome-wide microsatellite genotyping. The availability of the complete mouse genome sequence will have an enormous impact on the efficiency of these cloning efforts. Currently, major work is under way to develop necessary databases and cryoconservation archives for making the ENU mutagenesis–derived mutants available to the scientific community.

THE USE OF ENU MUTAGENESIS IN TOXICOLOGY

The phenotypic assays employed so far in the ongoing ENU mutagenesis projects are to a large degree influenced by the interests and capabilities of the labs involved. However, one of the important messages that has come out of these projects is that, for almost any phenotype that can be scored with a robust, cost-efficient, and reliable assay, mutants can be isolated. There are many assays and endpoints that are of high interest to toxicologists. Increased or decreased susceptibility and resistance to toxic compounds are among these. However, it is also the dissection of pharmacological mechanisms that is attracting increasing interest. Mutants with abnormal absorption, distribution, metabolism, or excretion (ADME) of drugs or toxic chemicals can provide important insight into the molecular mechanisms of individual drug efficacy or toxicity. Mouse ADME mutants isolated from ENU screens could be a great tool for human toxicogenetics and pharmacogenetics. Currently, the mouse is not used as intensively in toxicological research as it should. The rat, mainly for historical reasons, is still the major animal in toxicological risk assessment. Given that pharmacological and toxicological risk evaluation has to be based on the most updated knowledge, it is a question of time before the mouse takes over a major role in toxicology during the process of drug development. Although the rat will continue to be very important for specific questions, the advantage of the genetics of the mouse needs to be taken into consideration for future toxicological research.

OUTLOOK

Toxicology of the new millennium will profit tremendously from the progress currently made in genomics and proteomics.[42] With the availability of the complete human and mouse genome sequences within the next few years, DNA array technology will soon become a routine procedure in evaluating xenobiotic and drug responses.[43–45] Through functional genomics, the role of individual genes as well as the interaction of many genes within the genome will be studied in toxicology and pharmacology. Individual predisposition as opposed to the responses at the population level will move to the forefront of toxicology research.[46–48] Pretty soon, we will apply tools of complex system analysis to describe the consequences of toxic exposure to cells and organisms. Multigenic and multifactorial traits, genetic predisposition, global and genome-wide expression changes, and the integration of structure-activity relationships will all become integral components of toxicological hazard identification and risk assessment. A systematic production of new mouse mutants will facilitate to make the necessary rational and scientifically based decisions in future toxicological research.

REFERENCES

1. NÜSSLEIN-VOLHARD, C. & E. WIESCHAUS. 1980. Mutations affecting segment number and polarity in *Drosophila.* Nature **287:** 795–801.
2. PICK, L. 1998. Segmentation: painting stripes from flies to vertebrates. Dev. Genet. **23:** 1–10.

3. ORENIC, T.V. & S.B. CARROLL. 1992. The cell biology of pattern formation during *Drosophila* development. Int. Rev. Cytol. **139:** 121–155.
4. DRIER, E.A. & R. STEWARD. 1997. The dorsoventral signal transduction pathway and the rel-like transcription factors in *Drosophila*. Semin. Cancer Biol. **8:** 83–92.
5. WODARZ, A. & R. NUSSE. 1998. Mechanisms of Wnt signaling in development. Annu. Rev. Cell Dev. Biol. **14:** 59–88.
6. SHULMAN, J.M., N. PERRIMOON & J.D. AXELROD. 1998. Frizzled signaling and the developmental control of cell polarity. Trends Genet. **14:** 452–458.
7. IRVINE, K.D. 1999. Fringe, notch, and making developmental boundaries. Curr. Opin. Genet. Dev. **9:** 434–441.
8. BURKE, R. & K. BASLER. 1997. Hedgehog signaling in *Drosophila* eye and limb development-conserved machinery: divergent roles? Curr. Opin. Neurobiol. **7:** 55–61.
9. INGHAM, P.W. 1998. Transducing hedgehog: the story so far. EMBO J. **17:** 3505–3511.
10. PARISI, M.J. & H. LIN. 1998. The role of the hedgehog/patched signaling pathway in epithelial stem cell proliferation: from fly to human. Cell Res. **8:** 15–21.
11. MURONE, M., A. ROSENTHAL & F.J. DE SAUVAGE. 1999. Hedgehog signal transduction: from flies to vertebrates. Exp. Cell Res. **253:** 25–33.
12. GAILANI, M.R. & A.E. BALE. 1997. Developmental genes and cancer: role of patches in basal cell carcinoma of the skin. J. Natl. Cancer Inst. **89:** 1103–1109.
13. INGHAM, P.W. 1998. The patched gene in development and cancer. Curr. Opin. Genet. Dev. **8:** 88–94.
14. PADGETT, R.W., P. DAS & S. KRISHNA. 1998. TFGβ signaling, Smads, and tumor suppressors. Bioessays **20:** 382–390.
15. BIENZ, M. 1999. APC—the plot thickens. Curr. Opin. Genet. Dev. **9:** 595–603.
16. HAHN, H., L. WOJNOWSKI, G. MILLER & A. ZIMMER. 1999. The patched signalling pathway in tumorigenesis and development: lessons from animal models. J. Mol. Med. **77:** 459–468.
17. MORIN, P.J. 1999. Beta-catenin signaling and cancer. Bioessays **21:** 1021–1030.
18. FAVOR, J. 1996. The frequency of dominant cataract and recessive specific-locus mutations in mice derived from 80 or 160 mg ethylnitrosurea per kg body weight treated spermatogonia. Mutat. Res. **162:** 69–80.
19. MANSOURI, A., G. GOUDREAU & P. GRUSS. 1999. Pax genes and their role in organogenesis. Cancer Res. **59:** 1707s–1710s.
20. WALTERHOUSE, D.O., J.W. YOON & P.M. IANNACCONE. 1999. Developmental pathways: Sonic hedgehog-patched-GLI. Environ. Health Perspect. **107:** 167–171.
21. LAMMER, E.J., D.T. CHEN, R.M. HOAR, N.D. AGNISH, P.J. BENKE, J.T. BRAUN, C.J. CURRY, P.M. GERNHOFF, A.W. GRIX, JR., I.T. LOTT *et al.* 1985. Retinoic acid embryopathy. N. Engl. J. Med. **313:** 837–841.
22. SIMEONE, A., D. ACAMPORA, V. NIGRO, A. FAIELLA, M. D'ESPOSITO, A. STONAIUOLO, F. MAVILIO & E. BONCINELLI. 1991. Differential regulation by retinoic acid of the homeobox genes of the four HOX loci in human embryonal carcinoma cells. Mech. Dev. **33:** 215–227.
23. BONCINELLI, E., A. SIMEONE, D. ACAMPORA & F. MAVILIO. 1991. HOX gene activation by retinoic acid. Trends Genet. **7:** 329–334.
24. BALLING, R., G. MUTTER, P. GRUSS & M. KESSEL. 1989. Craniofacial abnormalities induced by ectopic expression of the homeobox gene Hox 1.1 in transgenic mice. Cell **58:** 337–347.
25. KESSEL, M., R. BALLING & P. GRUSS. 1990. Variations of cervical vertebrae after expression of a Hox 1.1 transgene in mice. Cell **61:** 301–308.
26. MING, J.E., E. ROESSLER & M. MUENKE. 1998. Human developmental disorders and the Sonic hedgehog pathway. Mol. Med. Today **4:** 343–349.
27. COOPER, M.K., J.A. PORTER, K.E. YOUNG & P.A. BEACHY. 1998. Teratogen-mediated inhibition of target tissue response to Shh signaling. Science **280:** 1603–1607.
28. INCARDONA, J.P., W. GAFFIELD, R.P. KAPUR & H. ROELINK. 1998. The teratogenic *Veratrum* alkaloid cycopamine inhibits Sonic hedgehog signal transduction. Development **125:** 3553–3562.
29. FAIELLA, A., M. WERNIG, G. CONSALEZ, U. HOSTICK, C. HOFFMANN, E. HUSTERT, E. BONCINELLI, R. BALLING & J.H. NADEAU. 2000. A mouse model for valproate terato-

genicity: parental effects, homeotic transformations, and altered HOX expression. Hum. Mol. Genet. **9:** 227–236.
30. CAPECCHI, M.R. 1997. Hox genes and mammalian development. Cold Spring Harbor Symp. Quant. Biol. **62:** 273–281.
31. FAVIER, B. & P. DOLLE. 1997. Developmental functions of mammalian Hox genes. Mol. Hum. Reprod. **3:** 115–131.
32. HRABÉ DE ANGELIS, M. & R. BALLING. 1998. Large scale ENU mutagenesis screens in the mouse: genetics meets genomics. Mutat. Res. **400:** 25–32.
33. BROWN, S.D. & J. PETERS. 1996. Combining mutagenesis and genomics in the mouse—closing the phenotype gap. Trends Genet. **12:** 433–435.
34. BROWN, S.D. & P.M. NOLAN. 1998. Mouse mutagenesis—systematic studies of mammalian gene function. Hum. Mol. Genet. **7:** 1627–1633.
35. RINCHIK, E.M. & D.A. CARPENTER. 1999. N-Ethyl-N-nitrosurea mutagenesis of a 6- to 11-cM subregion of the Fah-Hbb interval of mouse chromosome 7: complete testing of 4557 gametes and deletion mapping and complementation analysis of 31 mutations. Genetics **152:** 373–383.
36. BATTEY, J., E. JORDAN, D. COX & W. DOVE. 1999. An action plan for mouse genomics. Nat. Genet. **21:** 73–75.
37. RUSSELL, W.L., P.R. KELLY, P.R. HUNSICKER, J.W. BANGHAM, S.C. MADDUX & E.L. PHIPPS. 1979. Specific-locus test shows ethylnitrosurea to be the most potent mutagen in the mouse. Proc. Natl. Acad. Sci. U.S.A. **76:** 5918–5922.
38. JUSTICE, M. & V. BODE. 1986. Induction of new mutations in a mouse t-haplotype using ethylnitrosurea mutagenesis. Genet. Res. Camb. **47:** 187–192.
39. SHEDLOVSKY, A., T.R. KING & W.F. DOVE. 1988. Saturation germ line mutagenesis of the murine t region including a lethal allele at the quaking locus. Proc. Natl. Acad. Sci. U.S.A. **85:** 180–184.
40. RINCHIK, E.M., D.A. CARPENTER & P.A. SELBY. 1990. A strategy for fine-structure functional analysis of a 6- to 11-centimorgan region of mouse chromosome 7 by high-efficiency mutagenesis. Proc. Natl. Acad. Sci. U.S.A. **87:** 896–900.
41. JUSTICE, M.J., J.K. NOVEROSKE, J.S. WEBER, B. ZHENG & A. BRADLEY. 1999. Mouse ENU mutagenesis. Hum. Mol. Genet. **8:** 1955–1963.
42. RODI, C.P., R.T. BUNCH, S.W. CURTISS, L.D. KIER, M.A. CABONCE, J.D. DAVILA, M.D. MITCHELL, C.L. ALDEN & D.L. MORRIS. 1999. Revolution through genomics in investigative and discovery toxicology. Toxicol. Pathol. **27:** 107–110.
43. ROCKET, J.C. & D.J. DIX. 1999. Application of DNA arrays to toxicology. Environ. Health Perspect. **107:** 681–685.
44. SCHENA, M., D. SHALON, R. HELLER, A. CHAI, P.O. BROWN & R.W. DAVIS. 1996. Parallel human genome analysis: microarray-based expression monitoring of 1000 genes. Proc. Natl. Acad. Sci. U.S.A. **93:** 10614–10619.
45. AFSHARI, C.A., E.F. NUWAYSIR & J.C. BARRET. 1999. Application of complementary DNA microarray technology to carcinogen identification, toxicology, and drug safety evaluation. Cancer Res. **59:** 4759–4760.
46. INGELMAN–SUNDBERG, M. 1998. Functional consequences of polymorphism of xenobiotic metabolizing enzymes. Toxicol. Lett. **28:** 155–160.
47. LANG, M. & M. PELKONEN. 1999. Metabolism of xenobiotics and chemical carcinogens. IARC Sci. Publ. **148:** 13–22.
48. WORMHOUDT, L.W., J.N. COMMANDEUR & N.P. VERMEULEN. 1999. Genetic polymorphisms of human N-acetyltransferase, cytochrome P450, glutathione-S-transferase, and epoxide hydrolase enzymes: relevance to xenobiotic metabolism and toxicity. Crit. Rev. Toxicol. **29:** 59–124.

Molecular Genetic Control of Axis Patterning during Early Embryogenesis of Vertebrates

GARY C. SCHOENWOLF[a]

Department of Neurobiology and Anatomy, University of Utah School of Medicine, Salt Lake City, Utah 84132, USA

ABSTRACT: Formation of the axis and its subsequent patterning to establish the tube-within-a-tube body plan characteristic of vertebrates are initiated during gastrulation. In higher vertebrates (i.e., birds and mammals), gastrulation involves six key events: establishment of the rostrocaudal/mediolateral axis; formation and progression of the primitive streak and organizer; epiboly of the epiblast, ingression of prospective mesodermal and endodermal cells through the primitive streak, and migration of cells away from the primitive streak; regression of the primitive streak; establishment of the right-left axis; and formation of the tail bud. Over 50 years of study of these processes have provided a morphological framework for understanding how these events occur, and recent advances in imaging, microsurgical intervention, and cell tracking are beginning to elucidate the underlying cell behaviors that drive morphogenetic movements. Moreover, homotopic transplantation and dye microinjection studies are being used to generate high-resolution fate maps, and heterotopic transplantation studies are revealing the cell-cell interactions that are sufficient as well as required for mesodermal and ectodermal commitment. Additionally, the roles of the organizer and secondary signaling centers in establishing the body plan are being defined. With the advent of the molecular/genetic age, the molecular basis for axis formation is beginning to become understood. Thus, it is becoming clear that secreted growth factors/signaling molecules produced by localized signaling centers induce and pattern the axis, presumably through downstream activation of signal-transduction proteins and cascades of transcription factors.

INTRODUCTION

Axis patterning in vertebrate embryos involves a number of important developmental events. This process is initiated with gastrulation and culminates in the formation of the tube-within-a-tube body plan characteristic of vertebrate embryos. Below, I describe this body plan, provide a brief overview of gastrulation in higher vertebrates, describe fate maps and consider the organization of the blastoderm during gastrulation, discuss the timing of mesodermal commitment, describe the auxiliary system responsible for reconstitution of the organizer and the use of blastoderm isolates as model systems for understanding the role of the organizer and other signaling centers in axial patterning, and discuss our progress towards achieving a molecular-genetic under-

[a]Address for correspondence: Department of Neurobiology and Anatomy, University of Utah School of Medicine, 50 North Medical Drive, Salt Lake City, UT 84132. Voice: 801-581-6453; fax: 801-581-4233.
Schoenwolf@med.utah.edu

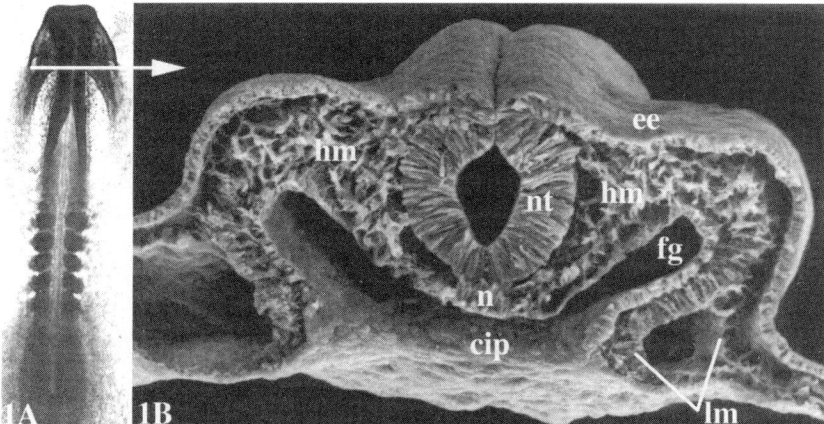

FIGURE 1. (A) Whole mount and (B) scanning electron micrograph of a transverse slice through the head of a stage-8 chick embryo showing the tube-within-a-tube body plan typical of vertebrate embryos. The arrow in part A indicates the level of the slice shown in part B. Terms: cip, cranial intestinal portal; ee, epidermal ectoderm; fg, foregut; hm, head mesenchyme; lm, lateral mesoderm; n, notochord; nt, neural tube (mesencephalon level).

standing of axis patterning. For my discussion, I will focus chiefly on these events as they occur in the chick embryo, which has been well studied.

THE TUBE-WITHIN-A-TUBE BODY PLAN

Vertebrate (actually chordate) embryos are characterized by a body plan consisting of a tube-within-a-tube configuration (FIG. 1). The outer tube of the tube-within-a-tube body plan is derived from ectoderm. The more lateral portion of the ectoderm (the epidermal ectoderm) remains on the surface of the embryo, forming the skin and the associated appendages, such as hair, feathers, and nails. Some of this ectoderm undergoes localized thickening to form placodes, such as the lens placode, the otic placode, the nasal placode, and the epibranchial placodes. The most medial portion of the ectoderm thickens to form the neural plate, the earliest rudiment of the adult central nervous system, which folds into a neural tube during the process of neurulation. The inner tube of the tube-within-a-tube body plan is derived from endoderm. This endoderm folds into the head of the embryo as the foregut, the caudal trunk of the embryo as the hindgut, and the remainder of the trunk as the midgut. The space between the inner and outer tubes of the tube-within-a-tube body plan is filled with mesoderm that ingressed into the interior of the embryo during gastrulation. This mesoderm eventually becomes subdivided into a number of mesodermal rudiments that differ in the head, trunk, and tail. Within the head, the mesoderm forms the prechordal plate, notochord, paraxial mesoderm (which segments partially into somitomeres), and lateral mesoderm, with the splanchnic mesodermal component of the latter forming the heart (i.e., the cardiac mesoderm) and the somatic mesodermal component forming the coelomic epithelium lining the body wall. The space between these two layers forms the pericardial cavity. Within the trunk, the mesoderm forms the notochord, paraxial mesoderm (which segments into somites), intermediate mesoderm, and lateral plate mesoderm (which, like the lateral mesoderm of the head, splits into somatic and splanchnic mesodermal layers separated by the coelom). Within the tail, the medialmost mesoderm forms the core of the tail bud, a mass of mesenchymal cells covered dorsally by epidermal ectoderm and ventrally by endoderm. More laterally, the mesoderm of the tail is organized as the lateral plate mesoderm, with its somatic and splanchnic mesodermal layers separated by a coelom.

The tube-within-a-tube body plan is progressively developed during stages of gastrulation, neurulation, cardiogenesis (i.e., formation of the heart), segmentation, and body folding. It has well-defined cardinal axes (i.e., rostrocaudal, dorsoventral, mediolateral, and right-left). A major question I will address is as follows: how is this body plan established? Although not completely understood, our progress in answering this question has been phenomenal in recent years. Below, I discuss some of the major areas of progress.

OVERVIEW OF GASTRULATION IN HIGHER VERTEBRATES

Formation of the body plan begins with gastrulation (for a recent review, see reference 1). Gastrulation in higher vertebrates (i.e., birds and mammals) often is considered to be initiated with the formation of the primitive streak, and the usual definition of gastrulation is the phase of development in which the embryo forms its three primary germ layers—the ectoderm, mesoderm, and endoderm. However, gastrulation actually involves a number of events in addition to the formation of the primitive streak and germ layers, including the establishment of the rostrocaudal/mediolateral axis, the formation of the organizer, the establishment of the right-left axis, and the formation of the tail bud. This latter process, which leads to so-called secondary body development, that is, the development of the caudal portion of the embryo from the tail bud (a derivative of Hensen's node and the rostral primitive streak), can be considered to be a continuation of gastrulation. Many of the events of gastrulation are illustrated in FIGURE 2.

Formation of the primitive streak is induced in the epiblast by a signal (perhaps the TGFβ family member Vg1)[2] produced by the caudal margin of the blastoderm (e.g., see reference 3). Such induction seems to occur progressively from caudal to rostral such that, as the primitive streak forms, it also elongates along the future midline of the embryo toward the future rostral end of the embryo. With formation of the primitive streak, two body axes become clearly defined: the rostrocaudal and the mediolateral. The dorsoventral axis is established earlier, prior to the onset of gastrulation; how it is established remains uncertain. Additionally, with establishment of the dorsoventral, rostrocaudal, and mediolateral axes, a fourth axis becomes evident: the right-left axis. However, at the time of primitive streak formation, this fourth axis has not yet become fixed, so embryos are still potentially bilaterally symmetric.

As formation of the primitive streak occurs, the epiblast initiates a spreading movement toward it (i.e., medially) called epiboly. As the epiblast cells spread toward the primitive streak, the medialmost cells enter the primitive streak, undergo an epithelial-to-mesenchymal transformation, and ingress into the interior of the em-

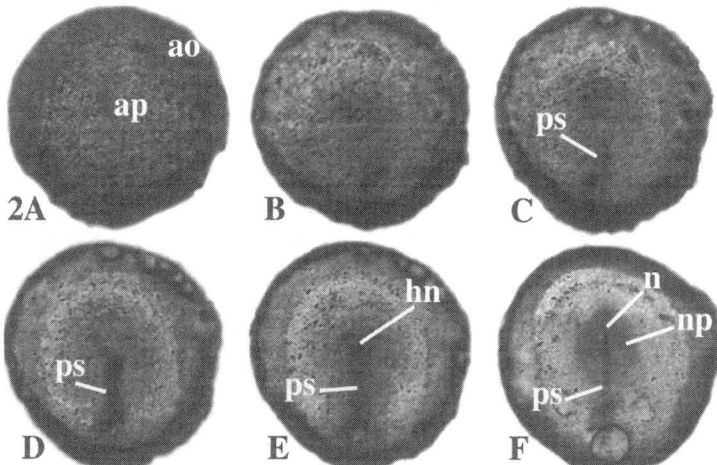

FIGURE 2. A series of frames from a time-lapse movie showing gastrulation in an avian embryo. The series was collected over the first 24 hours of incubation after the egg was laid. Frames are lettered in temporal sequence. The caudal end of the embryo is at the bottom, midline of each figure. Terms: ao, area opaca; ap, area pellucida; hn, Hensen's node; n, notochord; np, neural plate; ps, primitive streak.

bryo, where they migrate bilaterally to form two of the three primary germ layers, the mesoderm and endoderm (FIG. 3). This movement of cells toward, through, and away from the primitive streak can be likened to water flow from an upstream source, toward and over a waterfall, and then away from the fall where it flows downstream. After gastrulation has been completed, those epiblast cells that remained on the surface of the blastoderm constitute the third primary germ layer, the ectoderm.

The movement of prospective mesodermal and endodermal cells toward, through, and away from the primitive streak can be tracked by either microinjecting fluorescent dyes into embryos or grafting labeled cells from a donor embryo into an unlabeled host embryo. By following such labeled cells, their bilateral movements and their subsequent fates can be readily established (FIG. 4).

Cells contained within Hensen's node at the fully elongated primitive-streak stage exhibit a different migratory behavior than that just described (FIG. 5). These cells become sequestered within Hensen's node near the time of its formation and they progressively leave this reservoir-like structure to form the midline rudiments of the developing embryo: the floor plate of the neural tube, the notochord, and the mid-dorsal endoderm of the gut. Rather than migrating bilaterally, such cells of Hensen's node undergo an intercalation toward the midline, undergoing a convergent-extension movement (i.e., resulting in a reduction in the diameter of the notochord and a concomitant and proportional increase in its length). As these cells leave Hensen's node, they also continue to divide mitotically, with about half of them exhibiting rostrocaudally oriented mitotic spindles, thereby positioning themselves to facilitate the rostrocaudal elongation of the forming midline.[4]

As the midline rudiments are laid down, the rostral half of the primitive streak undergoes regression. Regression is a caudalward displacement that eventually posi-

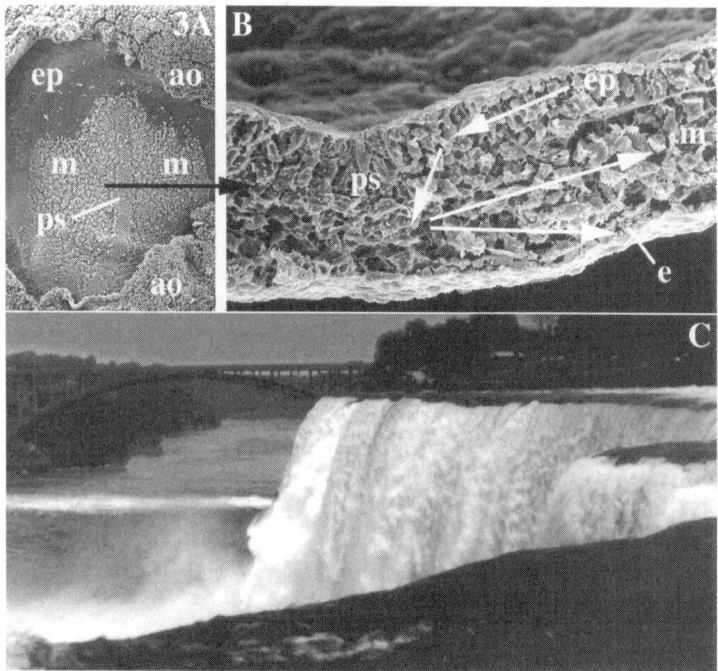

FIGURE 3. (A) Scanning electron micrograph of a chick blastoderm in which the primitive streak (ps) and ingressed mesodermal mantle (m) are viewed *en face* after removal of the endodermal layer. The embryo is at the stage illustrated in FIGURE 2E. The basal surface of the epiblast is partially visible (ep). The caudal end of the embryo is at the bottom, midline of the figure. The arrow in part A indicates the level of the slice shown in part B. Terms: ao, yolk-ladened cells of the area opaca. **(B)** Scanning electron micrograph of a transverse slice through the blastoderm at the stage illustrated in FIGURE 2E. The arrows indicate the directions of migration of cells toward, into, and away from the primitive streak (ps). Terms: ep, epiblast; e, endoderm; m, mesoderm. **(C)** Niagara Falls as shown in a 1956 photograph taken by one of the author's parents on a family vacation. With the exception of the prospective notochordal cells contained within Hensen's node, the movement of cells toward, into, and away from the primitive streak occurs in a manner similar to that of water going toward and over the falls, and then flowing downstream. Thus, a constant turnover of cells occurs throughout most of the primitive streak.

tions Hensen's node and persisting remnants of the immediately more caudal primitive streak at the caudal end of the embryo, where they form the tail bud. The tail bud is a mesenchymal cluster of cells expressing many of the same genes expressed during gastrulation (e.g., *Brachyury*, see below) and giving rise to the caudal portion of the embryo, namely, the lumbosacral and tail neural tube (spinal cord), neural crest, and somites (but not the caudal notochord, which grows into the caudal body from more rostral levels), through a process called secondary body development.[5–9] Thus, the caudal portion of the body develops differently than the head and trunk, and the manner in which this area is induced and patterned (i.e., organized) remains largely unknown.

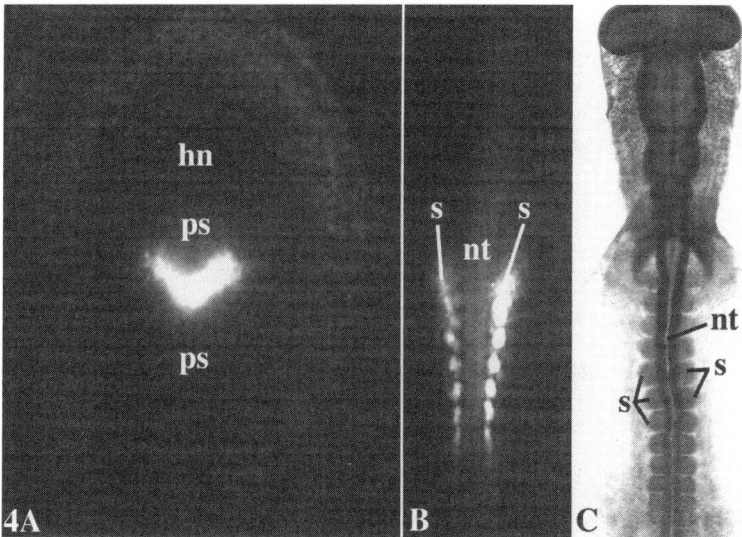

FIGURE 4. Fate mapping by following fluorescent dyes microinjected into the primitive streak (ps). **(A)** Two hours after injection of dye into the cranial one-third of the primitive streak (caudal to Hensen's node; hn), cells are beginning to migrate bilaterally. The caudal end of the embryo is at the bottom, midline of the figure. **(B)** At sacrifice 24 hours after injection, labeled cells have migrated bilaterally, populating the paraxial mesoderm of the trunk and subsequently forming the somites (s) flanking the neural tube (nt). **(C)** Whole mount at a stage similar to that shown in part B to demonstrate better the anatomy of the embryo at the time of sacrifice.

During early gastrulation, the embryo appears morphologically to be bilaterally symmetric. The first indication of the development of asymmetry appears as Hensen's node initiates its regression. With regression, the node changes shape from symmetrical to asymmetrical, and genes expressed by Hensen's node (e.g., Sonic hedgehog) also become asymmetrically localized. Asymmetric gene expression within Hensen's node occurs as a result of asymmetric signaling (for a review, see reference 10). For example, asymmetric expression of Sonic hedgehog in Hensen's node is induced by right-sided expression of the Activin receptor (and presumably right-sided Activin signaling), and left-sided expression of Sonic hedgehog in turn induces left-sided expression of nodal, a member of the TGFβ family of secreted proteins. Nodal is directly involved in some unknown manner in establishing asymmetry during subsequent development of the heart (i.e., right-sided looping) and gastrointestinal system (i.e., intestinal rotation during its return from the umbilical cord to the peritoneal cavity).

FATE MAPS AND ORGANIZATION OF THE BLASTODERM

Relatively high-resolution fate maps exist for many stages of gastrulation of higher vertebrates (FIG. 6). At the fully elongated primitive-streak stage,[11,12] the chick

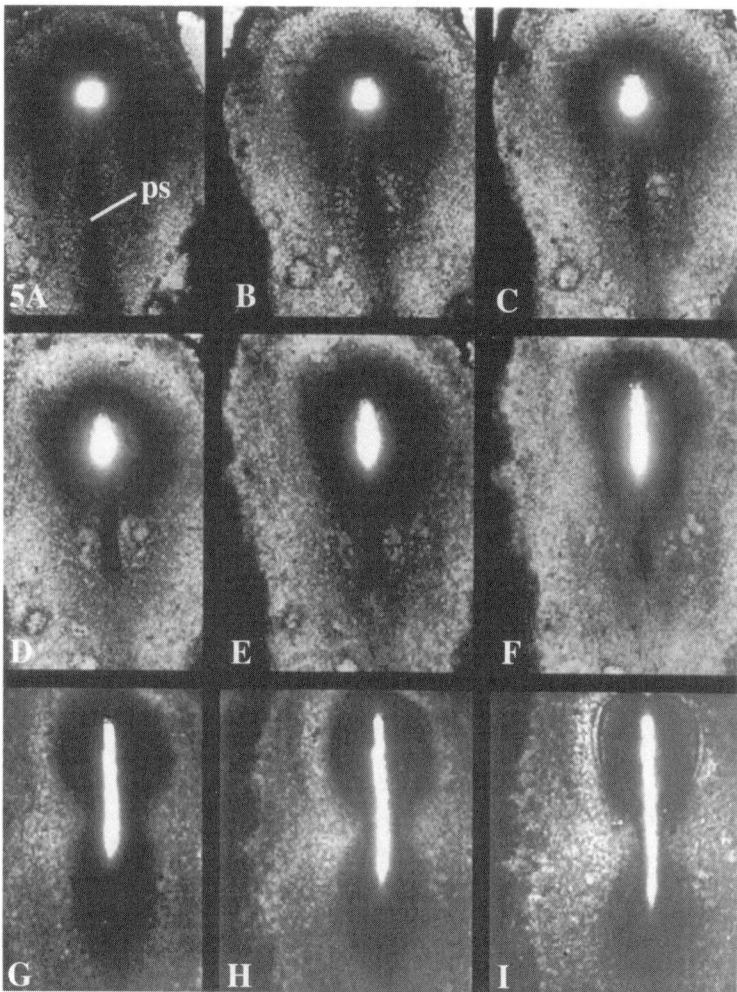

FIGURE 5. A series of frames from a time-lapse movie showing the convergent-extension movements characteristic of midline cells derived from Hensen's node (i.e., the floor plate of the neural tube, the notochord, and mid-dorsal endoderm of the gut). Hensen's node, from a fluorescently labeled donor embryo, was transplanted homotopically and isochronically in place of the unlabeled Hensen's node of the host. Frames are lettered in temporal sequence. The caudal end of the embryo is at the bottom, midline of each figure. Terms: ps, primitive streak.

epiblast is subdivided into prospective epidermal ectoderm, otic placodes, neural plate, and mesoderm, with surprisingly large areas of overlap among the cells of the prospective otic placodes, medial epidermal ectoderm, and lateral neural plate. The prospective endoderm is restricted to Hensen's node and the remainder of the primitive streak. The prospective mesoderm occupies both the medial epiblast (caudal to the prospective neural plate) and the primitive streak. At the fully elongated

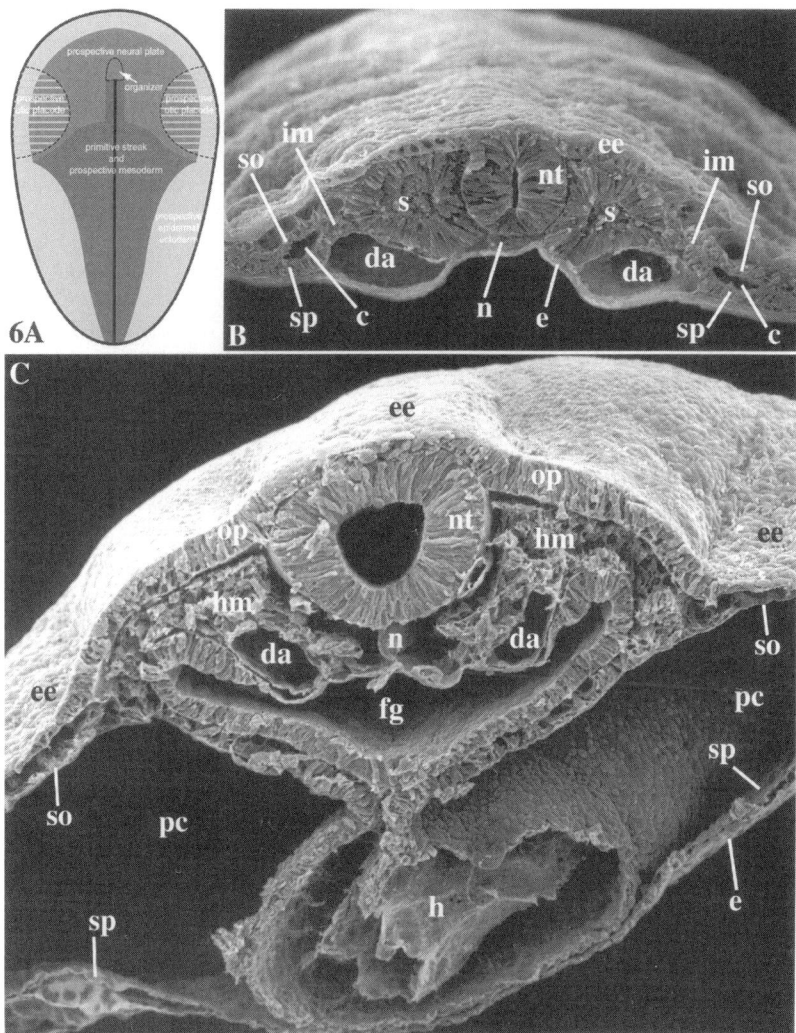

FIGURE 6. (A) Prospective fate map of the chick embryo blastoderm at the fully elongated primitive-streak stage. (B) Mesodermal subdivisions of the trunk derived 24 hours later from cells migrating through the fully elongated primitive streak as seen in a scanning electron micrograph of a transverse slice through the trunk. Terms: c, coelom; da, dorsal aorta; e, endoderm; ee, epidermal ectoderm; im, intermediate mesoderm; n, notochord; nt, neural tube; s, somite; so, somatic mesodermal component of the lateral plate mesoderm; sp, splanchnic mesodermal component of the lateral plate mesoderm. (C) Mesodermal subdivisions of the head derived 24 hours later from cells migrating through the early to midprimitive streak as seen in a scanning electron micrograph of a transverse slice through the head. Terms: da, dorsal aortae; e, endoderm; ee, epidermal ectoderm; fg, foregut; h, heart; hm, head mesenchyme; n, notochord; nt, neural tube (hindbrain); op, otic placode; pc, pericardial cavity; so, somatic mesodermal component of lateral mesoderm; sp, splanchnic mesodermal component of lateral mesoderm.

primitive-streak stage, the prospective mesoderm contributes principally to the trunk mesoderm (with the exception of some of the mesoderm derived from Hensen's node and the most rostral primitive streak). Prospective mesodermal cells ingress through the primitive streak in a rostral-to-caudal order that presages their medial-to-lateral position within the mesodermal mantle after they have ingressed. Thus, the notochord is derived from the most rostral part of the primitive streak (i.e., Hensen's node), the paraxial (i.e., somitic) mesoderm ingresses more caudally (i.e., about 125–750 μm caudal to the rostral border of Hensen's node), the intermediate mesoderm more caudally (i.e., at the interface between prospective somitic and lateral plate mesoderm), the lateral plate mesoderm more caudally (i.e., about 750–1000 μm caudal to the rostral border of Hensen's node), and the extra-embryonic mesoderm more caudally (i.e., 1000 μm caudal to the rostral border of Hensen's node to the caudal end of the primitive streak).

As the primitive streak is forming and progressing (i.e., elongating rostrally), it contributes cells principally to the head mesoderm, of which the cardiac mesoderm is considered initially a component of, and the extra-embryonic mesoderm. As at the fully elongated primitive-streak stage, prospective mesodermal cells ingress through the early to mid-primitive streak in a rostral-to-caudal order that presages their medial-to-lateral order within the mesodermal mantle.[13] Thus, within the head, the prechordal plate mesoderm is derived from the rostral part of the primitive streak, the paraxial (i.e., somitomeric) mesoderm ingresses more caudally, and the lateral mesoderm (including the cardiac mesoderm, which originates from its splanchnopleuric component) originates more caudally (i.e., between 125 and 750 μm caudal to the rostral border of Hensen's node). The remainder of the primitive streak contributes cells to the extra-embryonic mesoderm. Furthermore, most of the endoderm derives from the primitive streak at the early to mid-primitive-streak stage.

Additionally, within the region of the early to mid-primitive streak that forms the heart mesoderm, the future rostrocaudal subdivisions of the straight-heart tube are arrayed in series. Thus, the outflow tract of the heart is located at the rostral end of the heart-forming region of the primitive streak, and the inflow tract is located at the caudal end of this region. Because the paired heart rudiments fuse together in the midline in rostral-to-caudal sequence, with the rostral ends of the paired rudiments oriented more medially and the caudal ends oriented more laterally, the rostrocaudal position of prospective cardiac mesodermal cells within the primitive streak (like those of other types of prospective mesodermal cells within the primitive streak at either the early to mid-primitive-streak stage or the fully elongated primitive-streak stage) presages their mediolateral position (which quickly transforms to rostrocaudal position with fusion to form the straight-heart tube).

MESODERMAL COMMITMENT

Whether cells with a particular prospective fate are committed to that fate is not revealed by conventional fate mapping techniques. To determine whether such cells are committed, groups of cells are transplanted heterotopically, that is, to a foreign site within the embryo. Additionally, cells can be transplanted heterochronically (e.g., from the primitive streak at the fully elongated primitive-streak stage to the primitive streak at the early to mid-primitive-streak stage), which places them in a heterotopic position. Such experiments reveal that essentially all cells within the primitive streak at the fully elongated primitive-streak stage have not yet become committed.[14,15] Thus, such cells change their fates when placed heterotopically, adapting to their new environment. However, one group of cells provides an exception: the prospective notochordal cells of Hensen's node at the fully elongated primitive-streak stage. These cells undergo self-differentiation when placed heterotopically, forming an ectopic notochord.

HOW IS THE TUBE-WITHIN-A-TUBE BODY PLAN ESTABLISHED?

As discussed above, a number of complex morphogenetic events occur during formation of the tube-within-a-tube body plan. These include gastrulation, neurulation, regionalization of the ectoderm/mesoderm/endoderm, and body folding. How are these events coordinated or choreographed so that a body plan of the proper size, shape, and proportion is formed? Although details remain unclear, what is clear is that the organizer plays a central role in this process. All vertebrate embryos have an organizer (FIG. 7). In each of the four vertebrate model systems, the organizer is a localized homologous and analogous region (for reviews, see references 16–18). In zebrafish the organizer is called the shield (or embryonic shield); in *Xenopus* it is called the dorsal lip of the blastopore; in the chick it is called Hensen's node (or the primitive knot); and in mouse it is called the node. The organizer has several important characteristics, including its unique ability to induce and pattern a secondary embryo when grafted to an extra-embryonic site. Moreover, the organizer expresses a number of secreted growth factors/signaling molecules, as well as several types of transcription factors (FIG. 8). Genes expressed within the organizer may also be expressed in other areas of the primitive streak (FIGS. 8A and 8D) and/or in its derivatives (e.g., Sonic hedgehog in the floor plate of the neural tube, the notochord, and the mid-dorsal endoderm of the gut; see FIG. 10B later). The organizer also has the ability to pattern the mesoderm (i.e., dorsalize it) and to induce the neural plate (for a recent review, see reference 19). Although details remain sketchy and species differences may exist, the organizer dorsalizes by inhibiting Wnt signaling through the secretion of "soluble Wnt receptors" such as FRZ-B and other frizzled-related pro-

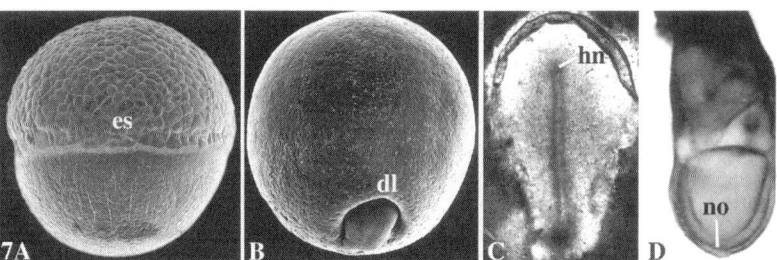

FIGURE 7. Gastrula stages of the four vertebrate models showing the organizer: (**A**) zebrafish; (**B**) *Xenopus*; (**C**) chick; (**D**) mouse. The organizer is known by different names in the four organisms: es, embryonic shield; dl, dorsal lip of the blastopore; hn, Hensen's node; no, node.

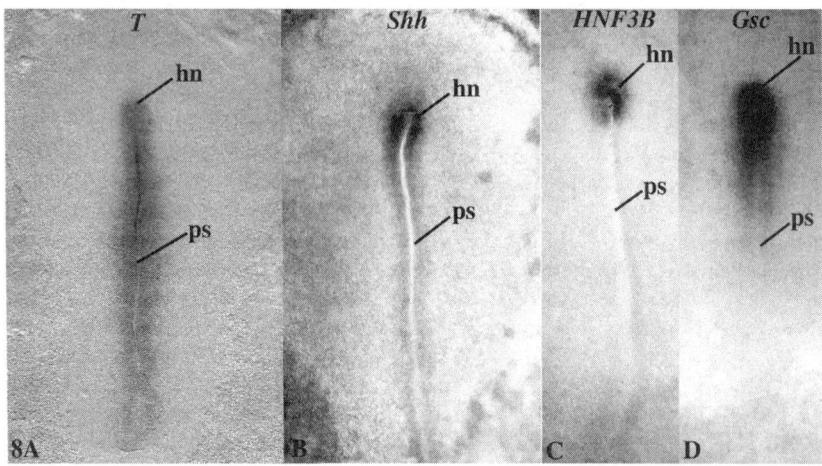

FIGURE 8. Whole-mount *in situ* hybridization of the chick blastoderm at the fully elongated primitive-streak stage. (**A**) The transcription factor *Brachyury* (*T*) labels the entire primitive streak (ps), including Hensen's node (hn). (**B**) The secreted factor *Sonic hedgehog* (*Shh*) labels Hensen's node (hn), but not the remainder of the primitive streak (ps). (**C**) The fork-head-related transcription factor, *HNF3β*, labels Hensen's node (hn), but not the remainder of the primitive streak (ps). (**D**) The transcription factor *Goosecoid* (*Gsc*) labels Hensen's node (hn) and also the rostral one-third of the primitive streak (ps).

teins (i.e., the SFRPs). Similarly, the organizer induces the neural plate by inhibiting BMP signaling through the secretion of BMP inhibitors such as noggin and chordin (BMP-4 is produced by the epidermal ectoderm; FIG. 9).

The precise role of the organizer in establishing the body plan along its rostrocaudal extent remains unclear. In some vertebrate embryos (e.g., the mouse), the organizer may be only a trunk organizer (or a trunk-tail organizer), acting in concert with a separate head organizer (the so-called anterior visceral endoderm) that is responsible for inducing and patterning the head.[20] In other vertebrates, tissues derived from the organizer might subsume this role (e.g., the prechordal plate in birds).[21]

The organizer gives rise to rudiments that become secondary signaling centers. For example, the organizer forms the midline rudiments of the embryo (the floor plate of the neural tube, the notochord, and the mid-dorsal endoderm), rudiments that like Hensen's node also secrete Sonic hedgehog (FIG. 10). Through the secretion of Sonic hedgehog, these rudiments act as secondary signaling centers to pattern the dorsoventral axes of the neural tube and somites (e.g., see references 22 and 23), in combination with other molecules secreted more dorsally (e.g., Wnt-1 from the dorsal neural tube and BMP-4 from the epidermal ectoderm).

THE AUXILIARY SYSTEM AND BLASTODERM ISOLATES AS MODEL SYSTEMS

In avian embryos, the organizer is present at early stages of gastrulation, when the primitive streak first forms. Despite being present so early, an auxiliary system

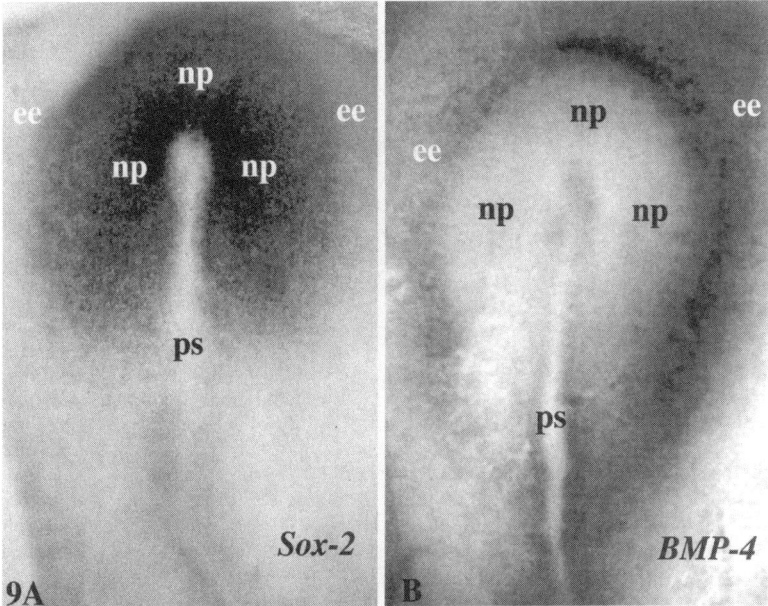

FIGURE 9. (**A**) Whole-mount *in situ* hybridization with the transcription factor *Sox-2* showing labeling throughout the neural plate (np). Terms: ee, epidermal ectoderm; ps, primitive streak. (**B**) Whole-mount *in situ* hybridization with the secreted factor *BMP-4* showing labeling at the neural plate (np)–epidermal ectodermal (ee) interface, as well as in the caudal epiblast and primitive streak (ps).

is present in the avian embryo as late as at the fully elongated primitive-streak stage that allows the organizer to reconstitute if ablated.[24–26] The normal function of this system is unknown, but the fact that it exists provides a fortunate experimental model system to explore how the organizer is formed and patterned, as well as indicating the role of the organizer in establishing the tube-within-a-tube body plan.

The auxiliary system seems to be inactive in the intact embryo because the normal organizer acts as a suppressor to prevent the unnecessary activation of the auxiliary system.[2,24] The auxiliary system consists of two main components (FIG. 11): a single midline inducer that occupies at least the middle rostral one-third of the primitive streak and extends into the flanking blastoderm; and paired responders, bilateral regions of the epiblast that in the presence of the inducers (and in the absence of the normal organizer) can reconstitute ectopic organizers. Thus, blastoderm isolates consisting of responders with or without inducers, or inducers with or without responders, can serve as model systems for studying the formation and patterning of the body plan. We have used such isolates to show that the inducer acts upon the responder to reconstitute an organizer[26] capable of self-differentiating notochord.[24] In addition, fully patterned body plans are reconstituted in lateral blastoderm isolates containing both inducer and responder, but not in isolates containing either one alone.[27] Moreover, omitting the inducer from isolates shows that the body plan is not prepatterned in lateral blastoderm isolates; rather, reconstitution of the body plan re-

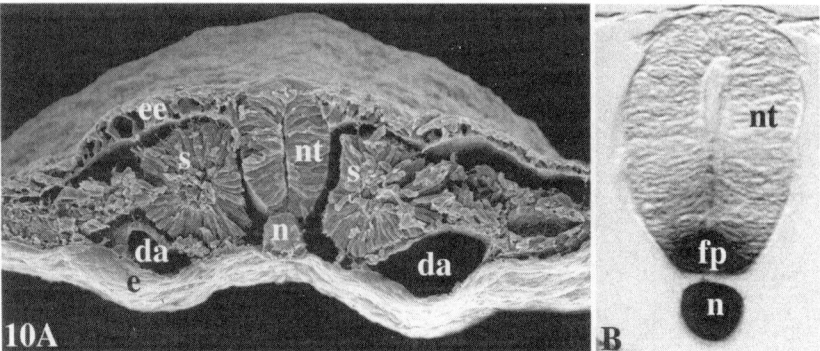

FIGURE 10. Secondary signaling centers are derived from Hensen's node. Hensen's node forms a number of structures, including midline ectodermal (floor plate of the neural tube), mesodermal (notochord), and endodermal (mid-dorsal gut) derivatives. **(A)** Scanning electron micrograph of a transverse slice through the trunk of a stage-10 chick embryo. Terms: da, dorsal aorta; e, endoderm; ee, epidermal ectoderm; n, notochord; nt, neural tube (spinal cord); s, somite. **(B)** Transverse section through the trunk of a chick embryo processed for whole-mount *in situ* hybridization for *Sonic hedgehog* at a stage comparable to that shown in part A. Note that *Sonic hedgehog* labels the notochord (n) and floor plate (fp) of the neural tube (nt), as well as the mid-dorsal endoderm (not shown).

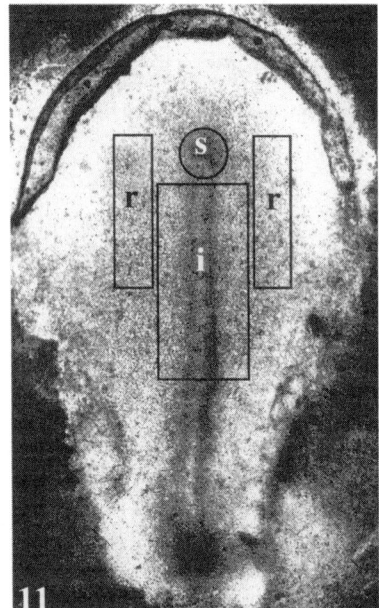

FIGURE 11. Schematic representation of the auxiliary system. In the intact embryo, Hensen's node acts as a suppressor (s), preventing the auxiliary system from becoming active. After ablation of the suppressor, the inducer (i), which spans the rostral half of the primitive streak and extends into the adjacent epiblast, acts upon the bilateral responders (r)—areas of epiblast corresponding to approximately the region of the caudal prospective neural plate—to induce new organizers.

quires reconstitution of the organizer and such reconstitution is sufficient to establish a fully patterned body plan.[27]

TOWARDS A MOLECULAR-GENETIC UNDERSTANDING OF GASTRULATION

The ultimate goal of research on axial formation and patterning is to determine the tissue, cellular, and molecular events involved in formation of the body plan. Considerable progress has been made in reaching a tissue and cellular level of understanding. In recent years, we have begun to gain a molecular understanding as well. This understanding has been achieved mainly by cloning vertebrate genes based on their homology to invertebrate (fly and worm) genes known to play a role in early development (i.e., as assessed through mutational analysis). As discussed above, we now know some of the molecular candidates acting in primitive streak induction, neural induction, patterning of the early neural tube, and establishment of right-left asymmetry. In most cases, our understanding is at a cursory level, often restricted only to the identity of secreted growth factors that initiate signaling. What occurs downstream of the initial signaling is known only in general terms. Thus, much remains to be learned about how gastrulation and axis patterning occur at the molecular level. Such information will likely be forthcoming, and sooner rather than later.

ACKNOWLEDGMENTS

My research was supported by NIH Grant No. NS 18112. I thank past and present members of my laboratory who provided the data upon which this brief review is largely based. FIGURE 7A was kindly provided by Robert E. Waterman, formerly of the University of New Mexico School of Medicine. I thank Eddy De Robertis, Brigid Hogan, Brian Houston, Robin Lovell-Badge, Ray Runyan, and Cliff Tabin for providing plasmids containing cDNA for the probes shown in FIGURES 8, 9, and 10B. I regret that space limitations preclude an exhaustive citation of the relevant literature. This manuscript is dedicated to Robert E. Waterman, a friend and mentor, on the occasion of his retirement.

REFERENCES

1. SCHOENWOLF, G.C. & J.L. SMITH. 1999. Gastrulation and early mesodermal patterning in vertebrates. *In* Methods in Molecular Biology: Developmental Biology Protocols. Volume 136, pp. 1–13. Humana Press. Totowa, NJ.
2. JOUBIN, K. & C.D. STERN. 1999. Molecular interactions continuously define the organizer during the cell movements of gastrulation. Cell **98:** 559–571.
3. BACHVAROVA, R.F., I. SKROMNE & C.D. STERN. 1998. Induction of primitive streak and Hensen's node by the posterior marginal zone in the early chick embryo. Development **125:** 3521–3534.
4. SAUSEDO, R.A. & G.C. SCHOENWOLF. 1993. Cell behaviors underlying notochord formation and extension in avian embryos: quantitative and immunocytochemical studies. Anat. Rec. **237:** 58–70.

5. SCHOENWOLF, G.C. 1977. Tail (end) bud contributions to the posterior region of the chick embryo. J. Exp. Zool. **201:** 227–246.
6. SCHOENWOLF, G.C. 1978. Effects of complete tail bud extirpation on early development of the posterior region of the chick embryo. Anat. Rec. **192:** 289–296.
7. SCHOENWOLF, G.C., N.B. CHANDLER & J. SMITH. 1985. Analysis of the origins and early fates of neural crest cells in caudal regions of avian embryos. Dev. Biol. **110:** 467–479.
8. CATALA, M., M.A. TEILLET & N.M. LE DOUARIN. 1995. Organization and development of the tail bud analysed with chick-quail chimera system. Mech. Dev. **51:** 51–66.
9. CATALA, M., M.A. TEILLET, E.M. ROBERTIS & N.M. LE DOUARIN. 1996. A spinal cord fate map in the avian embryo: while regressing, Hensen's node lays down the notochord and floor plate, thus joining the spinal cord lateral walls. Development **122:** 2599–2610.
10. LEVIN, M. 1997. Left-right asymmetry in vertebrate embryogenesis. Bioessays **19:** 287–296.
11. SCHOENWOLF, G.C., V. GARCIA-MARTINEZ & M.S. DIAS. 1992. Mesoderm movement and fate during avian gastrulation and neurulation. Dev. Dyn. **193:** 235–248.
12. GARCIA-MARTINEZ, V., I.S. ALVAREZ & G.C. SCHOENWOLF. 1993. Locations of the ectodermal and non-ectodermal subdivisions of the epiblast at stages 3 and 4 of avian gastrulation and neurulation. J. Exp. Zool. **267:** 431–446.
13. GARCIA-MARTINEZ, V. & G.C. SCHOENWOLF. 1993. Primitive-streak origin of the cardiovascular system in avian embryos. Dev. Biol. **159:** 706–719.
14. GARCIA-MARTINEZ, V. & G.C. SCHOENWOLF. 1992. Positional control of mesoderm movement and fate during avian gastrulation and neurulation. Dev. Dyn. **193:** 249–256.
15. INAGAKI, T., V. GARCIA-MARTINEZ & G.C. SCHOENWOLF. 1993. Regulative ability of the prospective cardiogenic and vasculogenic areas of the primitive streak during avian gastrulation. Dev. Dyn. **197:** 57–68.
16. GOULD, S.E. & R.M. GRAINGER. 1997. Neural induction and antero-posterior patterning in the amphibian embryo: past, present, and future. Cell. Mol. Life Sci. **53:** 319–338.
17. HARLAND, R. & J. GERHART. 1997. Formation and function of Spemann's organizer. Annu. Rev. Cell Dev. Biol. **13:** 611–667.
18. SMITH, J.L. & G.C. SCHOENWOLF. 1998. Getting organized: new insights into the organizer of higher vertebrates. Curr. Top. Dev. Biol. **40:** 79–110.
19. ZORN, A.M. 1997. Cell-cell signalling: frog frizbees. Curr. Biol. **7:** R501–R504.
20. BEDDINGTON, R.S.P. & E.J. ROBERTSON. 1998. Anterior patterning in mouse. Trends Genet. **14:** 277–284.
21. KNOETGEN, H., C. VIEBAHN & M. KESSEL. 1999. Head induction in the chick by primitive endoderm of mammalian, but not avian origin. Development **126:** 815–825.
22. FAN, C.M. & M. TESSIER-LAVIGNE. 1995. Patterning of mammalian somites by surface ectoderm and notochord: evidence for sclerotome induction by a hedgehog homolog. Cell **79:** 1175–1186.
23. TANABE, Y. & T.M. JESSELL. 1996. Diversity and pattern in the developing spinal cord. Science **274:** 1115–1123.
24. YUAN, S., D.K. DARNELL & G.C. SCHOENWOLF. 1995. Identification of inducing, responding, and suppressing regions in an experimental model of notochord formation in avian embryos. Dev. Biol. **172:** 567–584.
25. PSYCHOYOS, D. & C.D. STERN. 1996. Restoration of the organizer after radical ablation of Hensen's node and the anterior end of the primitive streak in the chick embryo. Development **122:** 3263–3273.
26. YUAN, S. & G.C. SCHOENWOLF. 1998. *De novo* induction of the organizer and formation of the primitive streak in an experimental model of notochord reconstitution in avian embryos. Development **125:** 201–213.
27. YUAN, S. & G.C. SCHOENWOLF. 1999. Reconstruction of the organizer is both sufficient and required to re-establish a fully-patterned body plan in avian embryos. Development **126:** 2461–2473.

Genetic Basis of Susceptibility to Environmentally Induced Neural Tube Defects

RICHARD H. FINNELL,[a,b,c] JANEE GELINEAU–VAN WAES,[b,c] GREGORY D. BENNETT,[c] ROBERT C. BARBER,[b] BOGDAN WLODARCZYK,[b,d] GARY M. SHAW,[e] EDWARD J. LAMMER,[f] JORGE A. PIEDRAHITA,[g] AND JAMES H. EBERWINE[h]

[b]*Center for Human Molecular Genetics, University of Nebraska Medical Center, Omaha, Nebraska 68198-5455, USA*

[c]*Department of Cell Biology and Anatomy, University of Nebraska Medical Center, Omaha, Nebraska 68198-6395, USA*

[d]*Department of Pharmacology and Toxicology, National Veterinary Research Institute, Pulawy, Poland*

[e]*California Birth Defects Monitoring Program, Oakland, California 94606, USA*

[f]*Division of Medical Genetics, Children's Hospital, Oakland, California 94609, USA*

[g]*Department of Veterinary Anatomy and Public Health, Texas A&M University, College Station, Texas 77843-4458, USA*

[h]*Department of Pharmacology, University of Pennsylvania School of Medicine, Philadelphia, Pennsylvania 19107, USA*

ABSTRACT: Neural tube defects (NTDs) are among the most common of all human congenital defects, with multifactorial etiologies comprising both environmental and genetic components. Several murine model systems have been developed in an effort to elucidate genetic factors regulating expression of NTDs. Strain-dependent differences in susceptibility to teratogenic insults and altered patterns of gene expression observed within the neuroepithelium of affected embryos support the hypothesis that subtle genetic changes can result in NTDs. Since several affected genes are folate-regulated, transgenic knockout mice lacking a functional folate receptor were developed. Nullizygous embryos died *in utero* with significant morphological defects, supporting the critical role of folic acid in early embryogenesis. While epidemiological studies have not established an association between polymorphisms in the human folate receptor gene and NTDs, it is known that folate supplementation reduces infant NTD risk. Continued efforts are therefore necessary to reveal the mechanism by which folate works and the nature of the gene(s) responsible for human NTDs.

[a]Address for correspondence: Center for Human Molecular Genetics, 985455 Nebraska Medical Center, Omaha, NE 68198-5455. Voice: 402-559-5397; fax: 402-559-4001.
rfinnell@unmc.edu

INTRODUCTION

Neural tube defects (NTDs) are common congenital malformations that occur when the embryonic neural tube, which ultimately forms the brain and spinal cord, fails to properly close during the first few weeks of development. Anencephaly, or the absence of the brain, is invariably fatal and results from a failure of the anterior neural folds to properly fuse (for review, see reference 1). Spina bifida is the incomplete development of the posterior neural tube, with a protrusion of neural tissue through an opening in the vertebral arches. The severity of NTDs can range from craniorachischisis, where the entire neural tube remains open, to a lesion limited to a single vertebral level. These defects affect approximately 1 per 1000 live-born infants.[2] Including those pregnancies that are electively terminated, approximately 4000 pregnancies per year or 12 pregnancies per day in the United States are affected by an NTD. As such, they are among the most common of all human birth defects, yet their etiologic basis and embryology remain poorly understood.

Neural tube defects appear to be etiologically heterogeneous.[3] For the most part, empirical risk figures, together with numerous clinical studies, indicate that NTDs are of a multifactorial origin, having both a genetic and an environmental component.[4–6] It has been well documented that there is a significantly higher prevalence of consanguinity among the parents of infants with NTDs, suggesting a clustering of liability genes within families. Furthermore, once a woman has had one affected infant, the recurrence risk of her having another infant with an NTD is increased by at least 3-fold above that of the general population. Finally, siblings of affected individuals have at least a 10-fold increased risk of having an NTD as compared to the general population.[4,7,8] These observations support a prominent role for genetically inherited components in the occurrence of NTDs.

In terms of environmental factors contributing to the prevalence of NTDs, there have been several agents identified over the years that are capable of increasing the risk for these malformations in genetically susceptible fetuses. These factors include—but are not limited to—the following: retinoids,[9] pesticides,[10] and a variety of occupational exposures to organic solvents[11,12] and ionizing radiation[13,14] (for review, see reference 15). Several environmental contaminants such as vinyl chloride, water nitrates, and disinfection by-products have been proposed as potential causative agents, although the data have not consistently substantiated these claims.[16–25]

There are additional environmental agents for which a compelling body of literature has developed. The adverse effects of maternal hyperthermia on embryonic development have been widely appreciated for at least 30 years. Although it has been argued that humans are homeothermic and are therefore able to withstand wide fluctuations in temperature, the literature suggests that elevations as small as 1.5°C to 2.5°C in the maternal core temperature is sufficient to disrupt normal morphogenesis. Such temperature elevations are not uncommon in humans, resulting from either a pathogenic agent inducing a febrile episode or an environmental exposure to high exogenous temperature, such as associated with certain occupational environments or recreational saunas/hot tubs. There are a number of anecdotal reports in the clinical literature supporting these conclusions. For example, Miller and colleagues[26] noted that 7 out of 63 anencephalic pregnancies had a positive history for maternal hyperthermia (>38.9°C), which represents a 100-fold increased risk when compared to the general, nonfebrile population risk. Layde and colleagues[27] observed a highly significant association between first-trimester maternal fever and spina bifida, but not with anencephaly. Erickson[28] examined the parents of 4900 infants with major congenital malformations, as well as the parents of 300 unaffected neonates, and observed a highly significant association between a maternal febrile illness and CNS malformations, including both anterior and posterior NTDs. Thus, clinical, epidemiological, and experimental animal data support the hypothesis that an elevation of maternal core temperature by as little as 1.5–2.5°C during critical periods of neural tube closure (NTC) can alter normal morphogenesis and result in an NTD (for review, see reference 29).

The anticonvulsant medications, carbamazepine (Tegretol®, Ciba-Geigy, NY) and valproic acid (Depakene®, Abbott Laboratories, Abbott Park, IL), have also been shown to be associated with an increased risk for posterior NTDs in both human studies and experimental animal models.[30–36] It has been estimated that 1–2% of all infants exposed to valproic acid during early pregnancy will have spina bifida, a 20-fold increased prevalence over that observed in the general population.[32] For carbamazepine, the risk for exposed infants presenting with an NTD has variously been described as being between 0.5% and 1%.[33,37,38] In a Dutch study of the offspring of epileptic women, two-thirds of the 34 NTD cases had been exposed *in utero* to valproic acid, while nearly a fifth of the cases received carbamazepine monotherapy.[34] Clearly, these two pharmaceutical compounds are human teratogens capable of inducing NTDs in genetically susceptible infants.

Finally, a large number of heavy metals have been suspected of producing NTDs in exposed infants.[11,12] While the experimental animal literature consistently demonstrates that sodium arsenate is a risk factor for NTDs and other congenital malformations,[39,40] the human literature is more uncertain. In the few human studies that have been described, prenatal exposure to arsenic has been associated with multiple adverse outcomes, including NTDs (for review, see reference 41). In general, there is abundant evidence supporting the hypothesis that environmental factors, including physical agents, pharmaceuticals, or industrial pollutants, are capable of inducing NTDs in humans. The above-mentioned environmental compounds do not represent an exhaustive list and other such agents may have a similar teratogenic potential. The important point is that this evidence makes a strong case for NTDs being multifactorial events that have multiple genetic contributions and are subject to a variety of environmental modulations.

Given that isolated NTDs are transmitted in a multifactorial fashion with both genetic and environmental components to their etiology, the goal of our research program has been to utilize animal model systems in order to ask questions concerning the underlying genetic factors regulating susceptibility to NTDs. This review article details our efforts to arrive at a number of candidate genes for further evaluation in human epidemiological studies.

MOUSE NEURAL TUBE DEFECT MODELS

Hyperthermia-Induced Neural Tube Defects

In order to have sufficient numbers of embryos with which to examine altered patterns of gene expression, it is necessary to have experimental paradigms that con-

TABLE 1. The effect of maternal hyperthermia treatment on the number of implants, resorptions, live-born fetuses, exencephalic fetuses, and exencephalic litters

Strain	Treatment day	No. litters	Implants (mean ± SEM)	Resorptions (%)	Live-born	No. exencephaly (%)	No. exencephalic litters (%)
DBA/2J	Control[a]	10	6.7 ± 0.56	26.9	49	0 (0)	0 (0)
	8:0	10	5.8 ± 0.55	43.0	33	0 (0)	0 (0)
	8:12	10	5.8 ± 0.61	53.4	27	0 (0)	0 (0)
	9:00	14	5.5 ± 0.51	26.0	57	0 (0)	0 (0)
C57BL/6J	Control[a]	8	5.0 ± 0.78	10.0	36	0 (0)	0 (0)
	8:0	15	6.9 ± 0.27	22.3	80	8 (10.0)	8 (53.3)
	8:12	14	6.7 ± 0.38	38.3	58	1 (1.7)	1 (7.1)
	9:00	10	5.4 ± 0.65	13.0	47	0 (0)	0 (0)
SWR/J	Control	10	9.4 ± 0.92	4.3	90	0 (0)	0 (0)
	8:0	10	9.6 ± 0.58	43.8	54	4 (7.4)	1 (10)
	8:12	14	10.1 ± 0.50	7.9	139	19 (13.7)	5 (33)
	9:00	10	9.0 ± 0.73	11.1	80	4 (5.0)	2 (20)
LM/Bc	Control	12	9.8 ± 0.48	6.8	109	0 (0)	0 (0)
	8:0	13	8.1 ± 0.50	44.8	58	1 (1.7)	1 (7.7)
	8:12	14	9.9 ± 0.31	9.4	123	17 (13.6)	7 (50)
	9:00	14	9.4 ± 0.44	6.1	124	1 (0.8)	1 (7.1)
SWV	Control	10	12.6 ± 0.56	7.9	116	1 (0.9)	1 (10)
	8:0	11	11.8 ± 1.18	36.2	86	1 (1.1)	1 (10)
	8:12	10	13.6 ± 0.37	22.1	106	47 (44.3)	9 (90)
	9:00	10	12.5 ± 0.43	3.2	121	1 (0.8)	1 (10)

[a]Control data for day 8:12 at 38°C.

sistently reproduce the desired lesions. We have selected two different mouse model systems that have been useful in producing mammalian embryos with anterior NTDs. The first of these systems involves using the physical agent heat to induce maternal hyperthermia. Utilizing a simple procedure of partially submerging restrained mice in a 43°C circulating water bath, it is possible to elevate maternal core temperatures in a reproducible fashion. When pregnant females of several different inbred murine strains were subjected to a 10-minute water-bath exposure during the period of NTC [gestational day (GD) 8.5–10], it was possible to produce varying degrees of exencephaly.[42] The frequency of exencephalic fetuses produced by this procedure was both strain- and time-dependent. When pregnant dams from various strains were treated on GD 8.5, there was a hierarchy of susceptibility to induced NTDs, ranging from the completely resistant (0%) DBA/2J strain to the highly sensitive (44.3%) SWV strain (TABLE 1). The LM/Bc and SWR/J strains displayed a modest sensitivity to heat-induced NTDs (13.6%). When the C57BL/6J dams were treated at GD 8.5, the embryos were almost completely resistant to the heat treatment; however, if the dams were treated 12 hours earlier, on GD 8.0, the frequency was increased to 10% (TABLE 1). Clearly, the SWV strain is unique in its response to the teratogenic treatment. This variation in the response frequencies to an identical

TABLE 2. Percent exencephaly after hyperthermia treatment on day 8:5 in reciprocal crosses

Strain of dam	Strain of sire		
	SWV	LM/Bc	C57BL/6J
SWV	44.3[a]	9.3	5.2
LM/Bc	11.0	13.6	2.2
C57BL/6J	11.0	7.0	1.7

[a] $p < 0.05$; significantly higher response frequency than all other genotypes.

TABLE 3. Beginning and end of each closure under control conditions

Closure	DBA/2J day/hours	LM/Bc day/hours	SWV/SD day/hours
CL 0	8:06	8:18	8:22
CL I	8:16–9:08	8:13–9:01	8:20–9:14
CL II	8:21–9:09	8:21–9:04	9:00–9:12
CL III	8:21–9:10	8:21–9:06	9:00–9:13
CL IV	9:02–9:11	9:00–9:08	9:02–9:14
Complete	9:11	9:08	9:14
Treatment (43°C)	9:12	9:20	10:06
Total delay (h)	1	12	16
% NTDs (43°C)	0	13.6	44.3

environmental insult suggests that there is a strong genetic component in determining susceptibility to heat-induced exencephaly.[42]

In order to determine the mode of inheritance for the hyperthermia-induced NTD sensitivity trait, a series of reciprocal genetic crosses between strains of high (SWV), intermediate (LM/Bc), and low (C57) sensitivity were initiated. The results from these diallelic crosses demonstrate that the high response rate of the SWV strain is rapidly lost in F_1 hybrids when outcrossed to either the LM/Bc or C57 strains (see TABLE 2). The fact that the F_1 fetuses had response frequencies similar to the low sensitivity parental strains suggests that the genetic basis for the high susceptibility to heat-induced NTDs involves only a few recessive genes that may be unique to the SWV strain. Equally important from these studies was the finding that it was the embryo's genotype, and not that of the mother, that was the critical factor in determining susceptibility to hyperthermia-induced exencephaly.[42]

In terms of the three different inbred mouse strains, there is a very strong association between the length of time that NTC is delayed and susceptibility to NTDs. In the completely resistant DBA/2J strain under control conditions, embryos begin NTC around GD 8:06 and all embryos complete NTC by GD 9:11 (TABLE 3). However, when exposed to the hyperthermia treatment, NTC is delayed by 1 hour and embryos do not complete NTC until GD 9:12. In contrast, the highly NTD-sensitive SWV strain embryos normally initiate NTC by GD 8:22, 16 hours after the DBA/2J embryos, and complete this process by GD 9:14, which is only 3 hours later than control DBA/2J embryos (TABLE 3). However, when the SWV embryos are exposed

TABLE 4. The effect of maternal valproic acid treatment on maternal weight gain[a] **and the number of implants, resorptions, viable fetuses, exencephalic fetuses, and exencephalic litters**

Strain	Treatment day	No. litters	No. implants (mean ± SEM)	Resorptions (%)	No. viable fetuses	No. exencephaly (%)	No. exencephalic litters (%)
DBA/2J	Control[b]	6	8.67 ± 0.49	25	39	0 (0)	0 (0)
	8:06	10	6.10 ± 0.83	32.8	41	0 (0)	0 (0)
	8:12	12	6.00 ± 0.71	31.9	49	0 (0)	0 (0)
	8:18	7	5.71 ± 0.64	30	28	0 (0)	0 (0)
LM/Bc	Control	14	8.93 ± 0.50	5.6	118	0 (0)	0 (0)
	8:06	13	9.00 ± 0.64	3.2	122	20 (16.4)	7 (53.9)
	8:12	11	8.54 ± 0.34	3.2	91	18 (19.8)	7 (63.6)
	8:18	15	8.87 ± 0.36	4.5	127	7 (5.5)	6 (40)
SWV	Control	7	12.00 ± 0.38	6.0	79	0 (0)	0 (0)
	8:06	12	11.42 ± 0.54	17.5	113	17 (15)	6 (50)
	8:12	10	11.50 ± 0.76	15.7	97	34 (35)	8 (80)
	8:18	14	12.00 ± 0.41	17.3	139	33 (23.7)	10 (71.4)

[a]Weight gained from day 0 until sacrifice on GD 15:12.
[b]Control data for day 8:12 vehicle injection.

to teratogenic heat treatments, NTC is delayed to GD 10:06 in those embryos that are capable of completing closure, a delay of 16 hours from control embryos. In the moderately sensitive LM/Bc strain, 14% of the heat-treated fetuses will exhibit NTDs. In these mice, the neural tube will normally close by GD 9:08 hours. However, when the dam is treated at 43°C, there is a 12-hour delay in the length of time it takes for the neural tube to close. LM/Bc embryos that are heat-treated do not complete NTC until day 9:20. This significant difference in the time that it takes the embryos to close their neural tubes following teratogenic insult is consistent with their genetically determined sensitivity (TABLE 1). Understanding the genetic regulation of these responses is essential in identifying potential candidate genes conferring sensitivity (or resistance) to environmentally induced NTDs.

Valproic Acid–Induced Neural Tube Defects

A second teratogenic agent that has been used to learn more about gene-environment interactions as they relate to NTD susceptibility is the antiepileptic drug, valproic acid (VPA, Depakene®). This widely prescribed drug is associated with a 1–2% rate of NTDs in humans.[30–32] When the same inbred mouse strains as previously described in the maternal hyperthermia study were treated with a single ip injection of VPA (600 mg/kg body weight) on GD 8:12, we consistently observed the same hierarchy of susceptibility as was noted in the hyperthermia studies (see TABLE 4). The peak sensitivity to VPA-induced NTDs occurred when the drug was administered on GD 8:12. At that time, 19.8% of the exposed LM/Bc fetuses had NTDs, as compared with 35% of the SWV fetuses. The response frequency in the SWV strain could be increased to 100% with a second ip injection, 6 hours later, at GD 8:18 (Craig *et al.*, personal communication). As the treatment (environment) was held constant, the observed differences in NTD response frequency strongly suggest an underlying genetic contribution.

One potential mechanism by which VPA may exert its teratogenic effects is via altered folate metabolism. When folinic acid was coadministered with teratogenic concentrations of VPA, there was a significant reduction in the frequency of NTDs in Han:NMRI inbred mice.[43–45] While the total folate concentrations in either the dam or the embryos remained constant in response to the VPA treatment, there were significant alterations in the concentrations of selected formylated tetrahydrofolates (THFs).[44,45] Specifically, VPA reduced the concentration of both 5- and 10-formyl-THFs, as well as the 5-CH_3-THF metabolites. This decrease in the formylated THFs could be the result of a VPA-induced block in the interconversion of THF and the formylated metabolites by the enzyme glutamate formyltransferase.[44,45] When these metabolites were measured in VPA-exposed embryos from the NTD-sensitive (SWV) and resistant (DBA/2J) strains, there were significant differences in their metabolic profiles. Specifically, there was an 86–92% inhibition of the 5-CHO-THF and 5-CH_3-THF metabolites in the SWV embryos, while the DBA/2J embryos had no alterations in their 5-CH_3-THF concentrations and only a 50% inhibition in the 5-CHO-THF metabolite. This alteration in the production of specific folate metabolites may adversely affect purine biosynthesis, which could have significant consequences on the embryo's ability to synthesize DNA. Similarly, it may also result in a reduction in the rate of DNA methylation, which could lead to a lack of essential gene expression during critical periods of NTC, resulting in the development of the NTD.[46,47]

Gene Expression Studies in Mouse NTD Model Systems

Having identified inbred mouse strains that are either highly sensitive or highly resistant to a variety of both physical and chemical agents known to induce NTDs, experiments were designed to understand how the inbred mouse strains might differ in their response to the teratogens at both the biochemical and molecular levels. Specifically, our interest was in identifying those genetic processes that regulate the expression of anterior NTDs in the genetically sensitive mice. The experimental strategy involved identifying loci in the mice with expression patterns that were altered by the maternal teratogenic treatment and subsequently determining how this altered expression translated into abnormal neural development.

In the past, the problem in studying alterations in gene expression in response to teratogenic treatment has been the limited availability of sufficient quantities of embryonic material from which to isolate mRNA and ultimately develop cDNA libraries. With the advent of newer molecular biological approaches such as *in situ* transcription and antisense (aRNA) amplification, it was possible to circumvent these problems and examine gene expression directly in developing embryos. The experimental protocols for these types of gene expression studies have been previously described in some detail.[39,40,46–48] Briefly, staged embryos from both control or teratogen-treated dams were harvested at selected time points, generally GD 8:18, 9:0, and 9:12. The neural tube tissue is teased away from the remainder of the embryo using tungsten needles under a Wild M8 (Heerbrugg, Switzerland) dissecting microscope. The desired tissue is primed with an unlabeled oligo-dT-T7 amplification oligonucleotide for several hours at 37°C. This incubation is followed by the addition of reverse transcriptase and both labeled and unlabeled deoxynucleotides.[49,50] This reaction copies endogenous poly A$^+$ mRNA into cDNA along with the T7 promoter, while preserving the anatomical distribution of the cDNA transcripts, allowing studies to be conducted within specific regions of any structure in the developing embryo. The *in situ* transcribed cDNAs are made double-stranded by self-priming followed by a brief S1-nuclease treatment and blunt ending with T4 DNA polymerase and the Klenow fragment. The double-stranded cDNA is used as a template for the synthesis of amplified, antisense RNA (aRNA) following the addition of T7 RNA polymerase and ribonucleotides. This aRNA, whose abundance is increased several thousand-fold after a single round of amplification, has a high degree of fidelity to the original mRNA population in the embryonic neuroepithelium.

Gene transcriptional activity within the neuroepithelium of developing embryos, both within and between the two inbred mouse strains exposed to teratogenic concentrations of VPA, was compared by analyses of variance. This was accomplished by first calculating and comparing the means between control and VPA treatment groups for each time point and strain, calculating the means of the differences between the two treatment groups, and then contrasting these mean differences for significance ($p < 0.05$) across strains. Several cell cycle checkpoint genes including *bcl-2* and *p53* were evaluated for changes in VPA-induced expression, and these data can be seen in FIGURE 1. The overall expression of these genes was downregulated in response to the VPA treatment in the SWV embryos collected at GD 8:18, although these changes were not statistically significant (FIG. 1; $p > 0.05$). In contrast, the VPA treatment significantly upregulated the expression of both *bcl-2* and *p53* at GD 8:18 in the LM/Bc embryos (FIG. 1; $p < 0.05$). The relative expression was increased by 2- to 3-fold over that observed in the control embryos (FIG. 1). Furthermore, the level of expression in the VPA-treated LM/Bc embryos differed significantly from the expression observed in the SWV embryos for these two genes at GD 8:18 (FIG. 1; $p < 0.05$). In terms of growth factor genes, the expression of *bdnf*

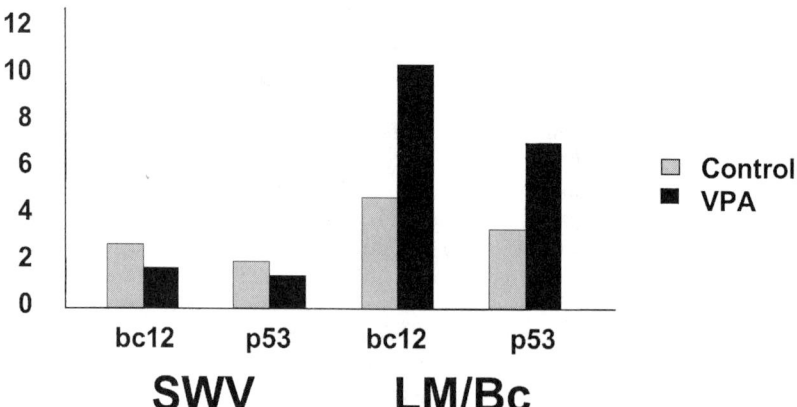

FIGURE 1. Cell cycle regulatory genes evaluated for changes in VPA-treated expression (GD 8:18 embryos).

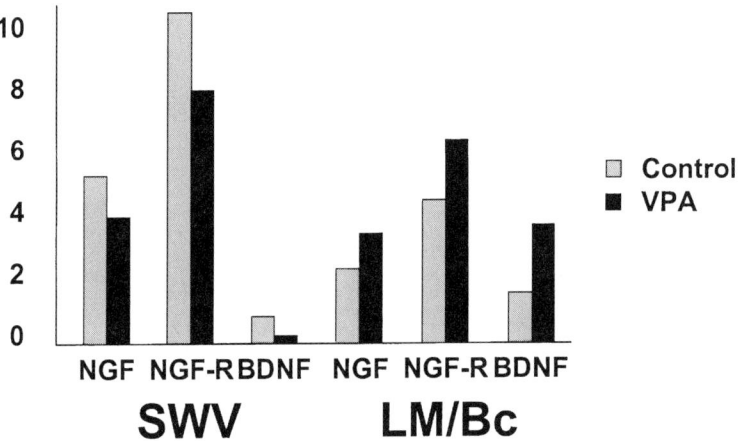

FIGURE 2. Expression of growth factor genes induced by VPA treatment (GD 8:18 embryos).

(brain-derived neurotrophic factor), *ngf* (nerve growth factor), and its receptor (*ngf-R*) were all significantly induced by the VPA treatment in the neuroepithelium dissected from the LM/Bc embryos at GD 8:18, which is 6 hours after treatment (FIG. 2). The teratogenic treatment induced expression of some of these growth factors by 2- to 3-fold. By contrast, exposure to a teratogenic dose of VPA failed to induce any significant alterations of these three genes in the neuroepithelium collected from SWV embryos (FIG. 2).

Finally, the changes in expression patterns for three folate pathway related genes can be seen in FIGURE 3. Although the mean expression level of *Folbp1* significantly decreased ($p < 0.05$) in response to VPA treatment in the SWV embryos at GD 8:18 compared to controls, the transcriptional activity of this gene remained significantly higher in these embryos than in the LM/Bc embryos ($p < 0.05$). The transcriptional activity of the *Folbp2* gene, however, remained significantly higher in the LM/Bc embryos compared to the level of expression seen in the SWV embryos ($p < 0.05$). Furthermore, the mean expression levels of the *MTHFR* gene were significantly increased in response to VPA treatment in the LM/Bc embryos compared to controls ($p < 0.05$; FIG. 3). This increase in transcriptional activity of *MTHFR* persisted among the LM/Bc embryos at each collection time point compared to the SWV embryos ($p < 0.05$).

In general, it appeared that teratogenic concentrations of VPA had a differential effect on the expression of several genes that are important to normal embryonic development. The gene expression data collected to date suggest that subtle, collective changes in several molecules, each of which by themselves may be developmentally harmless, together produce the adverse phenotypic changes that may result in the observed NTDs. Clearly, cell cycle and growth factor genes are involved, and these changes may well be folate-responsive. Taken in light of the recent observation in

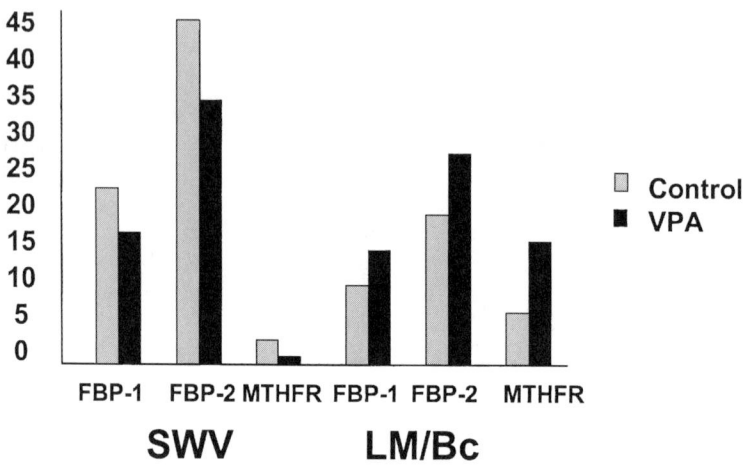

FIGURE 3. Expression of three folate pathway genes induced by VPA treatment (GD 8:18 embryos).

human epidemiological studies that folic acid supplementation could modify NTD risk, subsequent experiments were focused on the folate binding proteins as candidate genes for NTDs.[46,47]

FOLATE RECEPTOR ALPHA STUDIES

We raised the hypothesis that embryos with a subtle mutation in the FRα gene would be compromised in their ability to harvest sufficient folate from the placenta to ensure an adequate supply during embryogenesis and thus be at risk for an NTD or other congenital malformation.[46,47] This hypothesis was examined in both an animal model system and a human epidemiological investigation.

Folate Binding Protein-1 Knockout Mouse Model

Based upon the proposed function of the folate receptor, we sought to determine if it might be involved in maternal to fetal folate transport by inactivating the mouse folate receptors (*Folbp1*). Using homologous recombination in embryonic stem cells,[51] we produced embryos with a reduced ability to internalize folate. Crosses between mice heterozygous for the *Folbp1* gene deletion produced small litters compared with the wild-type controls. The surviving *Folbp1* progeny were physically indistinguishable and developed into apparently healthy adults. When the survivors were genotyped, there were no nullizygous embryos, indicating it was an embryonic lethal. In order to collect nullizygous embryos, the heterozygous crosses were collected at different gestational stages during early embryogenesis. The *Folbp1* nullizygous (−/−) embryos collected in this manner were found to have severe morphogenetic abnormalities and died *in utero* by GD 10.

Histologic examination of transverse sections of GD 8:12 nullizygous embryos revealed dramatic defects in the neuroepithelium. In the cephalic neural tube, neither the forebrain nor the optic vesicles were formed and the neuroepithelium was of very limited thickness. At the level of the midbrain, the neuroepithelium of both the basal and alar plates was also limited to less than two cells in thickness. The migration of the neural crest cells was adversely affected and only small aggregates of cells were identified within the mesenchyme in the region of the first branchial arch. In addition, there was no evidence of neural cell condensations lateral to the alar plate where the trigeminal ganglia normally develop. The neuroepithelial defect observed in the forebrain continued caudally. At the level of the otic placode, the neural tube remained widely flared and thinned, and the ectoderm forming the otic pit was thin and poorly defined. Caudal to the otic pit, the wild-type embryo's neural tube was closed, but the mutant's neuroepithelium remained open.

The targeted disruption of the *Folbp1* gene altered critical embryological events in nullizygous embryos that were incompatible with normal morphogenesis. This observation strongly supports the hypothesis that the folate receptor gene product is essential for intrauterine viability. *Folbp1* supplies the proper amount of folate to tissues at critical times during embryogenesis by concentrating it and delivering it to the cytoplasm of epithelialized cells.[52] A deficiency in plasma folate could secondarily result in elevated fetal homocysteine levels, which may be teratogenic.[53] The abnormalities occurring in embryos lacking *Folbp1* affirm that the high-affinity uptake of folate by cells is critically important to the folate homeostasis of the developing embryo. These results suggest that *Folbp1* plays a critical role in folate homeostasis during development and that functional defects in the homologue (FRα) of *Folbp1* may contribute to similar defects in humans.

Folate Receptor Alpha Human Epidemiological Investigations

In humans, folate receptors are encoded by a family of genes with three functional loci (α, β, and γ) and a pseudogene organized in tandem orientation on chromosome 11q13.[54,55] The predominant cell types that express FRα are epithelia that separate fluid spaces with different 5-MeTHF concentrations, including the proximal tubule brush border, the choroid plexus, the placenta, the lung, and the thyroid.[56–58] FRα possesses the highest affinity for the physiological form of folate, 5-MeTHF, and is the only member of the folate receptor gene family that would be near saturation at normal folate concentrations.[56,59] The genomic sequence of the FRα locus is slightly over 2 kb in length, including the 5′ and 3′ untranslated regions (UTRs). Given the importance of the receptor-mediated transport mechanism and the epidemiological evidence suggesting that folic acid is an important environmental factor modulating NTD risks, we hypothesized that human genetic variation of FRα that compromises expression or protein function might be associated with an increased risk for an NTD. We tested this hypothesis by searching for molecular genetic variation of the FRα gene among a large group of fetuses or infants with NTDs.

DNA analysis was conducted on whole blood spotted onto Guthrie cards, collected from newborn infants who were participants in two population-based case-control

TABLE 5. Study I: single-strand conformation analysis (SSCP) of the human folate receptor

Exon	Sample numbers	Result
3	cases = 163 controls = 902	1065 wt
5	cases = 126 controls = 393	519 wt
6	cases = 22 controls = 82	104 wt

NOTE: wt = homozygous for wild-type gene sequence.

studies conducted by the California Birth Defects Monitoring Program (CBDMP). Detailed descriptions of the case-control study have been previously published.[8,60,61] A protocol for the individual studies was approved by the State Committee for the Protection of Human Subjects. Fetuses or infants with spina bifida were ascertained by reviewing medical records, including prenatal diagnostic records, at all hospitals and genetic service providers for infants delivered in California counties (all except Los Angeles, Riverside, and Ventura) and whose mothers gave their residences as California. Eligible were live-born infants and fetuses diagnosed with spina bifida among the total cohort of 1,052,343 births between January 1987 and December 1988 and between June 1989 and May 1991. Control births were randomly selected from each surveillance area hospital in proportion to the hospital's estimated contribution to the total population of live-born infants in a given month from June 1989 to May 1991 or were randomly selected from all infants born alive during 1987–1988. The control infants had no apparent congenital malformations.

Residual blood specimens taken in the newborn period for PKU screening were the source of DNA from cases and controls. Live-born case and control infants were matched to the stored blood specimens. Blood spots were obtained and then stored at −80°C until genomic DNA was extracted using the Puregene DNA extraction kit (Gentra Systems, Minneapolis, MN) as per the manufacturer's instructions. The investigation of FRα as an NTD candidate locus was carried out in two parts. For study I, over 700 CBDMP blood spots were extracted and processed by SSCP for mutational analysis. The sample set for study II consisted of a group of 180 CBDMP blood spots, stratified into classes by maternal folate status (with or without multivitamin containing folic acid supplementation) and pregnancy outcome (normal or spina bifida–affected). The three exons of interest (III, V, and VI) of the 5-MeTHF receptor gene were amplified with primer sequences designed to span the entire exon sequence, yielding products ranging in size from 131 bases to 279 bases. The protocols have been previously published in detail.[62]

Study I

The results of the SSCP screening analysis of exons III, V, and VI of the FRα gene are summarized in TABLE 5. The number of samples examined for each exon varied considerably, with the emphasis placed on exons V and VI as these two regions of the

TABLE 6. Study II: dideoxy fingerprinting (ddF) analysis of the human FRα locus

Exon	Folate supplementation	Pregnancy outcome	Sample size	Result (wt = wild type)
3	+	control	60	60 wt
	+	case	39	39 wt
	−	control	60	60 wt
	−	case	60	60 wt
4	+	control	60	60 wt
	+	case	39	39 wt
	−	control	60	60 wt
	−	case	60	60 wt
5	+	control	60	60 wt
	+	case	39	39 wt
	−	control	60	60 wt
	−	case	60	60 wt
6	+	control	60	60 wt
	+	case	39	39 wt
	−	control	60	60 wt
	−	case	60	60 wt

coding sequence are believed to be the most important to the protein's function. Although over 2000 samples were analyzed (33% cases and 67% controls), there were no individuals who were identified as having a polymorphism in this gene.

Study II

The results of the ddF analysis of exons III–VI of the FRα gene for 180 individuals stratified by maternal use, or nonuse, of vitamins containing folic acid and by pregnancy outcome are detailed in TABLE 6. As in the previous study, we found no polymorphisms utilizing the ddF approach. Thus, neither SSCP nor dideoxy DNA fingerprinting identified either polymorphisms or silent mutations in the coding region or intronic bases surrounding the intron-exon boundaries of the FRα locus.

This investigation was initiated to examine the potential association between the FRα gene and susceptibility to NTDs. We hypothesized that individuals with an uncommon gene variant for FRα will be at an increased risk for an NTD as a result of altered folate receptor function. These abnormal receptors would be less efficient at binding and providing available 5-MeTHF to the cytoplasm of the target cells at critical periods of development. Such decreased affinity may significantly compromise receptor saturation in the syncytiotrophoblast and neuroepithelium, thereby increasing the risk of embryonic folate deprivation. In the epidemiological studies described herein, we sought to determine if, in fact, polymorphisms did exist in the FRα gene, but failed to identify any polymorphisms in the coding region of this gene. This suggests that abnormalities in the FRα gene must be sufficiently rare and therefore not likely to contribute substantially to the population burden of NTDs.

There are several possible explanations for the lack of polymorphism observed within the FR. The most obvious possibility is that this gene is essential for normal developmental processes and any mutations result in embryonic lethality. Orr and Kamen[63] have identified a mutant version of the FR that appears to confer a dominant-negative phenotype. Three mutations in the open reading frame of FRα were discovered in a squamous cell carcinoma cell line that was unable to bind either folic acid or 5-MeTHF. Each of the mutant alleles was found to produce a protein incapable of binding folate. When a receptor-positive cell line containing a normal copy of the FR gene was transfected with a plasmid containing one of the mutant alleles, its ability to bind folate decreased significantly, although normal receptor production increased. The presence of such a dominant-negative mutation in tumor cells has important implications. It may not be necessary for an individual to possess two defective copies of the receptor gene to exhibit a negative phenotype with respect to folate accumulation. In this case, all nonsynonymous mutations arising within the locus would be exposed to strong negative selection. As a result, individuals lacking a functional copy of the FRα gene would not continue development to term. Furthermore, the aforementioned transgenic knockout mouse studies[51] support this conclusion.

SUMMARY

Utilizing a variety of experimental approaches and model systems, it has been possible to identify potential candidate genes that regulate sensitivity to complex human congenital malformations, such as NTDs. While it is clear that there could be multiple developmental pathways that lead to the formation of the same clinically important malformations, the interactions between environmental factors and target genes are critically important to the regulation of these developmental pathways. The evidence from the mouse model systems would suggest that multiple genes are involved, perhaps in an additive fashion, which can set the embryo on a path of abnormal neural development if the regulation of these genes is perturbed by exogenous factors. While there does not appear at this time to be one single major gene contributing to the risk for NTDs, the model systems have proven their worth in efficiently identifying candidate genes that can be further explored in human molecular epidemiological investigations.

ACKNOWLEDGMENTS

The studies described in this manuscript were supported in part by Grant Nos. DE11303, DE13613, ES07165, ES/HD35396, and P30-ES09106 from the National Institutes of Environmental Health Sciences; Grant No. NS31171 from the National Institutes of Health; as well as Grant Nos. FY97-0583 and FY98-893 from the March of Dimes Birth Defects Foundation. Its contents are solely the responsibility of the authors and do not necessarily represent the official views of the NIEHS, NIH. We appreciate the technical assistance of T. Biela, J. Woodings, and D. Dichoso for the care and well-being of the animals.

REFERENCES

1. HUNTER, A.G. 1993. Brain and spinal cord. *In* Human Malformations and Related Anomalies. Volume II, pp. 74–86. Oxford University Press. London/New York.
2. NAKANO, K.K. 1973. Anencephaly: a review. J. Ment. Defic. Res. **1:** 4–15.
3. HOLMES, L.B., S.G. Driscoll & L. Atkins. 1976. Etiologic heterogeneity of neural tube defects. N. Engl. J. Med. **294:** 365–369.
4. CAMPBELL, L.R., D.H. DAYTON & G.S. SOHAL. 1986. Neural tube defects: a review of human and animal studies on the etiology of neural tube defects. Teratology **34:** 171–187.
5. FRASER, F.C. & J.J. NORA. 1986. Genetics of Man, pp. 187–189. Lea & Febiger. Philadelphia.
6. ERICKSON, J.D. 1976. Racial variations in incidence of congenital malformations. Ann. Hum. Genet. **39:** 315–320.
7. ELWOOD, J.M., J. LITTLE & J.H. EELWOOD. 1992. Epidemiology and Control of Neural Tube Defects. Oxford University Press. London/New York.
8. SHAW, G.M., N.G. JENSVOLD & C.R. WASSERMAN. 1994. Epidemiologic characteristics of phenotypically distinct neural tube defects among 0.7 million California births, 1983–1987. Teratology **49:** 143–149.
9. LAMMER, E.J., S.T. CHEN & R.M. HOAR. 1985. Retinoic acid embryopathy. N. Engl. J. Med. **313:** 837–841.
10. WHITE, F.M.M., F.G. COHEN, G. SHERMAN & R. MCCURDY. 1988. Chemicals, birth defects, and stillbirths in New Brunswick: associations with agricultural activity. CMAJ **138:** 117–123.
11. HOLMBERG, P.C. 1979. Central-nervous-system defects in children born to mothers exposed to organic solvents during pregnancy. Lancet **2:** 177–179.
12. BRENDER, J.D. & L. SUAREZ. 1990. Paternal occupation and anencephaly. Am. J. Epidemiol. **131:** 517–521.
13. MATTE, T.D., J. MULINARE & J.D. ERICKSON. 1993. Case-control study of congenital defects and parental employment in health care. Am. J. Ind. Med. **24:** 11–23.
14. SEVER, L.E., N.A. HESOL, E.S. GILBERT & J.M. MCINTYRE. 1988. The prevalence at birth of congenital malformations in communities near the Hanford site. Am. J. Epidemiol. **127:** 243–254.
15. SEVER, L.E. 1995. Looking for causes of neural tube defects: where does the environment fit in? Environ. Health Perspect. **103**(suppl. 6): 165–171.
16. EDMONDS, L.D., C.E. ANDERSON, J.W. FLYNT & L.M. JAMES. 1978. Congenital central nervous system malformations and vinyl chloride monomer exposure: a community study. Teratology **17:** 137–142.
17. THERIAULT, G., H. ITURRA & S. GINGRAS. 1983. Evaluation of the association between birth defects and exposure to ambient vinyl chloride. Teratology **27:** 359–370.
18. ROSENMAN, K.D., J.E. RIZZO, M.G. CONOMOS & G.J. HALPIN. 1989. Central nervous system malformations in relation to two polyvinyl chloride production facilities. Arch. Environ. Health **44:** 238–282.
19. MONTELEONE-NETO, R., D. BRUNONI, R. LAURENTI, H.M. JORGE, S.L.D. GOTLIEB & M.L. LEBRAO. 1985. Birth defects and environmental pollution: the Cubatao example. Prog. Clin. Biol. Res. **163B:** 65–68.
20. DORSCH, M.M., R.K.R. SCRAGG, A.J. MCMICHAEL, P.A. BAGHURST & K.F. DYER. 1984. Congenital malformations and maternal drinking water supply in rural South Australia: a case-control study. Am. J. Epidemiol. **119:** 473–486.
21. ARBUCKLE, T.E., G.J. SHERMAN, P.H. COREY, D. WALTERS & B. LO. 1988. Water nitrates and CNS birth defects: a population-based case-control study. Arch. Environ. Health **43:** 162–167.
22. BECKMAN, L. 1978. The Ronnskar smelter—occupational and environmental effects in and around a polluting industry in Northern Sweden. Ambio **7:** 226–231.
23. BOLLIGER, C.T., P. VANZIGL & J.A. LOAW. 1992. Multiple organ failure with adult respiratory distress syndrome in homicidal arsenic poisoning. Respiration **59:** 57–61.
24. LUGO, G., G. CASSADY & P. PALMISANO. 1969. Acute maternal arsenic intoxication with neonatal death. Am. J. Dis. Child. **117:** 328–330.

25. ZIERLER, S., M. THEODORE, A. COHEN & K.J. ROTHMAN. 1988. Chemical quality of maternal drinking water and congenital heart disease. Int. J. Epidemiol. **17:** 589–594.
26. MILLER, P., D.W. SMITH & T.H. SHEPARD. 1978. Maternal hyperthermia as a possible cause of anencephaly. Lancet **1:** 519–521.
27. LAYDE, P.M., L.D. EDMONDS & J.D. ERICKSON. 1980. Maternal fever and neural tube defects. Teratology **21:** 105–108.
28. ERICKSON, J.D. 1991. Risk factors for birth defects: data from the Atlanta birth defects case control study. Teratology **43:** 41–51.
29. FINNELL, R.H., M. VAN WAES, G.D. BENNETT & J.H. EBERWINE. 1993. Lack of concordance between heat shock proteins and the development of tolerance to teratogen-induced neural tube defects. Dev. Genet. **14:** 137–147.
30. ROBERT, E. 1982. Valproic acid and spina bifida: a preliminary report—France. CDC Morb. Mortal. Wkly. Rep. **31:** 565–566.
31. ROBERT, E. & P. GUIBAUDY. 1982. Maternal valproic acid and congenital neural tube defects. Lancet **11:** 937.
32. LAMMER, E.J., L.E. SEVER & G.P. OAKLEY, JR. 1987. Teratogen update: valproic acid. Teratology **35:** 465–473.
33. ROSA, F.W. 1991. Spina bifida in infants of women treated with carbamazepine during pregnancy. N. Engl. J. Med. **324:** 674–677.
34. LINDHOUT, D., H. MEINARDI, J.W.A. MEIJER & H. NAU. 1992. Antiepileptic drugs and teratogenesis in two consecutive cohorts: changes in prescription policy paralleled by changes in pattern of malformations. Neurology **42**(suppl. 5): 94–110.
35. FINNELL, R.H. 1991. Genetic differences in susceptibility to anticonvulsant drug-induced developmental defects. Pharmacol. Toxicol. **69:** 223–227.
36. BJERKEDAL, T., A. CZEIZEL, J. GOUJARD, B. KALLEN, P. MASTROIACORA, N. NEVIN, G. OAKLEY & E. ROBERT. 1982. Valproic acid and spina bifida. Lancet **2**(8302): 1096.
37. LINDOUT, D., R.D.J.E. HOEPPENER & H. MEINARDI. 1984. Teratogenicity of antiepileptic drug combinations with special emphasis on epoxidation (of carbamazepine). Epilepsia **25:** 77–83.
38. LINDHOUT, D. & D. SCHMIDT. 1986. *In-utero* exposure to valproate and neural tube defects. Lancet **1**(8494): 1392–1393.
39. WLORDARCZYK, B., G.D. BENNETT, J. CALVIN, J.C. CRAIG & R.H. FINNELL. 1996. Arsenic induced changes in transcription factor gene expression: implications for abnormal neural development. Dev. Genet. **18:** 306–315.
40. WLORDARCZYK, B., G.D. BENNETT, J.A. CALVIN & R.H. FINNELL. 1996. Arsenic induced neural tube defects in mice: alterations in cell cycle gene expression. Reprod. Toxicol. **10:** 447–454.
41. SHALAT, S.L., D.R. WALKER & R.H. FINNELL. 1996. The role of arsenic as a reproductive toxin and particular attention to neural tube defects. J. Toxicol. Environ. Health **48:** 101–120.
42. FINNELL, R.H., S.P. MOON, L.C. ABBOTT, J.A. GOLDEN & G.F. CHERNOFF. 1986. Strain differences in heat-induced neural tube defects in mice. Teratology **33:** 247–252.
43. TROTZ, M., C. WEGNER & H. NAU. 1987. Valproic acid induced neural tube defects reduction by folinic acid in the mouse. Life Sci. **41:** 103–110.
44. WEGNER, C. & H. NAU. 1991. Diurnal variation of folate concentrations in mouse embryo and plasma: the protective effect of folinic acid on valproic acid–induced teratogenicity is time-dependent. Reprod. Toxicol. **5:** 465–471.
45. WEGNER, C. & H. NAU. 1992. Alteration of embryonic folate metabolism by valproic acid during organogenesis: implications for mechanism of teratogenesis. Neurology **42**(suppl. 5): 17–24.
46. HEFER, T., H.Z. JOACHIMS, D. CARLSON & R.H. FINNELL. 1998. Factors associated with the etiology of congenital craniofacial anomalies: I. An update. J. Isr. Med. Assoc. **135:** 209–213.
47. HEFER, T., H.Z. JOACHIMS, D. CARLSON & R.H. FINNELL. 1998. Factors associated with the etiology of congenital craniofacial anomalies: II. Molecular mechanisms. J. Isr. Med. Assoc. **135:** 286–291.
48. GELINEAU–VAN WAES, J., G.D. BENNETT & R.H. FINNELL. 1999. Phenytoin-induced alterations in craniofacial gene expression. Teratology **59:** 23–34.

49. EBERWINE, J.H., C.M. SPENCER, K. MIYASHIRO, S.A. MACKLER & R.H. FINNELL. 1992. cDNA synthesis *in situ*: methods and applications. Methods Enzymol. **216:** 80–100.
50. EBERWINE, J.H., H. YEH, K. MIYASHIRO, Y. CAO, S. NAIR, R. FINNELL, M. ZETTEL & P. COLEMAN. 1992. Analysis of gene expression in single live neurons. Proc. Natl. Acad. Sci. U.S.A. **89:** 3010–3014.
51. PIEDRAHITA, J.A., B. OETAMA, G.D. BENNETT, J. VAN WAES, S.W. LACEY, B.A. KAMEN, J.A. RICHARDSON, R.G. ANDERSON & R.H. FINNELL. 1999. Mice lacking the folic acid–binding protein are defective in early embryonic development. Nat. Genet. **23:** 228–232.
52. ANDERSON, R.G.W., B.A. KAMEN, K.G. ROTHBERG & S.W. LACEY. 1992. Potocytosis: sequestration and transport of small molecules by caveolae. Science **255:** 410–411.
53. STEEGERS-THEUNISSEN, R.P., G.H. BOERS, F.J. TRIJBELS, J.D. FINKELSTEIN, H.J. BLOM, C.M. THOMAS, G.F. BORM, M.G. WONTERS & T.K. ESKES. 1994. Maternal hyperhomocysteinemia: a risk factor for neural-tube defects? Metab. Clin. Exp. **43:** 1475–1480.
54. LACEY, S.W., J.M. SANDERS, K.G. ROTHBERG, R.G. ANDERSON & B.A. KAMEN. 1989. Complementary DNA for the folate binding protein correctly predicts anchoring to the membrane by glycosyl phosphatidylinositol. J. Clin. Invest. **84**(2)**:** 715–720.
55. RAGOUSSIS, J., G. SENGER, J. TROWSDALE & I.G. CAMPBELL. 1992. Genomic organization of the human folate receptor genes on chromosome 11q13. Genomics **14:** 423–430.
56. ROSS, J.F., P.K. CHAUDHURI & M. RATNAM. 1994. Differential regulation of folate receptor isoforms in normal and malignant tissues *in vivo* and in established cell lines. Cancer **73**(9)**:** 2432–2443.
57. WEITMAN, S.D., R.H. LARK, L.R. CONEY, D.W. FORT, V. FRANSCA, V.R. ZURAWSKI & B.A. KAMEN. 1992. Distribution of the folate receptor GP38 in normal and malignant cell lines and tissues. Cancer Res. **52:** 3396–3401.
58. WEITMAN, S.D., A.G. WEINBERG, L.R. CONEY, V.R. ZURAWSKI, D.S. JENNINGS & B.A. KAMEN. 1992. Cellular localization of the folate receptor: potential role in drug toxicity and folate homeostasis. Cancer Res. **52:** 6708–6711.
59. WILLIS, S.A., S.W. LACEY, S.D. WEITMAN, B.A. KAMEN & P.D. NISEN. 1992. Folate receptor gene expression is tissue-specific and temporally-regulated. Cancer Ther. Control **2:** 223–230.
60. SHAW, G.M., E.J. LAMMER, C.R. WASSERMAN, C.D. O'MALLEY & M.M. TOLAROVA. 1995. Risks of orofacial clefts in children born to women using multivitamins containing folic acid periconceptionally. Lancet **345:** 393–396.
61. WASSERMAN, C.R., G.M. SHAW, C.D. O'MALLEY, M.M. TOLAROVA & E.J. LAMMER. 1996. Parental cigarette smoking and risk for congenital anomalies of the heart, neural tube, or limb. Teratology **53:** 261–267.
62. BARBER, R.C., G.M. SHAW, E.J. LAMMER & K.A. GREER. 1998. Lack of association between mutations in the folate receptor-α gene and spina bifida. Am. J. Med. Genet. **76**(4)**:** 310–317.
63. ORR, R.B. & B.A. KAMEN. 1995. Identification of a point mutation in the folate receptor gene that confers a dominant negative phenotype. Cancer Res. **55:** 847–852.

Transient Modulation of Gene Expression in the Neurulation Staged Mouse Embryo

E. SIDNEY HUNTER III[a] AND PHILLIP HARTIG

Reproductive Toxicology Division, National Health and Environmental Effects Research Laboratory, United States Environmental Protection Agency, Research Triangle Park, North Carolina, USA

ABSTRACT: Transient modulation of gene expression in the embryo during early organogenesis will allow studies to be conducted that determine tissue- and stage-specific function(s) of genes. To achieve this goal, viral vectors and antisense oligodeoxynucleotides have been used to produce gain-of-function and loss-of-function models. Adenoviral transduction of whole embryos, embryonic heart and vasculature, and primary neural crest cell culture has been reported. The morphological consequences of overexpression or decreasing expression of selected genes have been evaluated using these tools. Gene-teratogen interaction studies have also been performed. The viral vectors appear to be important tools for modulating gene expression and hold great promise for future research.

Transient modulation of gene expression during specific stages of development or in selected tissues will facilitate our understanding of the function(s) of selected genes during development. Additionally, by using this approach, it will also be possible to test hypotheses regarding mechanisms leading to abnormal development and teratogenesis. Because we are interested in altering the function(s) of genes during only selected periods of development or in specific tissues, traditional gene "knockout" or "knock-in" approaches may not be appropriate to answer our questions since, in those models, gene modulation occurs throughout development and not selectively or specifically. Therefore, we have used *in vitro* developmental models, such as mouse whole embryo culture, in combination with antisense oligodeoxynucleotides (ODN) and viral vectors to achieve the goal of transient modulation of gene expression in the embryo or embryonic tissues. We have focused our research and this chapter on modulating gene expression during the developmental period of neurulation in mammalian embryos. This developmental stage encompasses many critical developmental processes, such as closure of the neural tube, neural crest cell development, and early cardiogenesis. Thus, understanding the function of genes and the possible consequences of disrupting gene function during neurulation addresses many important questions.

[a]Address for correspondence: Sid Hunter, MD#67, Developmental Biology Branch, RTD, NHEERL, U.S. EPA, Research Triangle Park, NC 27711. Voice: 919-541-3490; fax: 919-541-4017.

Hunter.sid@epa.gov

For purposes of simplicity, we have discussed viral vector transduction and antisense oligodeoxynucleotides separately. This chapter focuses on the approaches and techniques required for these studies and only briefly discusses the application of these approaches. The necessary information regarding techniques required for culturing whole embryos, organs, or cells is beyond the scope of this chapter.

VIRAL VECTORS

Viral vectors have been used to deliver genes to the neurulation staged mouse embryo,[1,2] developing embryonic heart and vasculature,[3,4] and primary cultures of neural crest cells (unpublished data). We began our studies to determine an effective method to overexpress selected genes in the whole embryo[1] by comparing plasmid DNA (pCMVb, ClonTech) and an E1- and E3-deleted recombinant adenovirus (AdCMVlacZ/sub360; Engelhardt et al., 1993). Both constructs contain a LacZ reporter gene under control of the cytomegalovirus early gene promoter with an SV40 polyadenylation signal. Subsequent studies have used a recombinant baculovirus containing a mammalian CMV promoter[5] and an E1/E4-deleted adenoviral vector [deletion in the E1 region and modified to contain only the orf6 in the E4 region (Ad2 ΔE1&ΔE4 orf6)],[6] both also expressing the LacZ reporter gene. These studies demonstrated that the adenovirus is a more effective tool than the plasmid or baculovirus for expressing the reporter gene in the embryo. Since it is not necessary for the adenovirus to integrate into the embryonic DNA before expression, functional protein is present within 4–6 hours after administration of the virus. This is a much shorter time than that obtained in a hybrid-retroviral vector in neurulation staged embryos, which required 12–24 hours for gene expression.[2] Thus, when it is critical for gene expression to occur during a short time window, with a high level of embryonic transduction, the adenovirus is currently the best vector available.

In addition to LacZ reporter constructs, we have also used a green fluorescent protein (GFP) expressing adenovirus[1] that makes it possible to observe gene expression in living embryos during development. Preliminary studies also suggest that laser confocal microscopic imaging of embryonic GFP expression can be performed. This imaging will allow for a more accurate understanding of which cells are transduced and their subsequent development. Additionally, an adenovirus has been constructed that contains an internal ribosome entry site that is able to express the selected gene of interest and GFP on one mRNA. Using this single viral construct, we have been able to monitor expression of the selected gene by observing GFP fluorescence.

The technique used to deliver the vector to the embryo requires injection of the adenovirus into the amnionic cavity, into other cavities, or directly into the early somite staged embryo. On day 9 of gestation (plug day = 1), early somite staged conceptuses are prepared for culture as previously described.[7] The delivery technique is similar to that used for antisense oligodeoxynucleotide microinjection reported by Sadler et al.[8] A pneumatic IM 300 Narishige microinjector (Narishige, Japan) and handheld microinjectors made of 1-mm glass needles pulled using a model P-87 Flaming/Brown micropipette puller (Sutter Instrument Co.) are used. Glass needles are broken by hand using watchmaker forceps. Needle tips are positioned in the amnionic cavity by traversing the visceral yolk sac and amnionic membrane.

Conceptuses are injected until the amnion is fully distended. Since the amnionic cavity volume varies with gestational age, this approach allows displacement of as much amnionic fluid as possible with the solution of interest and provides a consistent concentration of material to the embryo. In our studies, the mean injection volume was 756 nL.[1] We have injected hundreds of conceptuses and have shown that injection into the amnionic cavity does not disrupt normal development.

Adenoviruses can also be injected into other regions of the embryo as has been shown by Baldwin and colleagues,[3,4] who injected viruses into the pericardial space, the head fold, and the sinus venosus. When an adenovirus with a LacZ reporter gene and CMV promoter was injected into the sinus venosus, beta-galactoside activity was demonstrated in the endothelium of the vasculature. In contrast, when the same reporter gene was used with an RSV promoter, LacZ expression was predominately localized in the myocardium and pericardium. Thus, the tissue-specific expression of a reporter gene was dependent upon the promoter. We have injected a CMV-GFP adenovirus into the heart tube of 2–3 somite mouse embryos and also observed distribution of the GFP in the heart and vasculature.

Gaiano et al.[2] have performed viral infection of neurulation staged embryos in vivo by using an ultrasound backscatter microscopy system that allows visualization of the conceptus in utero. Using this imaging system, they injected a murine leukemia virus–based genome and vesicular stomatitus virus envelope hybrid (VSV pseudotype) into the amnionic cavity, infecting mitotically active cells with a human placental alkaline phosphatase reporter gene. Gaiano reported high levels of reporter gene expression in the brain and spinal cord at day 12.5 of gestation. Although the ability to perform gene transduction experiments in vivo holds great promise, high rates (60%) of embryo lethality and exencephaly (41% of surviving embryos) were observed in these studies.

Malformations produced by viral transduction are not unique to in vivo exposure to virus. We[1] observed severe malformations in early somite mouse embryos injected with adenovirus. Malformations (especially prosencephalic and pharyngeal arch deficiencies) were observed in embryos after administration of a high viral concentration (e.g., 5×10^{10} PFU/mL). Therefore, in all studies using the viral delivery system, it is critical to have appropriate controls and evaluate the potential for the vector to produce defects. Our preliminary results indicate that the Ad2 ΔE1&ΔE4 orf6 adenoviral vector is less toxic than the E1/E3-deficient adenoviral vector used in earlier studies.[1] However, the level of reporter gene expression may be more robust in the E1/E3-deficient vector. Thus, future generations of viral vectors with decreased toxicity and increased gene expression require development.

The research questions that have been asked using viral vectors with neurulation staged embryos have used several approaches. Some have focused on the morphological effects of gain-of-function studies produced by Sonic hedgehog,[2] p53,[9] and Msx-2 in chick embryos in ovo.[10] In another study, Leconte et al.[4] used an adenoviral vector to deliver an antisense fibroblast growth factor-2 (FGF-2) and observed a disruption of vasculogenesis in the embryo and yolk sac. To demonstrate that the effects were mediated by expression of the FGF-2 antisense, they coinjected an adenoviral construct expressing FGF-2 with the antisense FGF-2 construct and observed morphologically normal embryos, verifying that the antisense was responsible for the defects. Our laboratory[9] has shown that expression of p53 in the embryo does not produce dysmorphology, but that p53 overexpression increases the susceptibility of the embryo to the teratogenic effects of arsenite *in vitro*. Thus, gain-of-function, loss-of-function, and gene-teratogen interaction studies have been performed in neurulation staged embryos using viral transduction vectors.

Although not included in this chapter, it is useful to state that viral transduction of zygotes, preimplantation staged embryos, and fetuses has been the focus of much research. Using retroviruses to infect embryonic stem cells to create transgenic animals and using gene therapy tools to "treat" genetic diseases, such as cystic fibrosis, are only two examples of the many studies using viral vectors during the prenatal period. It has also been reported that intravenous administration of plasmid DNA (CAT or LacZ genes) in a Transfectam complex into day 8 or 9 pregnant mice will be expressed in the embryo, fetuses, and neonates.[11] Thus, in addition to gene therapy tools, there are additional methods for delivering exogenous genes to the neurulation staged embryo *in vivo*.

Future studies using viral vectors have tremendous potential. For applications specific to neurulation staged embryos, the utilization of next-generation vectors will likely reduce the embryo toxicity produced by adenoviruses. Refinements of imaging systems, such as the ultrasound system reported by Gaiano *et al.*,[2] will be necessary to facilitate future *in vivo* gene delivery studies. Additional work on promoter-specific tissue expression and techniques to better regulate temporal expression of genes will also be necessary to provide the best methods for understanding gene function during early embryogenesis.

ANTISENSE OLIGODEOXYNUCLEOTIDES

An antisense oligodeoxynucleotide (ODN) is a strand of nucleotides that are a reverse complement to a specific unique nucleotide sequence in the targeted mRNA molecule. One mechanism by which antisense ODNs decrease gene expression is by binding to the complementary sequence of the targeted mRNA, resulting in RNase H degradation of the targeted mRNA. Thus, antisense ODNs produce a decrease in the targeted mRNA, thereby reducing translation and production of protein and resulting in a loss-of-function model.

Antisense ODNs have been used extensively by developmental biologists and are now also being used to answer questions in the field of developmental toxicology. Karen Augustine[12] has written an excellent review on antisense ODNs, including information on their mechanisms for decreasing gene expression and their use in studies of abnormal development.

We have used antisense ODNs to downregulate gene expression in the neurulation staged embryo. The technique of intra-amnionic injection is the same as that described for delivery of viral vectors. A major difference to note between techniques is that, when we use either phosphodiester or phosphorothioate nucleotides, we complex the ODN with Lipofectamine to facilitate the uptake of ODN into the embryonic cells. Many studies have observed significant embryo toxicity following injection with high (~50–100 μM) concentrations of phosphorothioate ODNs. The dysmorphogenesis may be observed in mismatch or scrambled sequences with no known gene homology, suggesting that the effects are independent of the nucleotide sequence. Thus, appropriate ODN controls are critical for these experiments.

Another important consideration for antisense ODN experiments is the half-life of the protein in question. Since exposure to antisense ODN only produces a transient decrease in mRNA, if the protein has a long half-life, or if feedback mechanisms result in an upregulation of mRNA production, it may be difficult to produce a significant decrease in protein content using this approach. In contrast, if the gene in question is developmentally regulated or induced by exposure, then antisense ODNs may effectively prevent an accumulation or increase of protein content in the embryo.

We used antisense ODNs with a phosphodiester backbone (used because they have a short intracellular half-life) directed against Krox-20 or Pax-3 to determine if short-term disruption of these genes would produce dysmorphogenesis (unpublished observation). These constructs did not induce malformations in early somite staged mouse embryos. We have also used phosphorothioate ODNs because they are resistant to nuclease activity and have a longer intracellular half-life. Antisense ODNs directed against heat-shock proteins 70-1/3 (HSP 70-1/3) did not produce sequence-specific dysmorphogenesis. However, the HSP 70-1/3 antisense ODN increased the incidence and severity of arsenic-induced neural tube defects and blocked arsenite induction of the HSP.[13] These studies further establish the critical role of heat-shock proteins in modulating the embryonic response to developmental toxicants and demonstrate one use of antisense ODNs in understanding the mechanisms responsible for developmental toxicity.

Future studies using antisense ODNs will likely continue as next-generation ODNs with less toxicity and higher resistance to cellular degradation become available. We are excited about the possibility of directing ODNs to specific cells based on the presence of specific membrane receptors. In human melanoma cells, a dramatic intracellular increase in antisense ODN was associated with a folic acid–polylysine carrier.[14] Although there is no information regarding the application of this approach in the embryo, this may be an important advancement in ODN delivery.

In summary, there are a number of tools available to modify gene expression in the embryo and embryonic tissues during critical windows of development. Some of these tools are well established in the literature for the study of development and others are just beginning to be used to study the neurulation staged embryos. Further advancements of the tools continue with next-generation oligonucleotides and viral vectors being developed with the goal of decreasing toxicity. Thus, the future holds great promise for research in the area of modulating gene expression in the embryo during selected periods of development and in specific tissues.

DISCLAIMER

This manuscript has been reviewed by the National Health and Environmental Effects Research Laboratory, U.S. EPA and approved for publication. Approval does not signify that the contents necessarily reflect the views and policies of the Agency, nor does mention of trade names or commercial products constitute endorsement or recommendation for use.

REFERENCES

1. HARTIG, P.C. & E.S. HUNTER III. 1998. Gene delivery to the neurulating embryo during culture. Teratology **58:** 103–112.
2. GAIANO, N. *et al.* 1999. A method for rapid gain-of-function studies in the mouse embryonic nervous system. Nat. Neurosci. **2:** 812–819.
3. BALDWIN, H.S., C. MICKANIN & C. BUCK. 1997. Adenovirus-mediated gene transfer during initial organogenesis in the mammalian embryo is promoter-dependent and tissue-specific. Gene Ther. **4:** 1142–1149.
4. LECONTE, I. *et al.* 1998. Adenoviral-mediated expression of antisense RNA to fibroblast growth factors disrupts murine vascular development. Dev. Dyn. **213:** 421–430.
5. SHOJI, I. *et al.* 1997. Efficient gene transfer into various mammalian cells, including non-hepatic cells, by baculovirus vectors. J. Gen. Virol. **78:** 2657–2664.
6. WERSTO, R.P. *et al.* 1998. Recombinant, replication-defective adenovirus gene transfer vectors induce cell cycle dysregulation and inappropriate expression of cyclin proteins. J. Virol. **72:** 9491–9502.
7. SADLER, T.W. 1979. Culture of early somite mouse embryos during organogenesis. J. Embryol. Exp. Morphol. **49:** 17–25.
8. SADLER, T.W., E.T. LIU & K.A. AUGUSTINE. 1995. Antisense targeting of engrailed-1 causes abnormal axis formation in mouse embryos. Teratology **51:** 292–299.
9. HUNTER, E.S., III & P.C. HARTIG. 1999. p53 overexpression increases susceptibility of mouse embryos to chemical-induced malformations. Submitted.
10. TAKAHASHI, K. *et al.* 1998. Adenovirus-mediated ectopic expression of Msx2 in even-numbered rhombomeres induces apoptotic elimination of cranial neural crest cells *in ovo*. Development **125:** 1627–1635.
11. TSUKAMOTO, M. *et al.* 1995. Gene transfer and expression in progeny after intravenous DNA injection into pregnant mice. Nat. Genet. **9:** 243–248.
12. AUGUSTINE, K. 1997. Antisense approaches for investigating mechanisms of abnormal development. Mutat. Res. **396:** 175–193.
13. HUNTER, E.S., III & D. DIX. 1999. Heat shock proteins Hsp70-1 and Hsp70-3 are necessary and sufficient to prevent arsenite-induced dysmorphology in mouse embryos. Submitted.
14. GINOBBI, P. *et al.* 1997. Folic acid–polylysine carrier improves efficacy of c-myc antisense oligodeoxynucleotides on human melanoma (M14) cells. Anticancer Res. **17:** 29–35.

Queueing and Inventory Theory in Clinical Practice

Application to Clinical Toxicology

C. P. ARUN[a]

Department of Urology, Ayr Hospital, Ayr KA6 6DX, Scotland

INTRODUCTION

Queueing theory, or congestion theory as it is sometimes called, deals with probabilistic models of systems where service is required by a "customer." The concept of arrivals, service, and departure is central to this theory. FIGURE 1 is a schematic diagram of poisoning as a queueing system. Queueing theory has traditionally been employed to study problems in business and industry. Recently, it has been applied to various disciplines in the clinical medical sciences. The queue paradigm is useful to describe the operations underlying the pathophysiology of various situations encountered in clinical practice. It is proposed that queueing theory is universally applicable to the study of clinical toxicology. Along with its cousin, inventory control theory, it affords a fresh perspective on various clinical problems arising in clinical toxicology.

REVIEW OF THE LITERATURE

Recent years have seen a rise in the application of stochastic methods in analyzing clinical problems. More recently, queueing theory has been applied to the study of various physiological problems.[1,2] So far, the dynamics of inhalational toxins[3] and ethanol[4] have been studied using queueing theory. This paper could not be presented as initially proposed in the abstract since it was discovered subsequently that a couple of papers[3,4] had already appeared in the indexed literature. A general treatment of poisoning as a queueing and inventory problem has not been available so far. It is this modified topic that this paper will address.

POISONING AS A QUEUEING PROBLEM

Any poisoning may be viewed as the "congestion" of a system with a toxin. Arrivals may be slow, in small quantities (as, in say, homicidal administration of arsenic) or in bulk (e.g., suicidal intake of salicylates). The toxin demands the "service" of elimination or detoxification. If arrivals are less than the service rate, then

---

[a]Present address: Department of Urology, Arrowe Park Hospital, Wirral L49 5PE, England.
arunpeter@yahoo.com

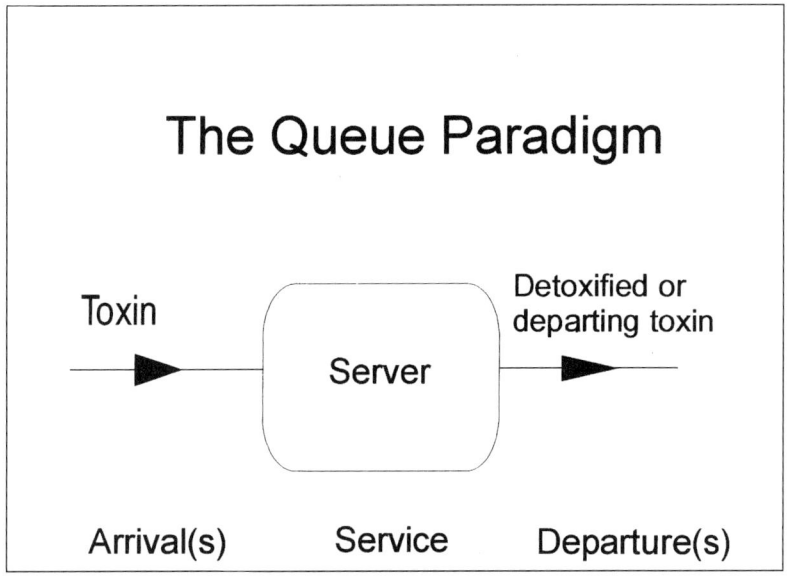

FIGURE 1. Schematic diagram of the handling of a poison as a queueing system. A quantity of toxin (customers) arrives at the server demanding the service of detoxification or elimination. After obtaining service, it departs the system.

the toxin can be satisfactorily dealt with. If, however, arrivals exceed the level of service provided, the system can be overwhelmed to the detriment of the organism. In therapeutic doses, aspirin finds application in a variety of conditions. Excessive intake (increased or bulk arrival) may result in poisoning (congestion). From a queueing standpoint, the treatment of poisoning may be viewed as involving the reduction or elimination of further arrivals, assisting in the service of detoxification and facilitating departure of the toxin. Using the example of aspirin again, further intake of aspirin must be stopped (reduce or eliminate arrivals), supportive therapy initiated to treat the systemic upset including fluid and electrolyte balance and acidosis, and elimination of the drug accelerated employing hemodialysis (to increase departures).

In certain cases of poisoning, it is also possible to employ antidotes (improve the service of dealing with the toxin).

POISONING AS AN INVENTORY PROBLEM

The concept of inventory has recently been introduced into physiology.[5] This concept is closely related to that of a "queue." In fact, probabilists group queues and inventories together under "stochastic storage processes." The body is known to hold "stocks" of various substances that are required for its effective functioning. Water, electrolytes, buffers, etc., are all conceptually "inventory". Certain poisons produce systemic upset by altering the level of "stocks" of various substances held in the

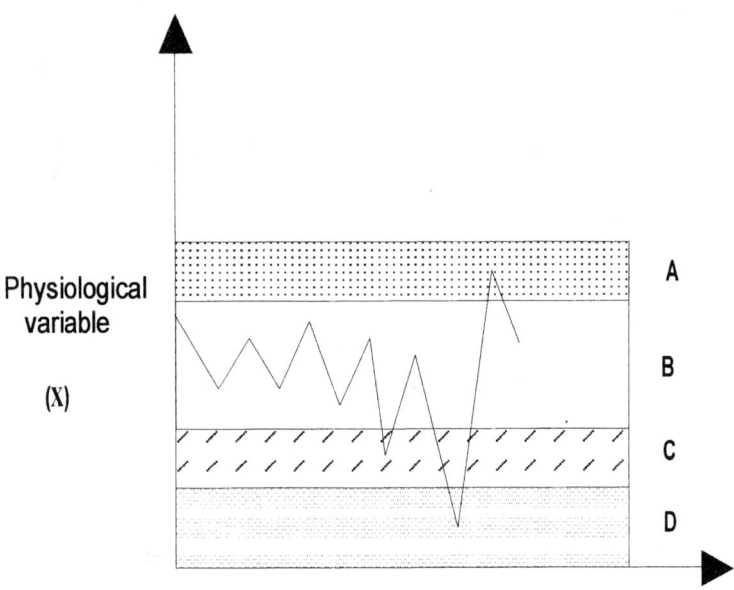

FIGURE 2. Certain poisons may alter a physiologic inventory towards excess or deficit, thereby disrupting homeostasis. In the diagram, the physiologic variable (*x*) that varies in health in the "normal" range (B) may, in a case of poisoning, be thrust towards an excess (A) or deficit (buffer stock range C or dangerously low level D).

body. Salicylates, for example, are known to produce metabolic acidosis by increasing the acid burden and a respiratory acidosis through hyperventilation. FIGURE 2 shows schematically how a physiologic variable (*x*) can be shifted to a state of excess or deficit as a result of the action of a poison. The mathematics of queues and inventories is a well-developed specialty and can help us to better analyze problems arising in the practice of clinical toxicology. A brief formulation of the queue and inventory paradigms follows.

A MATHEMATICAL FORMULATION OF THE PROBLEM

The Queueing Paradigm

Consider the arrivals of a poison as λ and the service of handling the toxin as μ. Clearly, if $\lambda > \mu$, there will be an accumulation of toxin within the body.

The Inventory Paradigm

Consider θ to be the "stock" of a physiological substance. In health, it varies within a certain range, $\theta \pm \alpha$. If a toxin causes a large shift in the quantity θ, then homeostasis is disrupted and life itself may be threatened. Therapy is aimed at restoring the body's inventories to their normalcy.

DISCUSSION

The queue and inventory paradigms help us to better describe and analyze various problems arising in clinical practice. Poisoning is yet another of those clinical situations lending itself to description using queueing and inventory control theory. It is reassuring to know that a set of mathematically founded theories are available to help us contend with problems in clinical toxicology for which, till now, only verbal descriptions were possible. In the new millennium, it is expected that mathematics and computer simulation will play an increasing role in various disciplines helping us treat various conditions in clinical medicine, including that of toxicology.

REFERENCES

1. ARUN, C.P. 1998. Queueing theory in clinical practice: application to the lower urinary tract. Presented at the Ninth IMA Conference on The Mathematical Theory of Biological Systems, Oxford.
2. ARUN, C.P. 1999. Queueing theory in clinical practice: application to the cardiovascular system. *In* Proceedings of the 1999 Summer Computer Simulation Conference, pp. 481–484. SCS Press. San Diego.
3. WU, G. 1998. Application of the queueing theory with Monte Carlo simulation to inhalation toxicology. Arch. Toxicol. **72**(6): 330–335.
4. WU, G. 1998. Application of queueing theory with Monte Carlo simulation to the study of the intake and adverse effects of ethanol. Alcohol Alcoholism **33**(5): 519–527.
5. ARUN, C.P. 1999. Physiological processes as problems of inventory management: a preliminary report. *In* Proceedings of the Fourth International Society for Inventory Research (ISIR) Summer School. University of Exeter Press. Exeter, England. In press.

The "Rodent Carcinogen" Dilemma

Formidable Challenge for the Technologies of the New Millennium

F. M. JOHNSON

Toxicology Operations Branch, Environmental Toxicology Program, National Institute of Environmental Health Sciences, Research Triangle Park, North Carolina 27709, USA

BACKGROUND

The NTP Rodent Bioassay (NTPRB) is a standardized test used to determine if a chemical is capable of causing cancer in rodents.[1] It is widely assumed that cancer-causing chemicals in rodents are also capable of causing cancer in humans.[2] While the NTPRB has many advocates, others have questioned its validity, primarily on the basis of the high doses used (e.g., cf. references 3–6).

In the early 1970s, Ames and colleagues discovered that many carcinogenic chemicals were mutagenic to special strains of *Salmonella*.[7,8] A number of other inexpensive mutation tests were also developed with the idea of applying them to the thousands of chemicals in the environment for which the mutagenic and carcinogenic potential was unknown.[9,10] The main objective of this effort was to find faster and cheaper alternatives for the rodent cancer tests.

The results from one group of tests, conducted by the National Toxicology Program, showed that no test (or combination of tests) predicted rodent carcinogenicity better than the Ames *Salmonella* test. However, *Salmonella* correctly predicted rodent carcinogenicity for only about 65% of chemicals.[11,12] Methods that are unable to predict chemical carcinogens accurately could conceivably do more harm than good to public health by restricting the use of safe chemicals while permitting entry of dangerous human carcinogens into the environment.[13] The quest for more accurate predictors of carcinogenicity remains a top priority item in the U.S. National Institutes of Health agenda.[14,15]

The present NIH strategy for gaining headway on the large backlog of untested chemicals is to use transgenic model systems as replacements for traditional long-term rodent bioassays.[14–25]

So far, the discordance rate for the transgenic approach is disappointingly high. Bucher,[23] for example, cites a discordance rate of 13/38 or a level of agreement of 66%, which is little different from the 65% shown by the *Salmonella* mutation test.[11,12] One possibility that could help explain the apparent lack of progress is genetic variability in the induced chemical-carcinogen response among rodents.

THE CHEMICAL CARCINOGEN/ANTICARCINOGEN RESPONSE "FINGERPRINT"

The tumor data can be extracted from the NTP reports and organized graphically to show which tissues demonstrated a statistically significant carcinogenic response following chemical exposure. TABLE 1 displays the resulting "fingerprint" for a sample of approximately 200 chemicals, identified by name and NTP technical report number. For this particular sample of chemical-exposed male F344 rats, there are 31 tissue/organ sites that demonstrate a capacity to show a carcinogenic or anticarcinogenic response. The full names of these tumor sites are given in a footnote at the bottom of the table.

The particular sites showing statistically significant ($p < 0.05$), chemically related carcinogenic (light letters on dark shading) or anticarcinogenic (dark letters on light shading) responses are indicated. Obviously, the number and kind of tissues involved in the carcinogenic response vary widely from one chemical to another. Female rats as well as male and female mice also show the same general kind of variation, but responses often vary between the sexes and species of rodents (data not shown).

A degree of uncertainty is associated with the "fingerprint" representation. Thus, some significant increases and decreases are possible artifacts that might not show up again in a repeated study of the same resolution. One might think of the uncertainty as "noise" that partially obscures the signal (i.e., the "true" carcinogenic and anticarcinogenic responses). Presumably, a less noisy fingerprint would appear similarly in character, but differ in detail. Many of the statistically significant increases and decreases depicted in TABLE 1 were not judged to be true chemically related effects by NTP and its peer review panels.[26]

The distribution of the data suggests the tumor response may be best explained by multiple, tissue-specific (more or less independently acting) factors. The fact that many structurally diverse chemicals can cause tissues to respond either positively or negatively would imply the existence of several chemically responsive determinants involved in the development or inhibition of cancer in each tissue.

Subtracting the number of decreases ("NDE" in TABLE 1) from the number of increases ("NIN") results in a term that reflects a sort of overall tumorigenic response: "I − D". On the positive end of the scale, increases exceed decreases, implying a relatively more harmful effect. On the negative end of the scale, decreases exceed increases, suggesting a less harmful effect of chemical exposure. Of course, this combination of terms is an oversimplification since it does not distinguish induced, rapidly lethal tumors from nonlethal tumors, which might have confounding effects on the overall distribution. Nevertheless, the overall response values provide another means to distinguish the effects of the different chemicals and help add insight into the chemical response fingerprint.

In TABLE 1, the overall tumorigenic response values were used as a basis for sorting the chemicals. Thus, chemicals associated with mostly decreases are located at the top of the table (dark letters on light shading) and those associated with mostly increases are at the bottom (light letters on dark shading). As one can see, most chemicals induced a combination of carcinogenic and anticarcinogenic effects. Such chemicals have been referred to as ambiguous[27] or Janus[28] carcinogens.

FIGURE 1 is a plot of survival (Y) versus strength of the response (X). These particular data are for low-dose-treated male rats and survival values are percent surviving after two years relative to control [(N treated alive/total N treated) ÷ (N control alive/total N control)] × 100. Values above 100 indicate a larger percentage of survivors in the chemical treated group than in the control group. As one can see, there is

TABLE 1. Summary of chemically related tumor increases and decreases by tissue/organ site in male F344 rats

TRN	CHEMICAL NAME	ROUTE	CALL	NIN[1]	NDE[2]	I-D[3]	BLA[4]	BRA	BON	ESO	FOR
446	1-TRANS-DELTA9-TETRAHYDROCANNABINOL	GAV	NE	0	5	-5					
322	PHENYLEPHRINE HYDROCHLORIDE	GAV	NE	0	4	-4					
424	O-BENZYL-P-CHLOROPHENOL	GAV	NE	0	4	-4					
293	HC BLUE 2	GAV	NE	0	3	-3					
299	C.I. DISPERSE BLUE 1	GAV	CE	2	5	-3	BLA				
305	CHLORINATED PARAFFINS: C23	FEED	NE	0	3	-3					
333	N-PHENYL-2-NAPHTHYLAMINE	FEED	NE	0	3	-3					
350	TRIBROMOMETHANE	GAV	SE	1	4	-3					
414	PENTACHLOROANISOLE	GAV	SE	1	4	-3					
217	DI(2-ETHYLHEXYL)PHTHALATE	FEED	P	1	3	-2					
219	2,6-DICHLORO-p-PHENYLENEDIAMINE	FEED	N	0	2	-2					
222	C.I. DISPERSE YELLOW 3	FEED	P	1	3	-2					
233	2-BIPHENYLAMINE HYDROCHLORIDE	FEED	N	0	2	-2					
242.284	DIALLYL PHTHALATE	GAV	NE	0	2	-2					
281	HC RED 3	FEED	NE	0	2	-2					
300	3-CHLORO-2-METHYLPROPENE	FEED	CE	2	4	-2					FOR
314	METHYL METHACRYLATE	FEED	NE	0	2	-2					
317	CHLORPHENIRAMINE MALEATE	GAV	NE	0	2	-2					
328	METHYL CARBAMATE	GAV	CE	1	3	-2					
348	ALPHA-METHYLDOPA SESQUIHYDRATE	FEED	NE	0	2	-2					
389	SODIUM AZIDE	GAV	NE	0	2	-2					
398	POLYBROMINATED BIPHENYLS	FEED	CE	1	3	-2					
426.2	SAFFLOWER OIL	GAV	NC	1	3	-2					
432	BARIUM CHLORIDE DIHYDRATE	WATER	NE	0	2	-2					
436	T-BUTYL ALCOHOL	WATER	SE	1	3	-2					
439	METHYLPHENIDATE HYDROCHLORIDE	FEED	NE	0	2	-2					
442	P-NITROBENZOIC ACID	FEED	NE	1	3	-2					
232	PENTACHLOROETHANE	GAV	E	1	2	-1					
235	ZEARALENONE	FEED	N	0	1	-1					
266	MONURON	GAV	CE	2	3	-1					
320	ROTENONE	GAV	EE	1	2	-1					
330	4-HEXYLRESORCINOL	GAV	NE	1	2	-1					
335	C.I. ACID ORANGE 3	GAV	NE	0	1	-1					
353	2,4-DICHLOROPHENOL	FEED	NE	0	1	-1					
354	DIMETHOXANE	GAV	NE	0	1	-1					
357	HYDROCHLOROTHIAZIDE	FEED	NE	0	1	-1					
379	2-CHLOROACETOPHENONE	INHAL	NE	0	1	-1					
380	EPINEPHRINE HYDROCHLORIDE	GAV	NT	0	1	-1					
395	PROBENECID	GAV	NE	0	1	-1					
403	RESORCINOL	GAV	NE	0	1	-1					
407	C.I. PIGMENT RED 3	FEED	SE	3	4	-1					
412	4,4'-DSDA (AMSONIC ACID)	FEED	NE	0	1	-1					
422	COUMARIN	GAV	SE	2	3	-1					
426.1	CORN OIL	GAV	NC	2	3	-1					
428	MANGANESE (II) SULFATE MONOHYDRATE	FEED	NE	0	1	-1					
429	DIETHYLPHTHALATE	SP	NE	0	1	-1					
431	BENZYL ACETATE	FEED	NE	0	1	-1					
208	FD & C YELLOW NO. 6	FEED	N	0	0	0					
211	C.I. ACID ORANGE 10	FEED	N	1	1	0					
212	DI(2-ETHYLHEXYL)ADIPATE	FEED	N	1	1	0					
214	CAPROLACTAM	FEED	N	1	1	0					
220	C.I. ACID RED 14	FEED	N	0	0	0					
221	LOCUST BEAN GUM	FEED	N	0	0	0					
223	EUGENOL	FEED	N	1	1	0					
224	TARA GUM	FEED	N	1	1	0					
225	D & C RED 9	FEED	P	2	2	0					
226	C.I. SOLVENT YELLOW 14	FEED	P	1	1	0					
227	GUM ARABIC	FEED	N	0	0	0					
230	AGAR	FEED	N	0	0	0					
236	D-MANNITOL	FEED	N	0	0	0					
237	1,1,1,2-TETRACHLOROETHANE	GAV	E	1	1	0					
247	L-ASCORBIC ACID	FEED	N	0	0	0					
250	BENZYL ACETATE	GAV	E	1	1	0					
255	1,2-DICHLOROBENZENE (o-DICHLOROBENZENE)	GAV	N	0	0	0					
257.2	DIGLYCIDYL RESORCINOL ETHER, STUDY 2	GAV	P	1	1	0					FOR
259	ETHYL ACRYLATE	GAV	P	1	1	0					FOR
263	1,2-DICHLOROPROPANE (PROPYLENE DICHLORIDE)	GAV	NE	0	0	0					
271	HC BLUE 1	GAV	EE	1	1	0					
272	PROPYLENE	FEED	NE	0	0	0					
274	TRIS(2-ETHYLHEXYL) PHOSPHATE	INHAL	EE	2	2	0					
275	2-CHLOROETHANOL (ETHYLENE CHLOROHYDRIN)	GAV	NE	0	0	0					
276	8-HYDROXYQUINOLINE	SP	NE	2	2	0					
282	CHLORODIBROMOMETHANE	GAV	NE	0	0	0					
289	BENZENE	GAV	CE	3	3	0					
296.1	TETRAKIS (HYDROXYMETHYL) PHOSPHONIUM SULFATE	GAV	NE	0	0	0					
296.2	TETRAKIS (HYDROXYMETHYL) PHOSPHONIUM CHLORIDE	GAV	NE	0	0	0					

TABLE 1. *Continued*

HMG	INT	KID	LIV	LUK	LUN	MAM	MES	NAS	ORA	PAA	PAI	PAR	PHE	PIT	PRE	SAL	SKO	SKS	SKK	SUB	SPL	TES	THC	THF	ZYM
			LIV			MAM				PAA				PIT								TES			
				LUK		MAM							PHE							SUB					
							MES								PRE		SKO		SKK				THC		
				LUK			MES				PAI		PHE	PIT								TES			
						MAM				PAA				PIT											
														PIT					SKK				THC		
	INT			LUK										PIT	PRE					SUB					
				LUK		MAM				PAA	PAI		PHE											
			LIV											PIT								TES	THC		
											PAI		PHE											
			LIV	LUK			MES																THC		
				LUK		MAM																			
						MAM													SKK						
				LUK									PHE						SKK			TES	THC		
														PIT	PRE										
				LUK																					
			LIV	LIV									PHE	PIT											
			LIV										PHE												
													PHE												
			LIV										PHE	PIT	PRE										
															PRE										
				LUK		MAM				PAA															
				LUK									PHE												
		KID									PAI			PIT										THF	
				LUK									PHE												
				LUK						PAA				PIT	PRE										
		KID												PIT						SUB					
																						TES			
		KID	LIV	LUK									PHE										THC		
																				SUB			THC		
												PAR													
				LUK																		TES	THC		
																						TES			
				LUK																					
				LUK																					
				LUK																					
									ORA														THC		
													PHE												
														PIT											
				LUK		MAM					PAI		PHE		PRE			SKS				TES			ZYM
														PIT											
		KID		LUK									PHE	PIT								TES			
			LIV	LUK						PAA			PHE							SUB					
													PHE										THC		
																			SKK						
			LIV	LUK																					
													PHE									TES			
																				SUB		TES			
					LUN																		THC		
											PAI											TES			
			LIV	LUK											PRE						SPL				
			LIV	LUK																					
			LIV											PIT											
										PAA												TES			
																							THC		
																	SKO								
			LIV	LUK																					
										PAA			PHE							SUB				THF	
			LIV	LUK	LUN																		THC		
									ORA				PHE	PIT				SKS					THC		ZYM

TABLE 1. Continued

TRN	CHEMICAL NAME	ROUTE	CALL	NIN[1]	NDE[2]	I-D[3]	BLA[4]	BRA	BON	ESO	FOR
307	EPHEDRINE SULFATE	INHAL	NE	0	0	0					
312.1	n-BUTYL CHLORIDE	INHAL	NE	0	0	0					
315	OXYTETRACYCLINE HYDROCHLORIDE	INHAL	EE	1	1	0					
327	XYLENES (MIXED)	GAV	NE	1	1	0					
334	2-AMINO-5-NITROPHENOL	GAV	SE	2	2	0					
336	PENICILLIN VK	GAV	NE	1	1	0					
338	ERYTHROMYCIN STEARATE	FEED	NE	1	1	0					
341	NITROFURANTOIN	FEED	SE	3	3	0			BON		
343	BENZYL ALCOHOL	GAV	NE	0	0	0					
346	CHLOROETHANE	INHAL	EE	1	1	0					
352	N-METHYLOLACRYLAMIDE	GAV	NE	2	2	0					
360	N-N-DIMETHYLANILINE	GAV	SE	1	1	0					
364	RHODAMINE 6G	FEED	EE	1	1	0					
365	PENTAERYTHRITOL TETRANITRATE	FEED	EE	1	1	0					
366	HYDROQUINONE	GAV	SE	2	2	0					
368	NALIDIXIC ACID	FEED	CE	2	2	0					
371	TOLUENE	INHAL	NE	0	0	0					
375	VINYL TOLUENE (MIXED ISOMERS)	INHAL	NE	0	0	0					
382	FURFURAL	GAV	SE	1	1	0					
387	dl-AMPHETAMINE SULFATE	FEED	NE	1	1	0					
392.1	CHLORINATED WATER	WATER	NE	0	0	0					
396	MONOCHLOROACETIC ACID	GAV	NE	0	0	0					
401	2,4,-DIAMINOPHENOL	GAV	NE	1	1	0					
404	5,5-DIPHENYLHYDANTOIN	FEED	EE	1	1	0					
408	MERCURIC CHLORIDE	GAV	SE	2	2	0					FOR
423	3,4-DIHYDROCOUMARIN	GAV	SE	2	2	0					
425	PROMETHAZINE HCL	GAV	NE	1	1	0					
427	TUMERIC OLEORESIN	FEED	NE	1	1	0					
433	TRICRESYL PHOSPHATE	FEED	NE	0	0	0					
435	4,4-THIOBIS(6-T-BUTYL-M-CRESOL)	FEED	NE	0	0	0					
438	BENZETHONIUM CHLORIDE	SP	NE	0	0	0					
207	CYTEMBENA	IP/IJ	P	1	0	1					
216	11-AMINOUNDECANOIC ACID	FEED	P	3	2	1	BLA				
229	GUAR GUM	FEED	N	1	0	1					
231	STANNOUS CHLORIDE	FEED	E	1	0	1					
238	ZIRAM	FEED	P	1	0	1					
243	TRICHLOROETHYLENE (WITHOUT EPICHLOROHYDRIN)	GAV	I	1	0	1					
245	MELAMINE	FEED	P	1	0	1					
248	4,4'-METHYLENEDIANILINE DIHYDROCHLORIDE	WATER	P	2	1	1	BLA				
252	GERANYL ACETATE	GAV	N	2	1	1					
253	ALLYL ISOVALERATE	GAV	P	2	1	1					
257.1	DIGLYCIDYL RESORCINOL ETHER, STUDY 1	GAV	P	1	0	1					FOR
261	CHLOROBENZENE	GAV	E	2	1	1					
267	PROPYLENE OXIDE	FEED	SE	1	0	1					
287	DIMETHYL HYDROGEN PHOSPHITE	FEED	CE	2	1	1					
298	DIMETHYL MORPHOLINOPHOSPHORAMIDATE	GAV	SE	2	1	1					FOR
303	4-VINYLCYCLOHEXENE	GAV	IS	2	1	1					
309	DECABROMODIPHENYL OXIDE	GAV	SE	2	1	1					
318	AMPICILLIN TRIHYDRATE	GAV	EE	2	1	1					
319	1,4-DICHLOROBENZENE	GAV	CE	1	0	1					
337	NITROFURAZONE	FEED	EE	3	2	1					
340	IODINATED GLYCEROL	GAV	SE	4	3	1					
344	TETRACYCLINE HYDROCHLORIDE	FEED	NE	2	1	1					
345	ROXARSONE	FEED	EE	1	0	1					
351	para-CHLOROANILINE HYDROCHLORIDE	GAV	CE	3	2	1					
358	OCHRATOXIN A	GAV	CE	1	0	1					
363	BROMOETHANE	INHAL	SE	3	2	1		BRA			
367	PHENYLBUTAZONE	GAV	EE	1	0	1					
369	ALPHA-METHYLBENZYL ALCOHOL	GAV	SE	2	1	1					
373	SUCCINIC ANHYDRIDE	GAV	NE	1	0	1					
377	CS2 (94% o-CHLOROBENZALMALONONITRILE)	INHAL	NE	2	1	1					
388	ETHYLENE THIOUREA (ETU)	FEED	CE	1	0	1					
393	SODIUM FLUORIDE	WATER	EE	2	1	1			BON		
394	ACETAMINOPHEN	FEED	NE	2	1	1					
406	GAMMA-BUTYROLACTONE	GAV	NE	1	0	1					
409	QUERCETIN	FEED	SE	1	0	1					
411	C.I. PIGMENT RED 23	FEED	EE	2	1	1					
415	POLYSORBATE 80	FEED	EE	1	0	1					
419	HC YELLOW 4	FEED	EE	1	0	1					
420.1	TRIAMTERENE	FEED	EE	1	0	1					
437	HEXACHLOROCYCLOPENTADIENE	INHAL	NE	1	0	1					
215	BISPHENOL A	FEED	E	3	1	2					
234	ALLYL ISOTHIOCYANATE	GAV	P	2	0	2	BLA				
251	2,4- & 2,6-TOLUENE DIISOCYANATE	GAV	P	2	0	2					
291	ISOPHORONE	GAV	SE	2	0	2					
304	CHLORENDIC ACID	GAV	CE	4	2	2					
306	DICHLOROMETHANE (METHYLENE CHLORIDE)	GAV	SE	3	1	2					
329	1,2-EPOXYBUTANE	INHAL	CE	2	0	2					

TABLE 1. *Continued*

HMG	INT	KID	LIV	LUK	LUN	MAM	MES	NAS	ORA	PAA	PAI	PAR	PHE	PIT	PRE	SAL	SKO	SKS	SKK	SUB	SPL	TES	THC	THF	ZYM
				LUK									PHE												
														PIT											
										PAA				PIT					SKK			TES			
														PIT						SUB		TES			
																						TES			ZYM
		KID		LUK											PRE					SUB		TES			
																	SKO						THC		
			LIV										PHE						SKK			TES			
				LUK																	SPL				
			LIV																SKK						
				LUK																					ZYM
		KID				MAM							PHE	PIT											
							MES							PIT	PRE							TES			
			LIV																						ZYM
																						TES			
						MAM																TES			
			LIV			MAM																			
				LUK										PIT										THF	
		KID												PIT	PRE							TES			
				LUK									PHE												
																		SKS				TES			
							MES																		
			LIV	LUK		MAM																	THC		
																				SUB			THC		
																							THC		
		KID																							
				LIV LUK																				THF	
		KID												PIT				SKS							
				LUK										PIT	PRE										
			LIV											PIT								TES			
								NAS																	
			LIV	LUN																					
				LUK										PIT				SKS							
				LUK														SKS				TES			
			LIV	LUK						PAA										SUB					
											PAI		PHE												
		KID																							
				LUK			MES								PRE		SKO					TES			
				LUK				NAS			PAI		PHE	PIT								TES		THF	
				LUK						PAA				PIT											
				LUK									PHE	PIT							SPL	TES			
		KID											PHE									TES			
		KID			LUN		MES						PHE												
		KID		LUK									PHE						SKK						
					LUN																	TES	THC		
																								THF	
				LUK										PIT						SUB		TES		THF	
							MES																		
		KID																							
		KID		LUK																SUB					
													PHE												
														PIT											
			LIV											PIT											
				LUK		MAM							PHE									TES			
				LUK																					
										PAA					PRE					SUB					
		KID													PRE							TES			
			LIV	LUN						PAA			PHE					SKS							
														PIT											
						MAM	MES																		
				LUN				NAS																	

TABLE 1. *Continued*

TRN	CHEMICAL NAME	ROUTE	CALL	NIN[1]	NDE[2]	I-D[3]	BLA[4]	BRA	BON	ESO	FOR
331	MALONALDEHYDE, SODIUM	GAV	CE	3	1	2					
361	HEXACHLOROETHANE	GAV	CE	2	0	2					
362	4-VINYL-1-CYCLOHEXENE DIEPOXIDE	SP	CE	3	1	2					
383	1-AMINO-2,4-DIBROMOANTHRAQUINONE	FEED	CE	4	2	2	BLA				
386	TETRANITROMETHANE	INHAL	CE	2	0	2					
392.2	CHLORAMINATED WATER	WATER	NE	2	0	2					
426.3	TRICAPRYLIN	GAV	NC	3	1	2					
430	C.I. DIRECT BLUE 218	FEED	SE	2	0	2					FOR
440.1	Ozone (2 year study)	INHAL	NE	2	0	2					FOR
440.2	OZONE	INHAL	NE	2	0	2					
240	PROPYL GALLATE	FEED	E	4	1	3					
269	1,3-DICHLOROPROPENE (TELONE II)	INHAL	CE	3	0	3					FOR
311	TETRACHLOROETHYLENE	SP	CE	3	0	3					
313.1	MIREX (FIRST STUDY)	GAV	CE	4	1	3					
316	DIMETHYLVINYL CHLORIDE (DMVC)	FEED	CE	4	1	3				ESO	FOR
321	BROMODICHLOROMETHANE	FEED	CE	4	1	3					
342	DICHLORVOS	GAV	SE	3	0	3					
347	D-LIMONENE	GAV	CE	4	1	3					
355	DIPHENHYDRAMINE HYDROCHLORIDE	FEED	EE	3	0	3		BRA			
356	FUROSEMIDE	FEED	EE	3	0	3		BRA			
370	BENZOFURAN	GAV	NE	3	0	3					
391	TRIS(2 CHLOROETHYL) PHOSPHATE	GAV	CE	4	1	3		BRA			
402	FURAN	GAV	CE	4	1	3					
228	VINYLIDENE CHLORIDE	GAV	N	4	0	4					
308	CHLORINATED PARAFFINS: C12	FEED	CE	4	0	4					
323	DIMETHYL METHYLPHOSPHONATE	FEED	SE	4	0	4					
339	2-AMINO-4-NITROPHENOL	GAV	SE	4	0	4					
359	8-METHOXYPSORALEN	GAV	CE	5	1	4					
378	BENZALDEHYDE	GAV	NE	4	0	4					
416	O-NITROANISOLE	FEED	CE	6	2	4	BLA				FOR
206	1,2-DIBROMO-3-CHLOROPROPANE	INHAL	P	5	0	5					
285	C.I. BASIC RED 9 MONOHYDROCHLORIDE	GAV	CE	6	1	5					
332	2-MERCAPTOBENZOTHIAZOLE	GAV	SE	5	0	5					
399	TITANOCENE DICHLORIDE	GAV	EE	5	0	5					FOR
447	ACETONITRILE	INHAL	EE	5	0	5					
210	1,2-DIBROMOETHANE (ETHYLENE DIBROMIDE)	INHAL	P	6	0	6					
372	3,3' DIMETHOXYBENZIDINE DIHYDROCHLORIDE	WATER	CE	7	0	7					
374	GLYCIDOL	GAV	CE	9	0	9		BRA			FOR
405	C.I. ACID RED 114	WATER	CE	9	0	9					
384	1,2,3-TRICHLOROPROPANE	GAV	CE	11	0	11					FOR
397	C.I. DIRECT BLUE 15	WATER	CE	11	0	11		BRA			

NOTE: A similar table that depicted only the statistically significant, chemically related increases was published previously.[29]

[1]NIN = number of tissue/organ sites showing statistically significant, chemically related tumor increases.

[2]NDE = number of sites showing statistically significant, chemically related tumor decreases.

[3]I − D = number of increases minus number of decreases.

[4]Abbreviations: BLA, urinary bladder tumors; BON, bone tumors; BRA, brain tumors; ESO, esophagus tumors; FOR, forestomach tumors; HMG, hemangioma/hemangiosarcoma; INT, intestine tumors (large and/or small intestine); KID, kidney tumors; LIV, liver tumors; LUK, leukemia; LUN, lung tumors; MAM, mammary gland tumors; MES, mesothelioma; NAS, nose/nasal cavity tumors; ORA, oral cavity tumors; PAA, pancreatic acinar cell tumors; PAI, pancreatic islet cell tumors; PAR, parathyroid tumors; PHE, adrenal pheochromocytoma; PIT, pituitary gland (pars distalis) tumors; PRE, preputial gland tumors; SAL, salivary gland tumors; SKK, skin tumors (keratoacanthoma); SKO, skin tumors (other tumor types); SKS, skin tumors (squamous cell papilloma/carcinoma); SPL, splenic sarcoma; SUB, subcutaneous tissue tumors; TES, testis tumors; THC, thyroid c cell tumors; THF, thyroid follicular cell tumors; ZYM, zymbal gland tumors.

TABLE 1. *Continued*

HMG	INT	KID	LIV	LUK	LUN	MAM	MES	NAS	ORA	PAA	PAI	PAR	PHE	PIT	PRE	SAL	SKO	SKS	SKK	SUB	SPL	TES	THC	THF	ZYM
											PAI		PHE	PIT										THF	
		KID											PHE												
															PRE		SKO	SKS					THC		
	INT	KID	LIV	LUK										PIT											
					LUN																	TES			
									ORA													TES			
			LIV	LUK						PAA															
									ORA																
																			SKK				THC		
				LUK	LUN																				
				LUK							PAI		PHE		PRE									THF	
			LIV										PHE												
		KID		LUK																		TES			
		KID	LIV										PHE	PIT										THF	
								NAS	ORA				PHE	PIT											
	INT	KID			LUN								PHE					SKS							
				LUK	LUN					PAA															
		KID		LUK														SKS		SUB		TES			
					LUN									PIT											
		KID												PIT											
						MAM								PIT								TES			
		KID		LUK										THC										THF	
			LIV	LUK							PAI				PRE				SKK						
											PAI		PHE							SUB		TES			
		KID	LIV	LUK						PAA															
		KID		LUK			MES						PHE												
		KID	LIV												PRE							TES			
		KID												PIT					SKK	SUB		TES			ZYM
	INT	KID					MES			PAA				PIT	PRE										
				LUK	LUN																				
			LIV	LUK			MES	NAS	ORA								SKO	SKS		SUB		TES		THF	ZYM
				LUK			MES			PAA			PHE		PRE							TES			
			LIV				MES			PAA												TES			
			LIV								PAI		PHE						SKK			TES		THF	
HMG							MES	NAS								SAL						TES			
	INT		LIV				MES		ORA						PRE		SKO	SKS				TES		THF	ZYM
	INT					MAM	MES										SKO	SKS	SKK			TES		THF	ZYM
			LIV		LUN				ORA				PHE				SKO	SKS				TES	THC		ZYM
	INT	KID	LIV						ORA	PAA					PRE		SKO	SKS				TES			ZYM
	INT		LIV	LUK					ORA				PHE		PRE									THF	ZYM

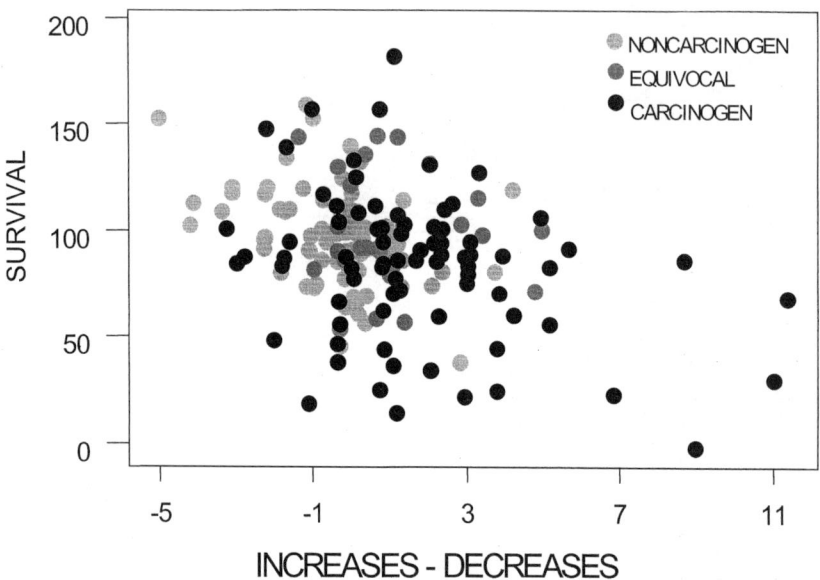

FIGURE 1. Plot of two-year survival (*Y*) versus overall tumorigenic effect (increases minus decreases) (*X*) for chemically treated male rats. Each dot represents a chemical classified as carcinogen, equivocal, or noncarcinogen (negative or no evidence).

some appearance of correlation between increasing tumorigenic response values and decreased survival, as one might have expected. Obviously, though, a few chemicals (≤10) at the extremes of the distribution contribute disproportionately to the effect. Somewhat surprising is the fact that many of the chemical exposures (including exposures to some chemicals classified as carcinogens) resulted in improved rather than worsened survival. Decreases in tumor incidence and increases in survival can sometimes be attributed to reduced caloric intake, which may occur when a chemical added to the feed makes the food unpalatable to the animals.[29] However, chemically related decreases are not limited to feed studies; that is, many chemicals administered by gavage also show chemically related decreases (TABLE 1).

The dots are shaded in FIGURE 1 to distinguish between chemicals classified as carcinogens (dark), equivocals (intermediate), and noncarcinogens (light). Although widely dispersed, the dots representing carcinogens are grouped somewhat more predominantly in the lower-right region of the plot, while dots representing the noncarcinogens are found to be somewhat more prevalent in the upper-left part of the graph. However, the two data clouds obviously overlap to a very large extent.

CARCINOGENIC, ANTICARCINOGENIC, OR AMBIGUOUS?

For chemicals tested in four sex-species groups in NTP studies, the proportion of chemicals testing positive in one, two, three, or four sex-species groups is over

50%.[30] However, even in one sex-species group, as shown here for tissue/organ sites in male rats, most chemicals are neither unanimously carcinogenic or anticarcinogenic nor entirely neutral. Most chemicals are Janus carcinogens, showing both a carcinogenic and anticarcinogenic effect. Across a large number of genotypes, the degree of ambiguity would presumably increase further, and an even larger proportion of tested chemicals would prove to be Janus carcinogens.

The underlying assumption in the predictive use of transgenic models is that they exhibit enhanced sensitivity to carcinogenic agents and reduce the complexity of identifying potential carcinogens.[17,31] If the carcinogenic response is the result of 100 or more independent acting genes, it is difficult to imagine a mechanism whereby it is possible for one or two special strains to reflect faithfully this diversity of carcinogenic action. Accordingly, it may not be wise to embrace the assumption uncritically.

The National Cancer Institute presently lists over 4500 different genes that are related to cancer.[32] Few of them have been tested for polymorphism in rodents or humans, but even if only a fraction prove to vary genetically it would provide for considerable individual variability in the chemical carcinogen response. Inbred strains of mice vary widely according to spontaneous tumor incidence, as well as by tumor cell type and the particular tissue/organ sites in which tumors develop.[33] This variation implies quite a high level of cancer-gene polymorphism in the populations from which the strains were developed and in animal populations in general. Many cases of strain-specific differences in the carcinogenic response to chemicals have also been described (e.g., nitrosamines).[34]

In natural populations, mutations whose only effect is to influence the rate at which tumors develop, and whose expression takes place only in the presence of a high-dose chemical, might not be affected by natural selection under most circumstances. Thus, the accumulation of such mutations over evolutionary time may account for the extensive variation observed in spontaneous and chemically induced tumors between inbred strains.

Having great genetic diversity, human populations would be expected to have a much larger assortment of susceptibility factors than a few laboratory rodent strains. Given this diversity, it may not be reasonable to expect the rodent response to mimic the human response to a chemical in every instance or even in most instances. For similar reasons, it may not be possible to find a cheaper, faster surrogate rodent test that responds like the rodent, which may explain why such efforts have proved unsuccessful for so long.

The data in TABLE 1 indicate the individual tissue/organ sites that responded to chemical exposure with an increased or decreased incidence of tumors in one genotype (male F344 rats). The data also represent nonresponsive tissues, that is, "control" tissues. Thus, one might contemplate using cDNA microarrays and applying them to tissues of chemically treated animals where a specific chemical exposure is already known to have a specific tumorigenic effect later in the life of the animals. Such work would have the potential of identifying the critical events in the beginning of the tumorigenic process, as well as the genes and allelic variants that confer susceptibility and resistance to chemically induced cancer. Eventually, it is conceivable that we will think of carcinogenic risk in terms of complex multilocus genotypes and functional groups of chemicals instead of chemicals simply classified as carcinogens, anticarcinogens, or noncarcinogens. Unfortunately, few if any humans may carry the same set of genes that characterize the carcinogenic/anticarcinogenic response of F344 rats to various chemicals. Predicting human effects from rodent responses, or from surrogate rodent tests, is thus likely to remain a formidable challenge well into the new millennium.

ACKNOWLEDGMENTS

I am indebted to Joseph Haseman for extracting the statistically significant chemically related increases and decreases from the NTP technical reports in the course of our earlier collaborative study.[29] I thank John Drake and James Huff for reviewing the manuscript.

REFERENCES

1. HUFF, J., J. HASEMAN & D. RALL. 1991. Scientific concepts, value, and significance of chemical carcinogenesis studies. Annu. Rev. Pharmacol. Toxicol. **31:** 621–652.
2. FUNG, V.A., J.C. BARRETT & J.E. HUFF. 1995. The carcinogenesis bioassay in perspective: application in identifying human cancer hazards. Environ. Health Perspect. **103:** 680–683.
3. LEWIS, D.F.V., C. IONNIDES & D.V. PARKE. 1998. Cytochromes P450 and species differences in xenobiotic metabolism and activation of carcinogen. Environ. Health Perspect. **106:** 633–641.
4. AMES, B.N. & L.S. GOLD. 1997. Environmental pollution, pesticides, and the prevention of cancer: misconceptions. FASEB J. **11:** 1041–1052.
5. REIZENSTEIN, P., B. MODAN & L.H. KULLER. 1994. The quandry of cancer prevention. J. Clin. Epidemiol. **47:** 575–581.
6. GORI, G.B. 1991. Are animal tests relevant in cancer risk assessment? A persistent issue becomes uncomfortable. Regul. Toxicol. Pharmacol. **13:** 225–227.
7. AMES, B.N. 1973. Carcinogens are mutagens: their detection and classification. Environ. Health Perspect. **6:** 115–118.
8. AMES, B.N., F.D. LEE & W.E. DURSTON. 1973. An improved bacterial test system for the detection and classification of mutagens and carcinogens. Proc. Natl. Acad. Sci. U.S.A. **70:** 782–786.
9. COMMITTEE 17. 1975. Environmental mutagenic hazards: mutagenicity screening is now both feasible and necessary for chemicals entering the environment. Science **187:** 503–514.
10. COMMITTEE 3. 1983. International commission for protection against environmental mutagens and carcinogens: regulatory approaches to the control of environmental mutagens and carcinogens. Mutat. Res. **114:** 174–216.
11. TENNANT, R.W., B.H. MARGOLIN, M.D. SHELBY, E. ZEIGER, J. HASEMAN, J. SPALDING, W. CASPARY, M. RESNICK, S. STASIEWICZ, B. ANDERSON & R. MINOR. 1987. Prediction of chemical carcinogenicity in rodents from *in vitro* genetic toxicity assays. Science **236:** 933–941.
12. ZEIGER, E., J.K. HASEMAN, M.D. SHELBY, B.H. MARGOLIN & R.W. TENNANT. 1990. Evaluation of four *in vitro* genetic toxicity tests for predicting rodent carcinogenicity: confirmation of earlier results with 41 additional chemicals. Environ. Mol. Mutagen. **16**(suppl. 18)**:** 1–14.
13. JOHNSON, F.M. & M.L. SNELL. 1986. Short-term tests are unable to distinguish between human carcinogens and noncarcinogens. Cancer Invest. **4:** 271–280.
14. OLDEN, K. 1999. NIEHS Fiscal Year 2000 Budget Request to the U.S. Congress (http://www.niehs.nih.gov/external/testimony.htm).

15. OLDEN, K. 2000. NIEHS Fiscal Year 2001 Budget Request to the U.S. Congress (http://www.niehs.nih.gov/external/fy2001/home.htm).
16. LEDER, A., A. KUO, R.D. CARDIFF, E. SINN & P. LEDER. 1990. v-Ha-ras transgene abrogates the initiation step in mouse skin tumorigenesis: effects of phorbol esters and retinoic acid. Proc. Natl. Acad. Sci. U.S.A. **87:** 9178–9182.
17. SPALDING, J.W., J. MOMMA, M.R. ELWELL & R.W. TENNANT. 1993. Chemical induced skin carcinogenesis in a transgenic mouse line (TG*AC) carrying a v-Ha-ras gene. Carcinogenesis **14:** 1335–1341.
18. TENNANT, R.W., J.E. FRENCH & J.W. SPALDING. 1995. Identifying chemical carcinogens and assessing potential risk in short-term bioassays using transgenic mouse models. Environ. Health Perspect. **103:** 942–950.
19. TENNANT, R.W., J. SPALDING & J.E. FRENCH. 1996. Evaluation of transgenic mouse bioassays for identifying carcinogens and noncarcinogens. Mutat. Res. **365:** 119–127.
20. YAMAMOTO, S., Y. HAYASHI, K. MITSUMORI & T. NOMURA. 1997. Rapid carcinogenicity testing system with transgenic mice harboring the human prototype c-HRAS gene. Lab. Anim. Sci. **47:** 121–126.
21. THOMPSON, K.L., B.A. ROSENZWEIG & F.D. SISTARE. 1998. An evaluation of the hemizygous transgenic Tg.AC mouse for carcinogenicity testing of pharmaceuticals. II. A genotypic marker that predicts tumorigenic responsiveness. Toxicol. Pathol. **26(4):** 548–555.
22. HOLDEN, H.E., R.E. STOLL, J.W. SPALDING & R.W. TENNANT. 1998. Hemizygous Tg.AC transgenic mouse as a potential alternative to the two-year mouse carcinogenicity bioassay: evaluation of husbandry and housing factors. Appl. Toxicol. **18:** 19–24.
23. BUCHER, J.R. 1998. Update on National Toxicology Program (NTP) assays with genetically altered or "transgenic" mice. Environ. Health Perspect. **106:** 619–621.
24. NTP. 1998. NTP Annual Program Plan (http://ntp-server.niehs.nih.gov/htdocs/98AP/8Carc.html#explore).
25. NTP. 1998. National Toxicology Board of Scientific Counselors Review: Summary Minutes (http://ntp-server.niehs.nih.gov/htdocs/Liason/BSC_Feb5.html).
26. NTP. 2000. National Toxicology Program Long Term Study Abstracts (http://ntp-server.niehs.nih.gov/htdocs/pub.html).
27. WEINBERG, A.M. & J.B. STORER. 1985. Ambiguous carcinogens and their regulation. Risk Anal. **5:** 151–156.
28. VON BORSTEL, R.C. & J.A. HIGGINS. 1998. Janus carcinogens and mutagens. Mutat. Res. **402:** 321–329.
29. HASEMAN, J. & F.M. JOHNSON. 1996. Analysis of National Toxicology Program rodent bioassay data for anticarcinogenic effects. Mutat. Res. **350:** 131–141.
30. JOHNSON, F.M. 1999. Carcinogenic chemical-response "fingerprint" for male F344 rats exposed to a series of 195 chemicals: implications for predicting carcinogens with transgenic models. Environ. Mol. Mutagen. **34:** 234–245.
31. SPALDING, J.W., J.E. FRENCH, S. STASIEWICZ, M. FUREDI-MACHACEK, F. CONNER, R.R. TICE & R.W. TENNANT. 2000. Responses of transgenic mouse lines p53(+/−) and Tg.AC to agents tested in conventional carcinogenicity bioassays. Toxicol. Sci. **53:** 213–223.
32. NCI. 2000. National Cancer Institute Cancer Gene List (http://lpg.nci.nih.gov/html-cgap/cgl/).
33. BULT, C.J., D.M. KRUPKE & J.T. EPPIG. 1999. Electronic access to mouse tumor data: the Mouse Tumor Biology (MTB) project. Nucleic Acids Res. **27:** 99–105.
34. LIJINSKY, W. 1993. Species differences in carcinogenesis. In Vivo **7:** 65–72.

Use of Bone Marrow Chimeras to Identify Cell Targets in the Immune System for the Actions of Chemicals

THOMAS A. GASIEWICZ,[a,b] T. SCOTT THURMOND,[b] J. ERIN STAPLES,[c] FRANCIS G. MURANTE,[b] AND ALLEN E. SILVERSTONE[c]

[b]*Department of Environmental Medicine, University of Rochester, Rochester, New York 14642, USA*

[c]*Department of Microbiology and Immunology, SUNY Health Sciences Center, Syracuse, New York 13210, USA*

INTRODUCTION

Since the immune system is essential to overall health status, there is concern over the potential ability of environmental and therapeutic agents to modulate immune function. The development of sensitive and meaningful markers of immunotoxicity to detect subtle, yet significant changes in health status is often difficult. This is hampered, at least in part, by the multicellular nature of the immune system and a lack of understanding of specific cell targets. This is true even when the specific receptor molecules with which these chemicals interact to cause toxicity are known. Both 2,3,7,8-tetrachlorodibenzo-*p*-dioxin (TCDD) and the estrogenic chemicals, diethylstilbestrol (DES) and β-estradiol (E2), are known to cause thymic atrophy and immune suppression. These chemicals act by binding to the aryl hydrocarbon (AhR) and estrogen (ER) receptors, respectively, to initiate signal transduction pathways. Yet, the actual cellular targets within the immune system are still unclear. These could be acting directly on the hemopoietic and/or supporting stromal cells in different ways to account for their effects. We have developed a strategy to identify the cellular targets in which these receptors must be activated to produce a particular immune system effect.

METHODS

Bone marrow cells are taken from AhR–[1] or ER–[2] null allele mice and are used to reconstitute, by tail vein injection, lethally irradiated animals containing these receptors.[3,4] This approach effectively creates mice that have stromal cells that are sensitive (+/+) to the actions of TCDD or E2, while the hemopoietic cells are insensitive (–/–). The converse experiment, that is, creating mice having +/+ hemopoietic and –/– stromal cells, is also performed. These chimeric mice are treated at 4 weeks

---

[a]Address for correspondence: Thomas A. Gasiewicz, Department of Environmental Medicine, University of Rochester Medical Center, Box EHSC, 601 Elmwood Avenue, Rochester, NY 14642. Voice: 716-275-7723; fax: 716-256-2591.
Tom_Gasiewicz@urmc.rochester.edu

TABLE 1. Consequences of TCDD treatment of chimeras

Chimera[a]	Thymic atrophy	Increased % CD44+/25−[b]	Decreased % CD4+/8+[b]	Increased % CD4−/8+[b]
+/+ → +/+	++	++	++	++
−/− → +/+	no effect	no effect	no effect	no effect
+/+ → −/−	++	++	++	++
−/− → −/−	no effect	no effect	no effect	no effect

[a]Donor mouse (and thus hemopoietic cells) indicated first; recipient second.
[b]The % of cells of the number remaining compared to vehicle-treated animals.

following radiation/reconstitution with TCDD (30 µg/kg, ip), E2 (5 mg/kg, sc), or olive oil. Results are compared to mice that contained both +/+ or −/− stromal and hemopoietic elements. Ten days after treatment, thymocyte and bone marrow cell suspensions are made, and mononuclear cells are counted and stained with fluorescent dye–conjugated monoclonal antibodies for assorted cell surface markers. Then, 10^5 or more fixed cells are analyzed on either a Becton-Dickinson FACScalibur Plus or FACScan flow cytometer using the LYSYS II program and CellQuest software.[3,4] Liver samples are prepared and analyzed as previously described.[5] Analyses for significance for tissue weight and cellular differences are performed using the two-tailed Student's t test for paired and unpaired variables.

RESULTS AND DISCUSSION

AhR Activation

When mice containing AhR−/− hemopoietic elements and AhR+/+ stromal elements were treated with TCDD, no signs of thymic atrophy were seen[3] (TABLE 1). In addition, there were no significant alterations in the phenotype of thymocytes as determined by analyses of CD4/8/3/44/25 markers.[3] These same results were also observed in chimeras containing both AhR−/− stromal and hemopoietic elements. In contrast, chimeric mice containing AhR+/+ hemopoietic and stromal elements (either chimeras or wild-type mice) and mice that had only AhR+/+ hemopoietic elements had significant declines in thymic weight and cell numbers after TCDD treatment. Phenotypic alterations included a reduction in the percentage of CD4+/8+ and CD44+/25+ cells and an increase in the percentage of CD44+/25− and CD4−/8+ cells.[3]

When bone marrow was examined, mice containing AhR+/+ hemopoietic and stromal elements or only AhR+/+ hemopoietic elements demonstrated increased percentages of c-kit+/Sca-1+ and c-kit−/Sca-1+ cells and decreased percentages of c-kit+/Sca-1− cells. However, animals containing both AhR−/− hemopoietic and stromal elements or only AhR−/− hemopoietic elements demonstrated none of these changes. The data indicate that TCDD-induced alterations to the thymus and bone marrow progenitor cells are dependent on AhR in hemopoietic cells.

TABLE 2. Consequences of E2 treatment of chimeras

Chimera	Thymic atrophy	Decreased % CD4+/8+	Increased % CD4+/8−	Increased % CD4−/8+
+/+ → +/+	++	++	++	++
−/− → +/+	++	++	++	++
+/+ → −/−	++	++	++	++
−/− → −/−	+/−	no effect	no effect	+

TCDD treatment also resulted in alterations in bone marrow B cell populations as defined by decreased pro/pre-B (B220lo/IgM−) and immature (B220lo/IgM+) cells. There was no effect on mature (B220hi/IgM+) cells. Treatment and analysis of the chimeric mice indicated that these B cell effects were dependent on AhR in both hemopoietic and stromal cells. Notably, analysis of control AhR−/− and AhR+/+ animals indicated that the AhR was necessary in both hemopoietic and stromal cells to maintain B cell phenotypic proportions. Increased pro/pre-B and immature B cells were consistently observed in AhR−/− animals.[6]

Finally, analysis of liver sections from these animals indicated that AhR activation in both stromal, that is, liver parenchymal cells, and hemopoietic cells contributed to hepatic lesions induced by TCDD.[5]

ERα Activation

Estradiol treatment to either wild-type or chimeric mice containing ERα in both hemopoietic and stromal elements resulted in significant thymic atrophy and alterations in thymocyte profiles as defined by decreased percentages of CD4+/8+ cells and increased percentages of CD4+/8− and CD4−/8+ cells (TABLE 2). Use of the chimeric mice containing ERα in either hemopoietic or stromal elements indicated that these alterations are dependent on the presence of ERα in both of these elements. Estradiol treatment also produced phenotypic alterations in bone marrow B cells as indicated by decreased percentages of pro/pre-B and immature B cells and increased percentages of mature B cells. These E2-induced changes were dependent on ERα signaling in both stromal and hemopoietic compartments.

Analysis of control ERα −/− and +/+ animals indicated that the presence of this receptor in stromal cells determines the size of the thymus. Thymic weight and cellularity in mice lacking ERα in stromal elements were less than 50% of this tissue from animals containing ERα in the stromal compartment. However, despite the decreased thymic cellularity, there were no differences in the relative percentages of CD4/8/3/44/25 cellular phenotypes. ERα also appeared to be necessary for B cell development since the relative percentages of pro/pre-, immature, and mature B cells were decreased in ER−/− animals.

CONCLUSIONS

These studies indicated that the use of chimeric animal models can identify cellular targets for the actions of immunomodulatory chemicals. Furthermore, these models can also be used to identify cells in which a particular receptor molecule has a normal function.

REFERENCES

1. FERNANDEZ-SALGUERO, P. *et al.* 1995. Immune system impairment and hepatic fibrosis in mice lacking the dioxin-binding Ah receptor. Science **268:** 722–726.
2. LUBAHN, D.B. *et al.* 1993. Alteration of reproductive function, but not prenatal sexual development after insertional disruption of the mouse estrogen receptor gene. Proc. Natl. Acad. Sci. U.S.A. **90:** 11162–11166.
3. STAPLES, J.E. *et al.* 1998. Thymic alterations induced by 2,3,7,8-tetrachlorodibenzo-*p*-dioxin are strictly dependent on aryl hydrocarbon receptor activation in hemopoietic cells. J. Immunol. **160:** 3844–3854.
4. STAPLES, J.E. *et al.* 1999. Estrogen receptor alpha is necessary in thymic development and estradiol-induced thymic alterations. J. Immunol. **163:** 4168–4174.
5. THURMOND, T.S. *et al.* 1999. Use of a chimeric Ah receptor knockout mouse model indicates that the presence of the Ah receptor in hematopoietic cells contributes to the hepatic lesions elicited by 2,3,7,8-tetrachlorodibenzo-*p*-dioxin. Toxicol. Appl. Pharmacol. **158:** 33–44.
6. THURMOND, T.S. *et al.* 2000. The aryl hydrocarbon receptor has a role in the *in vivo* maturation of murine bone marrow B lymphocytes and their responses to 2,3,7,8-tetrachlorodibenzo-*p*-dioxin. Toxicol. Appl. Pharmacol. **165:** 227–236.

The Effects of Lead on PKC Isoforms

ALDO A. COPPI, JACOB LESNIAK, DIANE ZIEBA,
AND FRANCIS A. X. SCHANNE[a]

College of Pharmacy and Allied Health Professions, St. John's University, Jamaica, New York 11439, USA

Lead toxicity continues to be a major health issue in the United States and a growing problem throughout the world. In the United States, lead affects a significant portion of preschool-age children, with those living in older urban areas at greater risk.[1] Lead poisoning is increasing in rapidly industrializing countries where there is little or no control over lead emissions or human exposure levels. Lead is a well-established neurotoxin. Exposure at various levels leads to mental retardation, cognitive impairments, maladaptive behavior, encephalopathy, and death.[1,2] Deficits in learning and memory are consistently associated with low levels of lead exposure both in human epidemiological studies and in experimentally treated animals.[1,2]

Protein kinase C (PKC) is a family of serine/threonine kinases, originally described for their calcium- and phospholipid-dependent activity.[3] As a major component of intracellular signal transduction, PKC mediates many kinds of cellular changes. PKC phosphorylates substrates upon its translocation to membranes with activation by diacylglycerol (DAG) and calcium (an important intracellular messenger).[3] In neurons, PKC plays an essential role in differentiation, development of cytoarchitecture, and alteration of the strength of synaptic connections between neurons.[4] Variations in the strength of synaptic connections between neurons have been hypothesized to be the physiological mechanism underlying learning and memory.[4]

Under normal physiologic conditions, calcium activates PKC in a concentration-dependent range from 10^{-7} to 10^{-4} M.[5] We have previously shown that lead can activate PKC at concentrations from 10^{-11} to 10^{-8} M, which is 1000 times less than the concentration of calcium required.[5,6] PKC appears to be the most sensitive target of lead identified to date. At least 11 distinct isoforms of PKC have been described, which share some structural components, but with some important differences among them.[3] The differences between the PKC isoforms can be attributed to their calcium-dependence. The conventional (cPKC) or calcium-dependent isoforms include PKC α, β-I, β-II, and γ. These require calcium for activation. Conversely, novel isoforms (nPKC), PKC δ, ε, and η, are calcium-independent kinases; hence, they do not require calcium for activation. Finally, the atypical isoforms (aPKC), PKC ζ and λ, do not require either calcium or DAG for activation. In the present study, we examined (1) the ability of lead to substitute for calcium in the activation of PKC isolated from rat brain, (2) the importance of a C2 domain for lead activation

---

[a]Corresponding author: Francis A. X. Schanne, College of Pharmacy and Allied Health Professions, St. John's University, 8000 Utopia Parkway, Jamaica, NY 11439. Voice: 718-990-5815; fax: 718-990-1877.
schannef@stjohns.edu

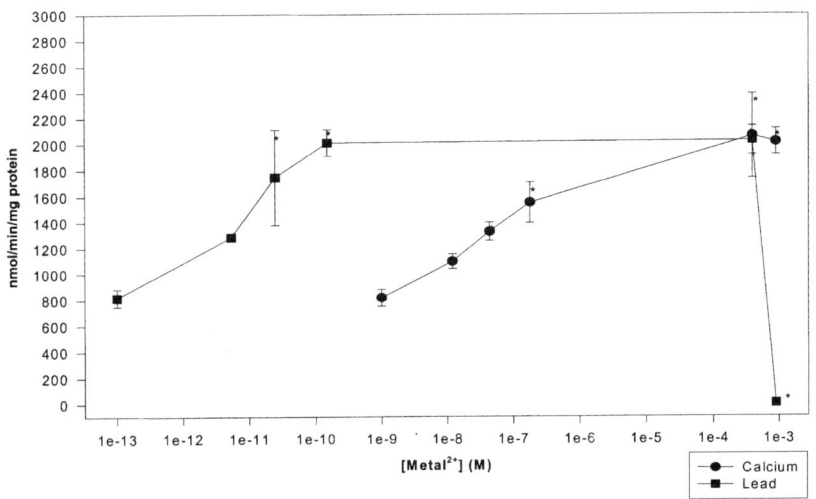

FIGURE 1. Brain homogenate activity with calcium chloride and lead acetate.

of PKC, and (3) the selective interactions of lead with individual isoforms of PKC in comparison to their interaction with calcium.

In part one of the study, a crude preparation of PKC from a 100,000g supernatant rat brain homogenate was examined. PKC activity was measured as the phosphatidylserine/DAG-dependent transfer of [γ-P^{32}]ATP to Histone H-1.[5] The specific metal-dependent activation of PKC was determined in the presence of specific concentrations of lead and calcium buffered by the divalent cation chelator 5F-BAPTA.[5] The specific free lead and calcium concentrations were determined using ^{19}F-NMR.[5] The results indicated activation with both lead and calcium. As shown in FIGURE 1, lead activated PKC at concentrations from 10^{-13} to about 4×10^{-4} M, while calcium activated at concentrations from 10^{-9} to about 4×10^{-4} M. However, lead at concentrations $> 4 \times 10^{-4}$ M inhibited PKC activity, while calcium did not.

In part two of the study, human recombinant PKC isoenzymes—conventionals (cPKC α, β-I, β-II, and γ) and novels (nPKC δ and ε)—were individually examined to determine the sensitivity and selectivity of these isoenzymes for activation and inhibition by lead and calcium. Each isoenzyme is treated in a similar manner as the brain homogenate preparation. As shown in FIGURE 2, a distinct sensitivity of PKC α for lead was revealed, activating the enzyme at concentrations from about 5×10^{-11} to about 4×10^{-4} M. Lead had little activating effect on PKC γ, but produced inhibition at concentrations $> 4 \times 10^{-11}$ M. Neither calcium nor lead activated PKC δ and ε. Lead inhibited PKC δ at concentrations $> 4 \times 10^{-4}$ M, while lead inhibited PKC ε at concentrations $> 4 \times 10^{-11}$ M.

These findings confirm the ability of lead to substitute for calcium in the activation of isolated PKC. Furthermore, the results confirm the importance of a C2 domain for the activation of PKC by lead due to the lack of activity observed with the nPKC isoforms. Finally, these data indicate that the range of lead concentrations necessary to activate and/or inhibit PKC is unique for each isoform. These findings

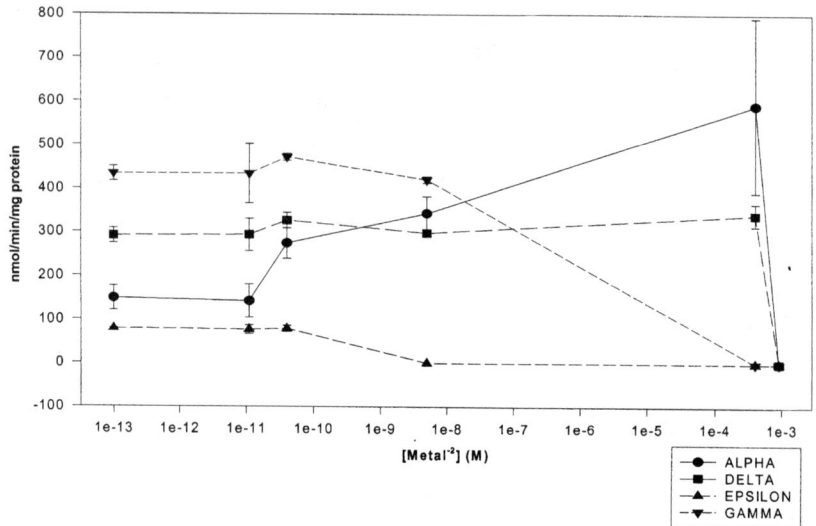

FIGURE 2. cPKC and nPKC activity with lead acetate.

suggest a complex pattern of PKC isoform activation and/or inhibition in lead poisoning at low to moderate lead exposure.

ACKNOWLEDGMENTS

This research was supported in part by NIH Grant No. ESO 9499 awarded to Francis A. X. Schanne.

REFERENCES

1. AGENCY FOR TOXIC SUBSTANCES AND DISEASE REGISTRY. 1988. The Nature and Extent of Lead Poisoning in Children in the United States: A Report to Congress. U.S. Department of Health and Human Services. Washington, D.C.
2. BELLINGER, D. & H.L. NEEDLEMAN. 1980. Neurodevelopmental effects of low level lead exposure in children. *In* Low Level Lead Exposure: The Clinical Implications of Current Research. Raven Press. New York.
3. NEWTON, A.C. 1995. Protein kinase C: structure, function, and regulation. J. Biol. Chem. **270:** 28495–28498.
4. BRESSLER, J.P. & G.W. GOLDSTEIN. 1991. Mechanism of lead neurotoxicity. Biochem. Pharmacol. **41:** 479–484.
5. LONG, G.J., J.F. ROSEN & F.A.X. SCHANNE. 1994. Lead activation of protein kinase C from rat brain. J. Biol. Chem. **269:** 834-837.
6. MARKOVAC, J. & G.W. GOLDSTEIN. 1988. Picomolar concentrations of lead stimulate brain protein kinase C. Nature **334:** 71–73.

Lead-Induced Activation of Protein Kinase C in Rat Brain Cortical Synaptosomes

CHRISTOPHER D. TOSCANO[a,b] AND FRANCIS A. X. SCHANNE[a,c]

[a]*Department of Pharmaceutical Sciences, College of Pharmacy and Allied Health Professions, St. John's University, Jamaica, New York 11439, USA*

Protein kinase C (PKC) is a calcium-activated, phospholipid-dependent Ser/Thr phosphotransferase that plays a role in signal transduction cascades, gene regulation, growth and development of cells, exocytosis of neurotransmitters, and neuronal plasticity.[1] It has been demonstrated using various cellular and subcellular models that submicromolar lead concentrations are able to activate PKC, presumably by acting as a calcium surrogate.[2–4] Even though these studies were able to demonstrate that lead does indeed activate PKC, they were not able to directly measure the free concentrations of lead and calcium needed for PKC activation. However, by using ^{19}F-NMR and the divalent cation chelator, 5,5'-difluoro-1,2-bis(2-aminophenoxy)ethane-N,N,N',N'-tetraacetic acid (5F-BAPTA), it is possible to measure the free lead and calcium concentrations needed to activate PKC.[5,6] The results of these experiments demonstrated that lead at free concentrations of 10^{-10} M is able to activate PKC, whereas calcium begins to activate PKC at free concentrations greater than 10^{-7} M.[5,6]

It has been demonstrated that low-level lead toxicity results in subtle nervous system defects such as cognitive and behavioral deficits.[7] The origins of these neurological effects are unknown and currently under investigation. It has also been demonstrated that one of the cellular targets for low-level lead toxicity is PKC.[2–6] Therefore, it is important to understand the involvement, if any, of PKC in the observed low-level lead-induced cognitive defects. To this end, we examined the effect of lead on PKC using rat brain cortical synaptosomes.[8]

In order to assay synaptosomal PKC activity and to control the intrasynaptosomal metal concentrations, an *in situ* assay of PKC activity was conducted in digitonin-permeabilized synaptosomes using 5F-BAPTA to buffer the free metal concentrations and ^{19}F-NMR to determine the free divalent cation concentrations. The maximal synaptosomal PKC activity in the absence and presence of 1 µM PMA was observed in digitonin-permeabilized synaptosomes at 4.2×10^{-4} M free calcium, whereas maximal lead-induced activation was observed to occur at 2.24×10^{-9} M free lead (FIGS. 1A and 1B). Even though lead-induced maximal activation occurs at concentrations that are 200,000 times lower than at maximal calcium activation, the maximal lead activation represents an enzyme activity that is 35% less than the

---

[b]Present address: Department of Environmental Health Sciences, Division of Toxicological Sciences, Johns Hopkins School of Hygiene and Public Health, Baltimore, MD 21205-2179.

[c]Corresponding author: Francis A. X. Schanne, Department of Pharmaceutical Sciences, College of Pharmacy and Allied Health Professions, St. John's University, 8000 Utopia Parkway, Jamaica, NY 11439. Voice: 718-990-5815; fax: 718-990-1877.

schannef@stjohns.edu

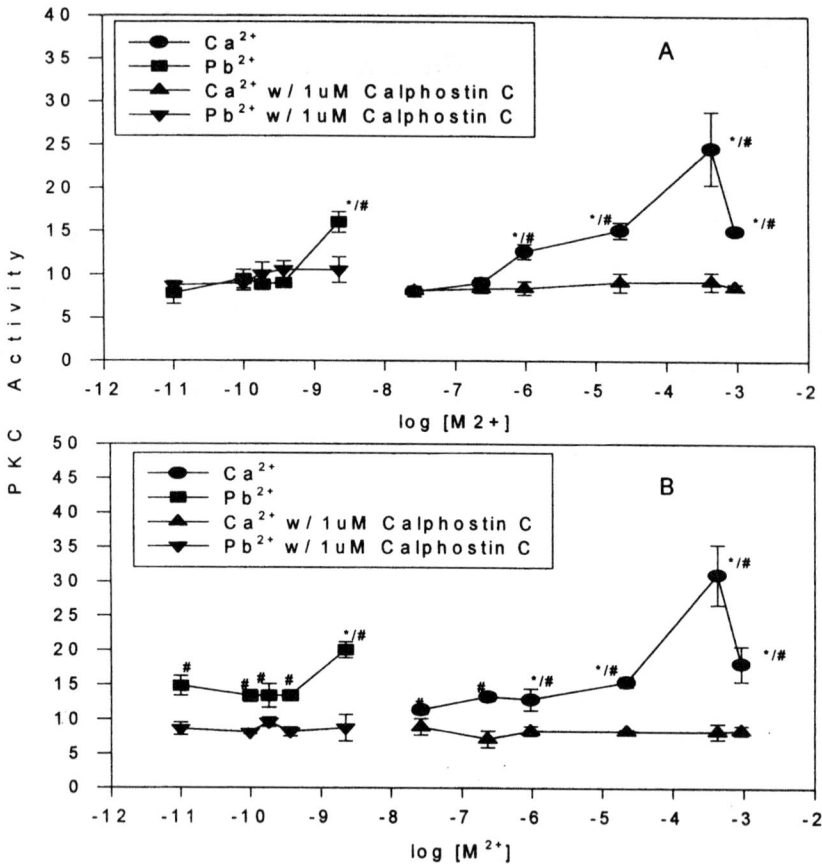

FIGURE 1. Synaptosomal PKC activity (nmol PO_4/10 min/mg) was assayed by incubation of the synaptosomes in a calcium-free Krebs-HEPES permeabilization buffer containing 50 µg/mL digitonin and 100 µg/mL leupeptin for 20 min at 30°C followed by the addition of the synaptosomes to the PKC activity assay. The final composition of each assay included 20 µg of synaptosomes, (**A**) no PMA or (**B**) 1 µM PMA, 1 µM okadaic acid, 100 µM [Ser^{25}]-PKC fragment 19–31 (Arg-Phe-Ala-Arg-Lys-Gly-Ser-Leu-Arg-Gln-Lys-Asn-Val), 500 µM ATP (75 nCi), and lead acetate or calcium chloride buffered with 2 mM 5F-BAPTA. After 10 min, the reaction was stopped with the addition of 25% trichloroacetic acid and an aliquot of the reaction mixture was spotted to a P81 phosphocellulose cation exchange filter, which was counted by liquid scintillation. Data are the means ± SD of two triplicate experiments. *Data points significantly different [ANOVA ($p < 0.05$); Dunnet's t test ($p < 0.05$)] from no added metal. #Data points significantly different ($p < 0.05$; Student's t test) from 1 µM calphostin C.

maximal calcium activation at 4.27×10^{-4} M. Whether the assay is conducted in the presence or absence of PMA, the observed activity is attributable to PKC due to the fact that calphostin C completely inhibits the observed metal- and PMA-dependent activity.

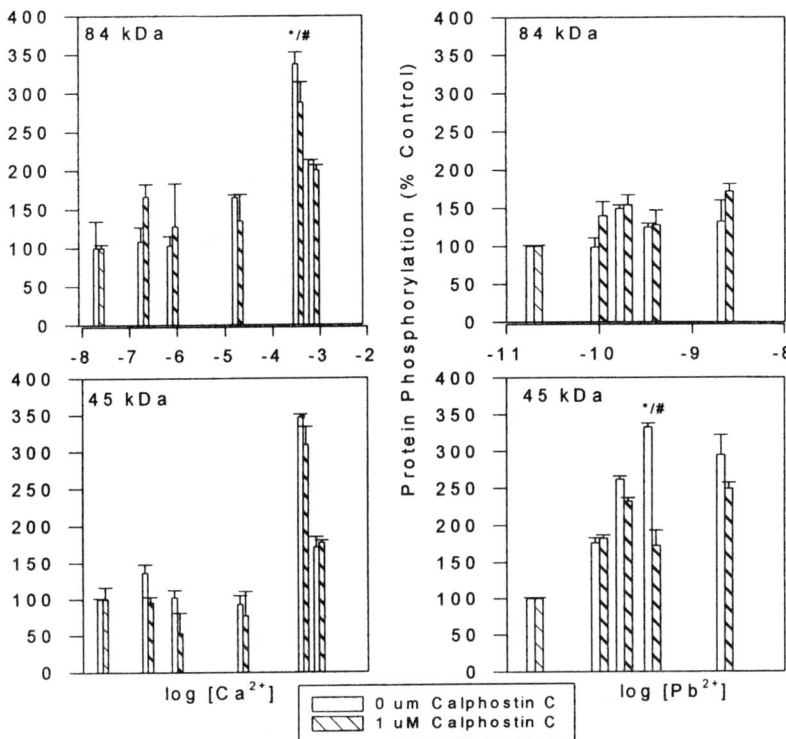

FIGURE 2. The phosphorylation of endogenous synaptosomal PKC substrates was assayed in permeabilized synaptosomes as detailed in FIGURE 1, except the reaction was stopped by the addition of SDS-PAGE sample buffer and no exogenous PKC substrate was added. After the addition of the sample buffer, the samples were loaded to a 10% SDS-PAGE gel. The proteins were separated by electrophoresis and the gels were exposed to X-ray film for 48 hours at $-20°C$. The intensity of the bands on the autoradiograph was analyzed using computerized densitometry. The assays were run in the presence and absence of 1 μM calphostin C, a selective and potent PKC inhibitor, in order to determine the contribution of PKC to the observed activity. Data are the means ± SD of three duplicate experiments. Percent control was calculated as intensity sample/intensity control × 100. *Data points significantly different [ANOVA ($p < 0.05$); Dunnet's t test ($p < 0.05$)] from no added metal. #Data points significantly different ($p < 0.05$; Student's t test) from 1 μM calphostin C.

No overall trends in calcium- or lead-induced phosphorylation of the 84- and 45-kDa proteins were observed in the endogenous phosphorylation densitometry experiments (FIG. 2). However, in the calcium-induced phosphorylation experiments, the phosphorylation of the 84-kDa protein was observed to significantly increase 250% over no added calcium in a PKC-mediated fashion at 4.2×10^{-4} M free calcium. Although there is a lack of an overall trend in lead-induced phosphorylation, a 250% lead-induced increase in PKC-mediated phosphorylation of the 45-kDa protein was observed at 3.65×10^{-10} M free lead.

The results obtained in this series of experiments correspond to the results observed in other accounts of lead-induced activation of PKC.[2-6] Therefore, it has been shown by this data set that presynaptic PKC is activated at concentrations of free lead comparable to that observed in other experimental models. This data set has also shown that lead-activated PKC is able to phosphorylate a physiological presynaptic substrate with a molecular weight of 45 kDa. This is an important observation since GAP-43, a major presynaptic PKC substrate involved in synaptic plasticity and neurotransmitter release, migrates on SDS-PAGE to a molecular weight of 45 kDa.[9] Thus, this is indirect evidence that PKC activated at nanomolar concentrations of free lead is able to phosphorylate GAP-43. Further investigation into the identity of the phosphorylated 45-kDa protein is needed before a definitive conclusion can be made. It is intriguing to consider the implications of lead-induced phosphorylation of GAP-43 since the phosphorylation of this protein appears to be essential for the induction of long-term potentiation.[10]

The free lead concentrations observed to result in PKC activation (10^{-10}–10^{-9} M) suggest the potential importance of this mechanism in low to moderate lead poisoning. The current definition of low to moderate blood lead is 10 to 50 µg/dL or 0.5 to 2.5×10^{-6} M.[7] At such blood lead concentrations, 98–99% has been found to be tightly associated with red blood cells and 1–2% of the lead in blood has been found in the plasma, while the cerebrospinal fluid was one-half the plasma concentration.[11] Thus, in low to moderate lead intoxication, neurons are bathed in 10^{-8} M lead. From this, it is reasonable to consider that intracellular free lead concentrations in the range of 10^{-10} to 10^{-9} M might occur in the presence of such extracellular concentrations. Therefore, the current findings as well as the findings of other investigators,[2-6] demonstrating the activation of PKC by extremely low concentrations of lead, may indeed be relevant to the etiology of low to moderate lead poisoning.

ACKNOWLEDGMENTS

This research was supported by a Sigma Xi, The Scientific Research Society Grant-in-Aid of Research, awarded to Christopher Dennis Toscano and by NIH Grant No. ESO 9499 awarded to Francis A. X. Schanne.

REFERENCES

1. OGITA, K., H. KOIDE, U. KIKKAWA, A. KISHIMOTO & Y. NISHIZUKA. 1990. The heterogeneity of protein kinase C in signal transduction cascade. *In* The Biology and Medicine of Signal Transduction. Raven Press. New York.
2. MARKOVAC, J. & G.W. GOLDSTEIN. 1988. Lead activates protein kinase C in immature rat brain microvessels. Toxicol. Appl. Pharmacol. **96:** 14–23.
3. TOMSIG, J.L. & J.B. SUSZKIW. 1995. Multisite interactions between lead and protein kinase C and its role in norepinephrine release from bovine adrenal chromaffin cells. J. Neurochem. **64:** 2667–2673.
4. BELLONI-OLIVI, L., M. ANNADATA, G.W. GOLDSTEIN & J.P. BRESSLER. 1996. Phosphorylation of membrane proteins in erythrocytes treated with lead. Biochem. J. **315:** 401–406.
5. SCHANNE, F.A.X., G.J. LONG & J.F. ROSEN. 1997. Lead-induced rise in intracellular free calcium is mediated through activation of protein kinase C in osteoblastic bone cells. Biochim. Biophys. Acta **1360:** 247–254.

6. LONG, G.J., J.F. ROSEN & F.A.X. SCHANNE. 1994. Lead activation of protein kinase C from rat brain. J. Biol. Chem. **269:** 834–837.
7. RUFF, H.A. & P.E. BIJUR. 1989. The effects of low to moderate lead levels on neurobehavioral functioning in children: toward a conceptual model. J. Dev. Behav. Pediatr. **10:** 103–109.
8. DUNKLEY, P.R., J.W. HEATH, S.M. HARRISON, P.E. JARVIE, P.J. GLENFIELD, J.A.P. ROSTAS & P.J. ROBINSON. 1988. A rapid Percoll gradient procedure for isolation of synaptosomes directly from an S1 fraction: homogeneity and morphology of subcellular fractions. Brain Res. **441:** 59–71.
9. DE GRAAN, P.N.E., A.B. OESTREICHER, P. SCHOTMAN & L.H. SCHRAMA. 1986. Protein kinase C substrate B-50 (GAP-43) and neurotransmitter release. *In* Progress in Brain Research. Volume 69. Elsevier. Amsterdam/New York.
10. RAMAKERS, G.M., P.N. DE GRAAN, I.J. URBAN, D. KRAAY, T. TANG, P. PASINELLI, A.B. OESTREICHER & W.H. GISPEN. 1995. Temporal differences in the phosphorylation state of pre- and postsynaptic protein kinase C substrates B-50/GAP-43 and neurogranin during long-term potentiation. J. Biol. Chem. **270:** 13892–13898.
11. MANTON, W.I. & J.D. COOK. 1984. High accuracy (stable isotope dilution) measurements of lead in serum and cerebrospinal fluid. Br. J. Ind. Med. **41:** 313–319.

Reactivities of the Skin-Sensitization Test in Guinea Pig (GPMT) as a Function of Three Parameters: Induction Doses (MID), Challenge Doses (SCD), and Direct Exposures (DED)

SATOSHI KITAJIMA,[a] JUNKO MOMMA, AND TOHRU INOUE

Cellular and Molecular Toxicology Division, National Institute of Health Sciences, Setagayaku, Tokyo 158-8501, Japan

In the phenomenon of chemical-induced skin sensitization, it remains unclear whether the dose needed for induction correlates directly with the dose that elicits a skin reaction. Furthermore, it is uncertain whether exposure to a continuous, very low level of the chemical or to a single high level is the most effective in induction. Similarly, it is not known which types of chemical exposure elicit a response more effectively, again whether at very low levels or at a high level.

Recently, we demonstrated a novel rule in the relationship between the levels of chemical exposures and a chemical-induced skin sensitization. This new formulation could lead to an index of the strength of chemicals as skin sensitizers. Our finding of the novel rule will be useful not only in practical immunotoxicological applications to predict possible skin sensitizers in humans, but also in understanding the fundamental immunology involved in sensitization. However, it will be necessary to clarify the immunological molecular mechanisms from which the new correlation formula arises.

Evaluating chemicals for their potential adverse effects on the human skin is accomplished by various skin-sensitization tests.[1] All the present assay systems are *in vivo* ones. Magnusson and Kligman[2] established the guinea pig maximization test (GPMT), which is a nonspecific test; the inclusion later of Freund's complete adjuvant (FCA) evoked a greater sensitization in the animals.

To explore whether a potential correlation exists between the results of the GPMT and the residual levels of chemicals in the causative products, we reassessed the data taken from eight chemicals that were evaluated by the GPMT together with records of their inclusion in commercial products.[3] All of the products have background data showing them as having induced accidental contact-sensitization in humans, possibly from the presence of the irritant chemicals in household appliances, clothes, and dyestuffs. These records classified the intensity of human sensitization as "highly significant", "significant", and "none". Nakamura *et al.*[3] introduced three parameters in their article, that is, the minimum induction dose (MID), the standard challenge dose (SCD), and the level of the chemical in the products (direct-exposure-

---

[a]Address for correspondence: Cellular and Molecular Toxicology Division, National Institute of Health Sciences, 1-18-1 Kamiyoga, Setagayaku, Tokyo 158-8501, Japan. Voice: 81-3-3700-9646; fax: 81-3-3700-9647.
satoshi@nihs.go.jp

dose = DED). [Terms: MID = the lowest induction dose under the maximum challenge, at which a skin reaction is least visible and still evaluable, in the GPMT; SCD = the challenge dose that produces "a modest skin reaction" after induction at the maximum nonirritating concentration; a modest skin reaction is adopted as the dose where the score is 1.0 on average, obtained from the dose-response curve between the scores and graded challenge doses in the GPMT; DED (direct-exposure-dose) = the possible levels of sensitizing chemicals remaining in commercial products, all of which are on record as having induced accidental contact-sensitization in humans.] Both MID and SCD are the parameters in the GPMT, and DED is closely related to the incidence of cases of human allergy.

Since the DED seemed to be independent from MID as well as from SCD, we plotted DED/MID and DED/SCD against each other for each of these groupings separately (FIG. 1). The groups diverged along curves that were hyperbolic in shape, in which the group on the abscissa and the other on the ordinate generally produced a constant product.

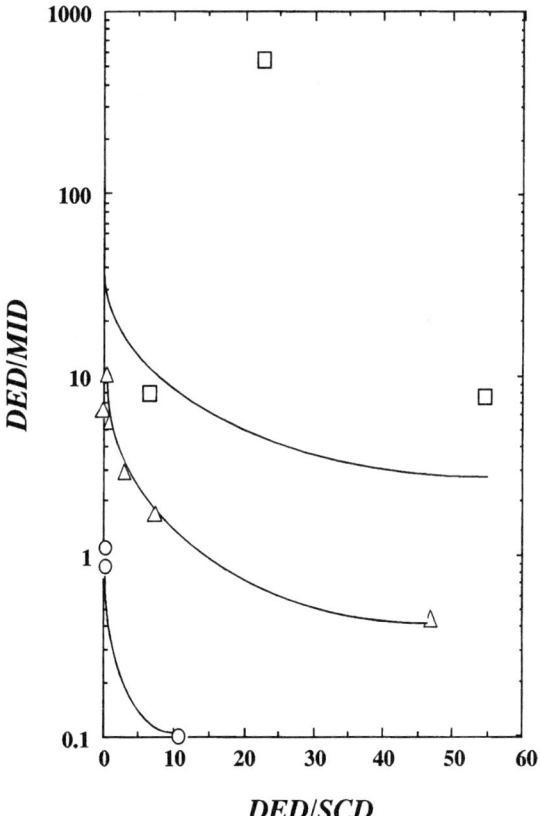

FIGURE 1. Correlation between the MID, SCD, and DED for human incidences (□: highly significant; △: significant; ○: none).

Several trials were made to seek a general function, and the following one was finally adopted for each group:

$$D = DED/(MID \cdot SCD) \qquad (1)$$

where D is a discrimination constant that is specific to each group along with a grade in intensity of human sensitization.

Accordingly, the D value for the grade of "highly significant (D4)" was calculated as 3.99 ± 2.61, which is highly distinguishable from the value of D1, "none", 0.00004 ± 0.00003. In addition, the D values for the other groups are also calculated as 0.026 ± 0.015 for "significant (D3)" and 0.0005 ± 0.0004 for "gray zone (D2)". In fact, each group, along with its grade in incidence of human cases, showed a split range of values.

Thus, we could demonstrate a novel rule of skin-sensitization intensity that corresponds to each grade. Since it is important for prediction of human sensitization to obtain the no-adverse-effect-level (NOAEL), the following formula was calculated, modified from equation 1:

$$R = DED = D \cdot (MID \cdot SCD). \qquad (1')$$

When D1 (for a nonsignificant level) is incorporated into the formula, the R1 calculated here is considered to be the NOAEL value.

From equation 1, the DED represents the chemical doses for continuous exposure on human skin. Thus, the equation indicates that continuous exposure doses should be linked directly to the single dose for both induction and elicitation, which are independent factors. If it is assumed that the mechanisms of skin sensitization are the same in humans and guinea pigs, and if D3 (for a significant level) is incorporated into the formula, the following equation was obtained, modified from equation 1:

$$DED = 0.026 \cdot (MID \cdot SCD). \qquad (2)$$

The reason why D3 is incorporated is that both MID and SCD are the standard dose for the induction and elicitation phase, respectively, and DED is the standard dose for continuous exposure.

REFERENCES

1. MAURER, T., A. ARTHUR & P. BENTLEY. 1994. Guinea-pig contact sensitization assays. Toxicology **93:** 47–54.
2. MAGNUSSON, B. & A.M. KLIGMAN. 1969. The identification of contact allergens by animal assay: the guinea pig maximization test. J. Invest. Dermatol. **52:** 268–276.
3. NAKAMURA, A., J. MOMMA, H. SEKIGUCHI et al. 1994. A new protocol and criteria for quantitative determination of sensitization potencies of chemicals by guinea pig maximization test. Contact Dermatitis **31:** 72–85.

Toxicity of Ethylene Glycol Metabolites in Normal Human Kidney Cells

K. E. McMARTIN[a] AND T. A. CENAC

Department of Pharmacology, Louisiana State University Health Sciences Center, Shreveport, Louisiana, USA

Ethylene glycol (EG) produces a toxic syndrome characterized by severe metabolic acidosis and acute renal failure, which can be fatal if untreated.[1] The toxicity of EG is linked with its metabolism to glycolic acid, which is responsible for the acidosis, and to oxalic acid. The latter is poorly soluble in the presence of calcium and the appearance of calcium oxalate crystals in the urine is used diagnostically.[1] The renal toxicity of EG has been related to the precipitation of oxalate crystals in the tubular lumen, leading to luminal blockage and compression-induced loss of glomerular filtration (renal failure). However, in transformed kidney cells, the oxalate ion induces cytotoxic damage,[2,3] which may explain the tubular necrosis that is noted in pathologic exams of EG-exposed kidneys. In our studies on the treatment of EG poisoning with fomepizole,[4] the mean plasma glycolate concentration in patients with renal failure was 21 mM, while that in patients without renal failure was 4 mM. Plasma oxalate levels were below the detectability limit (0.5 mM), while urine oxalate concentrations often reached 2 to 5 mM. These data suggest that the proximal tubule (PT) in EG-poisoned patients is exposed to much more glycolate than oxalate and that the cytotoxicity of glycolate needs to be studied. Therefore, we have compared the relative cytotoxicity of EG metabolites on HPT cells, which are primary cultures of normal human kidney cells, as opposed to transformed porcine and canine kidney cells.[2,3]

METHODS

HPT cells were grown to confluency in tissue culture flasks as outlined previously.[5] Cells were subcultured onto 24-well tissue culture plates and incubated at 37°C until the development of confluency. Cells were first rinsed with assay buffer (20 mM HEPES, pH 7.4, containing NaCl, KCl, $CaCl_2$, $MgCl_2$, D-glucose, and $NaHCO_3$); then, 1 mL of each substrate (in assay buffer) was added to separate wells, which were incubated for 0, 2, 4, and 6 hours at 37°C. Cells were treated with EG (0–25 mM), glycolate (0–25 mM), glyoxylate (0–5 mM), or oxalate (0–5 mM), that is, reasonable concentrations for each substance in human cases of EG poisoning.[1,4] In additional studies, the pH of the assay buffer was varied (6.5–7.4). After the incubations, assay buffer was aspirated, and the cells were rinsed and treated

---

[a]Address for correspondence: Kenneth McMartin, Department of Pharmacology, LSU Health Sciences Center, 1501 Kings Highway, Shreveport, LA 71130-3932. Voice: 318-675-7871; fax: 318-675-7857.

kmcmar@lsumc.edu

with the Live/Dead® reagent [2 μM calcein-AM and 4 μM ethidium homodimer-1 (EthD), from Molecular Probes, Eugene, OR]. The plates were incubated at room temperature for 45 min, and EthD fluorescence (RFU), as a measure of cell death, was quantitated using a fluorescence microplate reader. These RFU values were standardized by calculating the % cell death by the ratio of the EthD RFU for the treated sample to the EthD RFU for the sample after additional treatment to achieve 100% cell death (1 mL of 0.1% Triton). In these studies, the Live/Dead® assay determined whether any of the metabolites produced cell death or affected the viability of the HPT cells. LDH release is a standard assay for cytotoxicity assessment, but it was not used because glycolate adversely affects LDH activity measurements. In the Live/Dead® assay, viable cells contain intracellular esterase activity that converts the nonfluorescent, but permeable substrate, calcein-AM, to calcein, which is retained in live cells and produces a green fluorescence. EthD is impermeable to live cells, only entering cells with damaged plasma membranes, where it binds to nucleic acids, leading to a red fluorescence. Hence, this assay can be used to detect both viable cells and those with damaged membranes using fluorescence microscopy.

RESULTS

EG itself did not produce an increase in EthD fluorescence, indicating a lack of cytotoxicity. Glycolate in concentrations up to 25 mM (such levels are seen in patients with renal failure) did not affect the viability of HPT cells. The entry of glycolate, a weak acid, into cells is pH-dependent (lower pH, lesser ionization, greater uptake, and possibly greater toxicity). However, reducing the buffer pH to 6.5 did not produce any toxicity for glycolate. Glyoxylate, up to 5 mM, also failed to produce toxic effects on HPT cells, except when the buffer pH was lowered to 6.5. In contrast to these results, oxalate produced a time- and concentration-dependent increase in EthD fluorescence. At concentrations above 2 mM for 6 hours, oxalate produced a significant increase in % cell death (from $17 \pm 1\%$ to $33 \pm 5\%$ at 5 mM). These quantitative results were corroborated by fluorescence microscopy. Oxalate (5 mM, 6 h) produced dramatic increases in the number of dead cells (detection of red EthD fluorescence) and decreases in the number of viable cells compared to controls (detection of green calcein fluorescence). The toxic effects of oxalate were easily discerned using light microscopy with a Hoffman modulation contrast filter. The latter showed a loss of confluency and of normal morphology in the oxalate-treated HPT cells, as well as a possible presence of oxalate crystals intracellularly.

COMMENTS

These studies clearly show that oxalate induces a cytotoxicity in normal human kidney cells in culture, in concentrations similar to those observed in the urine of humans poisoned with EG. Hence, the oxalate levels in the tubular lumen of EG-poisoned patients are likely to contribute greatly to the acute tubular necrosis and renal failure observed in these cases. Although glycolate accumulates to much higher concentrations than oxalate, these studies suggest strongly that it does not play a role in the nephrotoxicity of EG.

REFERENCES

1. JACOBSEN, D. & K.E. MCMARTIN. 1986. Methanol and ethylene glycol poisonings: mechanism of toxicity, clinical course, diagnosis, and treatment. Med. Toxicol. **1:** 309–334.
2. SCHEID, C. et al. 1996. Oxalate toxicity in LLC-PK1 cells, a line of renal epithelial cells. J. Urol. **155:** 1112–1116.
3. HACKETT, R.L. et al. 1995. Alterations in MDCK and LLC-PK1 cells exposed to oxalate and calcium oxalate monohydrate crystals. Scanning Microsc. **9:** 587–596.
4. BRENT, J., K.E. MCMARTIN et al. 1999. Fomepizole for the treatment of ethylene glycol poisoning. N. Engl. J. Med. **340:** 832–838.
5. MCMARTIN, K.E. et al. 1992. Folate transport and binding by cultured human proximal tubule cells. Am. J. Physiol. **263:** F841–F848.

Cadmium-Induced Bioaccumulation in the Selected Tissues of a Freshwater Teleost, *Oreochromis mossambicus* (Tilapia)

A. USHA RANI[a]

Pesticide and Industrial Toxicology Center, Department of Zoology, Sri Venkateswara University, Tirupati 517 502 (A.P.), India

INTRODUCTION

In recent years, heavy metals discharged from industrial effluents have been a major source of pollution and have become a threat to all forms of life. Among the myriads of pollutants, cadmium (Cd^{++}) is a ubiquitous, nonessential heavy metal that possesses high toxicity to both humans and aquatic organisms.[1,2] A good deal of information is available on the toxic effects of Cd compounds on behavioral, physiological, biochemical, hematological, histological, reproductive, and teratological aspects of fish.[3–7] A very important biological property of metals is their tendency to bioaccumulate.[8] Cd, unlike other toxic pollutants, has the tendency to bioaccumulate in organisms. A number of biotic factors such as body size, maturity, sex, etc., influence the bioaccumulation.[9] This uptake of heavy metals is mostly tissue-specific and may even biomagnify in animals of higher trophic levels, including humans. It is this state of the art of the metal that is posing a threat to nontarget organisms of the trophic levels.

In this study, an attempt has been made to determine the possible uptake of cadmium and its residues in the selected tissues of the freshwater fish, *Oreochromis mossambicus (Tilapia)*, and also the tissue-specific type of Cd accumulation.

MATERIALS AND METHODS

Freshwater fish *Oreochromis mossambica* (10 ± 2 g) were collected from local ponds and were acclimated to laboratory conditions for a week under a natural photoperiod. Fish were fed *ad libitum* with powdered dry groundnut cake and were starved for 24 h before experimentation to avoid prandial effects.

Cadmium chloride (Analar grade) supplied by the British Drug House, India, was used as the metal toxicant in the experiment. The lethal limits were determined using the probit analysis of Finney[10] and the LC50 (48 h) was found to be 50 mg/L. Batches of 10 fish were exposed to sublethal concentrations [one-tenth of LC50 (48 h)] of Cd; that is, 5 mg/L for durations of 1, 15, and 30 days. A fourth group of 10 fish were maintained as controls in clean water. The ambient sublethal concentration of Cd

---

[a]Voice: 91 08574 50666, ext. 304; fax: 91 08574 25818.
asupatri@england.com

TABLE 1. Cadmium bioaccumulation in the selected tissues of *O. mossambicus*

S. no.	Tissue taken	Cd concentrations (ppm ± SD)			
		Control	1 day	15 days	30 days
1.	Gills	0.03 ± 0.001	0.05 ± 0.001 (66.6%)	0.30 ± 0.002 (900%)	1.0 ± 0.001 (3233%)
2.	Liver	0.2 ± 0.002	0.30 ± 0.002 (50%)	3.50 ± 0.001 (165%)	8.60 ± 0.53 (420%)
3.	Kidney	0.25 ± 0.001	0.80 ± 0.023 (220%)	5.60 ± 0.4 (2140%)	14.4 ± 1.4 (5640%)
4.	Intestine	0.0	0.01 ± 0.001	0.38 ± 0.02	0.85 ± 0.001
5.	Scales	0.0	0.005 ± 0.002	0.25 ± 0.01	0.70 ± 0.02

NOTE: Values are ppm ± SD of observations. Figures in parentheses represent the % change over control.

was renewed for every 24 h. After each time interval of sublethal exposure, the animals were taken from the container and washed in normal tap water to remove any medium from external body parts of the animal. Tissues like gills, liver, kidney, intestine, and scales were collected and weighed. Fifty mg of the tissue was taken in 10-mL-capacity airtight vials containing 5 mL of 3:2 nitric acid:perchloric acid mixture in which the actual digestion was carried out. The vials containing tissue samples were kept overnight for acid digestion. The acid sediment mixture was then slowly digested to near dryness on a controlled-temperature hot plate (temperature was kept below 120°C). The residue was dissolved in 5 mL of double-distilled water. The concentrations of Cd (in ppm) in the selected tissues were determined using an Atomic Absorption Spectrophotometer (Perkin-Elmer Model 2380).

RESULTS AND DISCUSSION

TABLE 1 shows the mean concentration of Cd (ppm) in the selected tissues like gills, liver, kidney, intestine, and scales of the freshwater fish, *O. mossambicus*. The amount of accumulation recorded in gills, liver, and kidney was significantly higher than that of control fish ($p < 0.001$). The level of metals examined was generally higher in kidney than in other tissues and markedly so for the 30-day exposure period (14.4 ppm). Intestine and scales showed much less accumulation of the metal (0.85 and 0.70 ppm, respectively). Liver also accumulated Cd at high levels (8.50 ppm), which was eight times greater than that in gills. As liver is the site for all metabolic activities and also is a good storage organ, there might be active accumulation sites for Cd. Bioaccumulation of Cd from water can take place either by passive diffusion through body surfaces or from water passing through the gills and subsequently through the body.[9] Therefore, the gills are in direct contact with the ambient, toxic medium and accumulation may take place by passive diffusion. According to Crespo *et al.*,[11] liver and spleen showed selective accumulation with regard to Cd and lead, with kidney exhibiting a higher heavy metal load in rainbow trout. In the present study, we could also observe a linear increase in the uptake of Cd by the tissues with an increased period of exposures. The parallelism between high-storage capacity for Cd in the excretory organs of fish and other mammals has led to the discovery of metalloproteins called "metallothioneins" in a variety of aquatic organisms. The presence of definitely characterized metallothioneins and metallothionein-like proteins has been reported to occur in marine crabs and fishes,[12,13] and it is assumed as a "protective detoxifying mechanism". Thus, in the present study, the high concentrations of Cd in kidney and liver suggest the possible formation of metallothioneins. The maximum accumulation in kidney reveals tissue specificity of Cd. Therefore, at Cd concentrations (5 ppm) of ambient waters, fish accumulate Cd and the Cd is not distributed uniformly in the body of the organism, but is selectively localized in different tissues.

REFERENCES

1. RAVERA, O. 1984. Cadmium in freshwater ecosystems (review). Experientia **40**: 1–14.
2. USHA RANI, A. & R. RAMAMURTHI. 1989. Histopathological alterations in the liver of freshwater teleost *Tilapia mossambica* in response to cadmium toxicity. Ecotoxicol. Environ. Safety **17**(no. 2): 221–226.
3. KOPP, S.J., T. GLOVEK, H.M. PERRY, JR., M. ERLANGRA & E.F. PERRY. 1982. Cardiovascular actions of cadmium at environmental exposure levels. Science **217**: 837–839.
4. WEISS, B. 1983. Behavioral toxicology of heavy metals. Neurobiol. Trace Elem. **2**: 1–50.
5. KAVIRAJ, A. 1983. Chronic effects of cadmium on the behavior, survival, growth, and reproductions of fish and on aquatic ecosystems. Environ. Ecol. **1**.
6. USHA RANI, A. & R. RAMAMURTHI. 1986. Effect of cadmium chloride on some aspects of physiology and histology in the freshwater teleost, *T. mossambica (Peters)*. Ph.D. thesis, S.V. University, Tirupati, India.
7. USHA RANI, A. & R. RAMAMURTHI. 1987. Effect of sublethal concentration of cadmium on oxidative metabolism in the freshwater teleost *Tilapia mossambica*. Indian J. Comp. Anim. Physiol.
8. WALDICHUK, M. 1974. Some biological concerns in heavy metal pollution. *In* Pollution and Physiology of Marine Organisms, pp. 1–57. Academic Press. New York.
9. RAY, S. 1984. Bioaccumulation of cadmium in marine organisms (a review). Experientia **40**: 14–23.
10. FINNEY, D.J. 1964. Probit Analysis. Second edition, p. 20. Cambridge University Press. London/New York.
11. CRESPO, S., G. NONNOTTE, D.A. COLIN, C. LERAY, L. NONNOTTE & A. AUBREE. 1986. Morphological and functional alterations induced in trout intestine by dietary cadmium and lead. J. Fish Biol. **28**: 69–80.
12. OLAFSON, R.W. & J.A.J. THOMPSON. 1974. Isolation of heavy metal binding proteins from marine vertebrates. Mar. Biol. **28**(2): 83–86.
13. OLAFSON, R.W., R.G. SIM & K.G. BOTO. 1979. Isolation and chemical characterization of the heavy metal binding protein, metallothionein, from marine invertebrates. Comp. Biochem. Physiol. **62B**: 407–416.

Concluding Remarks

ROBERT J. ISFORT

Research Division, Procter & Gamble Pharmaceuticals, Cincinnati, Ohio, USA

During the course of this conference, we have heard of many technologies that may be applicable and are being applied to toxicology. In particular, we heard presentations in the areas of genomics and proteomics—powerful new bioanalytical tools that provide a global and comprehensive scan of changes in the mRNA and protein phenotypes of a cell or tissue, resulting from a modulation of that biological sample; cell and organoid systems—advances in the culture of human cells and the creation of human tissues *in vitro* have opened the possibility of performing toxicology utilizing human samples; complex computer modeling—these technologies promise the utilization of complex computer modeling capabilities to create *in silico* biological systems, thus making *in silico* toxicology possible; and better animal models—if animals must be used for toxicological testing, they will be modified to have more humanlike responses, thus providing data that are more predictive of the human response. Several of these technologies are more upstream in terms of their application to toxicology and thus will require much effort to determine their potential usefulness and application to the field of toxicology, while other technologies are already in the validation stage.

During this meeting, I was struck by the fact that these technologies are being developed by industrial, academic, and governmental laboratories—an example of a truly cooperative effort. Finally, what do I think toxicology in the next millennium will look like? I believe there will continue to be a drive toward molecular and cellular tools; where animals must be used, they will be humanized in their responses in order to provide better information for assessing human risk. In my area of cancer toxicology, I believe the traditional rodent bioassay will no longer be used; instead, a collection of molecular, cellular, computer models and humanized animal tools will be used to provide better human risk assessment information both quicker and cheaper than that which is currently available. As other areas of toxicology including neurotoxicology, developmental toxicology, and immunotoxicology mature in terms of understanding of the underlying mechanisms of toxicity, I hazard a guess that development of tools based on these underlying principles will occur, thus improving the testing process. In short, the next millennium should be a dynamic and exciting time for the field of toxicology.

Index of Contributors

Aebersold, R., 33–47
Aleo, M.D., 171–187
Allard, J., 1–8
Anderson, N.L., 48–51
Andrews, D.L., 221–229
Arun, C.P., 284–287
Avery, M.J., 171–187

Balaban, D., 9–15
Balling, R., 239–245
Barber, R.C., 261–277
Beierschmitt, W.P., 171–187
Bennett, G.D., 261–277
Blanchard, A.P., 26–32
Blazka, M.E., 214–220
Bronaugh, R.L., 188–191
Bruccoleri, A., 214–220

Carvan, M.J., III, 133–147, 148–170
Cenac, T.A., 315–317
Copeland, C.B., 221–229
Coppi, A.A., 304–306
Crespi, C.L., 26–32
Cunningham, M.J., 52–67

Dalton, T.P., 133–147, 148–170
de Angelis, M.H., 239–245
Dong, L., 106–118
Drupa, C.A., 171–187
Durst, M., 9–15

Eberwine, J.H., 261–277

Figlewicz, D.A., 106–118
Finnell, R.H., 261–277
Fortner, J.H., 171–187
Fuhrman, S., 52–67

Gallucci, R.M., 214–220
Gasiewicz, T.A., 300–303

Gelineau–van Waes, J., 261–277
Gilbert, M.E., 119–132
Gilmour, M.I., 230–238
Gingeras, T.R., 9–15
Gygi, S.P., 33–47

Harris, C.C., 79–85
Hartig, P., 278–283
Heller, R.A., 1–8
Henney, J.E., 75–78
Hoffman, B.B., 9–15
Hollstein, M.H., 79–85
Holtzman, S., 68–74
Hu, J.-S., 9–15
Hunter, E.S., III, 278–283
Hussain, S.P., 79–85

Inoue, T., 312–314
Isfort, R.J., ix–x, 86–96, 321

Johnson, F.M., 288–299

Kaminski, N., 1–8
Kaplan, A.H., 171–187
Kerb, R., 9–15
Khurgin, E., 9–15
Kitajima, S., 312–314
Kitajima, T., 205–213
Kodavanti, P.R.S., 97–105

Lambert, A.L., 230–238
Lammer, E.J., 261–277
Lederberg, J., xi–xii
Lesniak, J., 304–306
Liang, S., 52–67
Luebke, R.W., 221–229
Luster, M.I., 214–220

Ma, J.-T., 9–15

Matheson, J.M., 214–220
Matsue, H., 205–213
McMartin, K.E., 315–317
Miller, V.P., 26–32
Mlodzienski, M., 106–118
Momma, J., 312–314
Mummert, M., 205–213
Murante, F.G., 300–303

Navetta, K.A., 171–187
Nebert, D.W., 133–147, 148–170

Osborne, R., 192–204

Perkins, M.A., 192–204
Piedrahita, J.A., 261–277

Rani, A.U., 318–320
Rhim, J.S., 16–25
Rist, B., 33–47
Robinson, M.K., 192–204

Schanne, F.A.X., 304–306, 307–311
Schoenwolf, G.C., 246–260
Seilhamer, J.J., 52–67

Selgrade, M.K., 230–238
Shaw, G.M., 261–277
Shepard, R.M., 171–187
Silverstone, A.E., 300–303
Simeonova, P.P., 214–220
Somogyi, R., 52–67
Staples, J.E., 300–303
Steiner, S., 48–51
Stresser, D.M., 26–32
Stuart, G.W., 133–147, 148–170

Takashima, A., 205–213
Thurmond, T.S., 300–303
Tilson, H.A., 97–105
Toscano, C.D., 307–311
Truong, V., 9–15
Turcotte, J.C., 106–118
Turner, S., 26–32

Walsh, C.M., 171–187
Ward, M.D.W., 230–238
Wlodarczyk, B., 261–277

Yucesoy, B., 214–220

Zieba, D., 304–306